Horizons in Medicine No. 5

Horizons in Medicine No. 5

EDITED BY

C. A. SEYMOUR PhD, FRCP
St George's Hospital Medical School,
University of London,
Cranmer Terrace, London

AND

A. P. WEETMAN MD, DSc, FRCP
Clinical Sciences Centre,
Northern General Hospital,
Herries Road, Sheffield

Royal College of Physicians of London

Blackwell Scientific Publications
OXFORD LONDON EDINBURGH BOSTON
MELBOURNE PARIS BERLIN VIENNA

Editorial Offices:
Osney Mead, Oxford OX2 0EL
25 John Street, London WC1N 2BL
23 Ainslie Place, Edinburgh EH3 6AJ
238 Main Street, Cambridge
Massachusetts 02142, USA
54 University Street, Carlton
Victoria 3053, Australia

Other Editorial Offices:
Librairie Arnette SA
1, rue de Lille
75007 Paris
France

Blackwell Wissenschafts-Verlag GmbH
Düsseldorfer Str. 38
D-10707 Berlin
Germany

Blackwell MZV
Feldgasse 13
A-1238 Wien
Austria

First published 1994

Set by Excel Typesetters Co., Hong Kong
Printed and bound in Great Britain
at the University Press, Cambridge

DISTRIBUTORS

Marston Book Services Ltd
PO Box 87
Oxford OX2 0DT
(*Orders*: Tel: 0865 791155
Fax: 0865 791927
Telex: 837515)

USA
Blackwell Scientific Publications, Inc.
238 Main Street
Cambridge, MA 02142
(*Orders*: Tel: 800 759-6102
617 876-7000)

Canada
Times Mirror Professional Publishing, Ltd
130 Flaska Drive
Markham, Ontario L6G 1B8
(*Orders*: Tel: 800 268-4178
416 470-6739)

Australia
Blackwell Scientific Publications Pty Ltd
54 University Street
Carlton, Victoria 3053
(*Orders*: Tel: 03 347-5552)

A catalogue record for this title is available from the British Library

ISBN 0-86542-815-8

Contents

PART 8: RESPIRATORY MEDICINE

PART 9: COLLAGEN VASCULAR DISEASE

List of contributors

R.N. ALLAN MD, FRCP, *Consultant Physician, Queen Elizabeth Hospital, Edgbaston, Birmingham B15 2TH*

P. BECK MA, MD, FRCP, *Consultant Physician, Llandough Hospital, Penarth, Near Cardiff, South Glamorgan CF6 1XX*

J.R. BENNETT MD, FRCP, *Consultant Gastroenterologist, Hull Royal Infirmary, Anlaby Road, Hull HU3 2ZJ*

C.M. BLACK MD, FRCP, *Consultant Rheumatologist, Department of Rheumatology, Royal Free Hospital, Pond Street, London NW3 2QG*

L.K. BORYSIEWICZ PhD, FRCP, *Professor of Medicine, University of Wales College of Medicine, Heath Park, Cardiff CF4 4XN*

C.G.D. BROOK MD, FRCP, *Professor of Paediatric Endocrinology, Endocrine Unit, The Middlesex Hospital, Mortimer Street, London W1N 8AA*

C.J. BULPITT MD, MSc, FFPM, FRCP, *Professor of Geriatric Medicine, Department of Medicine, Royal Postgraduate Medical School, Hammersmith Hospital, Du Cane Road, London W12 0NN*

C. BUNCH FRCP, *Clinical Reader in Medicine, Nuffield Department of Clinical Medicine, University of Oxford, Oxford OX3 9DU*

P.S. BURGE MD, FRCP, *Occupational Lung Disease Unit, East Birmingham Hospital, Bordesley Green East, Birmingham B9 5ST*

L.D.K. BUTTERY MSc, *Research Officer, Department of Histochemistry, Royal Postgraduate Medical School, Hammersmith Hospital, Du Cane Road, London W12 0NN*

D.A.S. COMPSTON PhD, FRCP, *Professor of Neurology, University of Cambridge Clinical School, Hills Road, Cambridge CB2 2QQ*

C.J. CORRIGAN MRCP, PhD, *Lecturer, Department of Allergy and Clinical Immunology, National Heart and Lung Institute, Dovehouse Street, London SW3 6LY*

P. CORRIS FRCP, *Consultant Physician, Clinical Senior Lecturer in Medicine, Department of Respiratory Medicine, Freeman Hospital, Newcastle-upon-Tyne NE7 7DN*

D. CROOK PhD, *Honorary Lecturer, Wynn Institute for Metabolic Research, 21 Wellington Road, London NW8 9SQ*

V. DUBOWITZ MD, PhD, FRCP, DCH, *Professor of Paediatrics, Department of Paediatrics and Neonatal Medicine, Royal Postgraduate Medical School, Hammersmith Hospital, Du Cane Road, London W12 0NN*

A.E. FLETCHER PhD, *Senior Lecturer in Epidemiology, London School of Hygiene and Tropical Medicine, Keppel Street, London WC1E 7HT*

R.S.J. FRACKOWIAK MA, MD, FRCP, *Professor of Clinical Neurology, MRC Cyclotron Unit, Hammersmith Hospital, Du Cane Road, London W12 0HS*

S. FRANKS MD, FRCP, *Professor of Reproductive Endocrinology, Department of Obstetrics and Gynaecology and Unit of Metabolic Medicine, St Mary's Hospital Medical School, Imperial College of Science, Technology and Medicine, London W2 1PG*

B.G. GAZZARD MA, MD, FRCP, *AIDS Unit Clinical Director, Chelsea and Westminster Hospital, Fulham Road, London SW10 9NH*

I.F. GODSLAND PhD, *Honorary Lecturer, Wynn Institute for Metabolic Research, 21 Wellington Road, London NW8 9SQ*

D.G. GRAHAME-SMITH FRCP, *Rhodes Professor of Clinical Pharmacology, MRC Clinical Pharmacology Unit, University Department of Clinical Pharmacology, Radcliffe Infirmary, Woodstock Road, Oxford OX2 6HE*

W.L. GREGORY BSc, MB BS, MRCP, *MRC Clinical Research Fellow, Pharmacogenetics Research Unit, Department of Pharmacological Sciences, The Medical School, Framlington Place, Newcastle-upon-Tyne NE2 4HH*

G.H. HALL MD, BSc, FRCP, *Chief Medical Officer, Medical Sickness Group, Pynes Hill, Exeter EX2 5SP*

M.C.S. HALL BMedSci, *Pharmacogenetics Research Unit, Department of Pharmacological Sciences, The Medical School, Framlington Place, Newcastle-upon-Tyne NE2 4HH*

T.A. HOWLETT MD, FRCP, *Consultant Physician and Endocrinologist, Leicester Royal Infirmary, Leicester LE1 5WW*

G.R.V. HUGHES MD, FRCP, *Consultant Rheumatologist, The Rayne Institute, St Thomas' Hospital, London SE1 7EH*

J.R. IDLE PhD, CChem, FRSC, *Professor of Pharmacogenetics, Pharmacogenetics Research Unit, Department of Pharmacological Sciences, The Medical School, Framlington Place, Newcastle-upon-Tyne NE2 4HH*

G. JACKSON FESC, FRCP, *Consultant Cardiologist, Guy's Hospital, St Thomas Street, London SE1 2RT*

D. JOHNSTON PhD, FRCP, *Professor of Clinical Endocrinology, Unit of Metabolic Medicine, St Mary's Hospital Medical School, Imperial College of Science, Technology and Medicine, London W2 1PG*

A.B. KAY PhD, FRCP, *Professor and Director, Department of Allergy and Clinical Immunology, National Heart and Lung Institute, Dovehouse Street, London SW3 6LY*

M.S. LENNARD PhD, *Senior Lecturer, The University Department of Medicine and Pharmacology, Section of Pharmacology and Therapeutics, The Royal Hallamshire Hospital, Glossop Road, Sheffield S10 2JF*

J.E. LENNARD-JONES MD, FRCP, FRCS, *Emeritus Professor of Gastroenterology; Consulting Gastroenterologist, Royal London Hospital and St Mark's Hospital, City Road, London EC1V 2PS*

C.M. LOCKWOOD FRCP, *Wellcome Reader in the School of Clinical Medicine and Honorary Consultant Physician, University of Cambridge, Department of Medicine, Addenbrooke's Hospital, Hills Road, Cambridge CB2 2SP*

L.M. LUXON BSc (Hons), FRCP, *Professor of Audiological Medicine, Institute of Laryngology and Otology, 330 Gray's Inn Road, London WC1X 8EE; The National Hospital for Neurology and Neurosurgery, Queen Square, London WC1N 3BG*

G.T. McINNES BSc, MD, FRCP (Glas), *Senior Lecturer and Honorary Consultant Physician, University Department of Medicine and Therapeutics, Gardiner Institute, Western Infirmary, Glasgow G11 6NT*

W.J. McKENNA MA, MD, FACC, FESC, FRCP, *Professor of Cardiology/Honorary Consultant Cardiologist, Department of Cardiological Sciences, St George's Hospital Medical School, Cranmer Terrace, London SW17 0RE*

C.A. MacREA BSc (Hons), MB ChB, MRCP, *Research Fellow, Department of Cardiological Sciences, St George's Hospital Medical School, Cranmer Terrace, London SW17 0RE; Division of Cardiology, Harvard Medical School, Boston, USA*

T.W. MEADE DM, FRCP, *Director, MRC Epidemiology and Medical Care Unit, Wolfson Institute of Preventive Medicine, The Medical College of St Bartholomew's Hospital, Charterhouse Square, London EC1M 6BQ*

J.M. POLAK DSc, MD, MRCP, FRCPath, *Professor of Endocrine Pathology and Head of the Department of Histochemistry, Royal Postgraduate Medical School, Hammersmith Hospital, Du Cane Road, London W12 0NN*

R. POUNDER MD, DSc(Med), FRCP, *Professor of Medicine, University Department of Medicine, Royal Free Hospital School of Medicine, Rowland Hill Street, London NW3 2QG*

S. ROBINSON MA, MRCP, *Lecturer in Endocrinology, Unit of Metabolic Medicine, St Mary's Hospital Medical School, Imperial College of Science, Technology and Medicine, London W2 1PG*

D.R. SPRINGALL MSc, PhD, *Senior Lecturer, Department of Histochemistry, Royal Postgraduate Medical School, Hammersmith Hospital, Du Cane Road, London W12 0NN*

G. STERN MD, FRCP, *Consultant Neurologist, Department of Neurology, The Middlesex Hospital, Mortimer Street, London W1N 8AA*

J.C. STEVENSON MB BS, FRCP, *Director, Wynn Institute for Metabolic Research, 21 Wellington Road, London NW8 9SQ; Honorary Consultant Physician and Senior Lecturer, National Heart and Lung Institute, Dovehouse Street, London SW3 6LY*

P.M. STEWART MB ChB, MD, MRCP, *MRC Senior Clinical Fellow and Honorary Consultant Physician, The University of Birmingham, Department of Medicine, Queen Elizabeth Hospital, Edgbaston, Birmingham B15 2TH*

J.R. STRADLING MD, FRCP, *Wellcome Senior Research Fellow, Osler Chest Unit, The Churchill Hospital, Headington, Oxford OX3 7LJ*

A.D. TOFT MD, FRCP (Edin), *Consultant Physician, Royal Infirmary, Edinburgh EH3 9YW*

M.J. WALPORT FRCP, *Professor, Rheumatology Unit, Department of Medicine, Royal Postgraduate Medical School, Hammersmith Hospital, Du Cane Road, London W12 0NN*

H.C. WATKINS BSc, MB BS, MRCP, *Lecturer, Department of Cardiological Sciences, St George's Hospital Medical School, Cranmer Terrace, London SW17 0RE; Research Fellow, Division of Cardiology, Harvard Medical School, Boston, USA*

A.J. WOOLCOCK AO, MD, FRACP, *Professor of Respiratory Medicine, Department of Medicine, University of Sydney, NSW 2006; Director, Institute of Respiratory Medicine, Page Chest Pavilion, Royal Prince Alfred Hospital, Camperdown, NSW 2050, Australia*

Preface

This volume of *Horizons in Medicine* records the thirtieth Advanced Medical Conference held at the Royal College of Physicians of London in February 1993. It has been an exciting and stimulating experience to organize this Conference and the contributions of the speakers to this book amply demonstrate the diversity and depth of the developments that were covered.

Discussion ranged from molecular mechanisms to practical management issues. As well as highlighting the new growth areas in cardiology, gastroenterology, endocrinology and neurology, there was a session devoted to aspects of medical management, reflecting the wider view physicians must take of their subject. Recent developments in clinical pharmacology were featured in another session and the Conference was completed by an update on collagen vascular diseases, whose protean manifestations are important for all in clinical medicine.

In addition, there were three outstanding lectures. Professor Frackowiak gave the Langdon-Brown Lecture and showed, using images of the human brain at work, the enormous potential of PET scanning. Professor Polak gave the Oliver Sharpey Lecture illustrating the myriad functions of nitric oxide, perhaps *the* molecule of the 1990s and Professor Woolcock gave a State of the Art Lecture on the likely cause of the troubling rise in asthma prevalence.

We are grateful not only to the authors of the contributions in the volume, but also to all of the College staff involved in running the Advanced Medicine Conference, and to the staff of the College Publications Department and of Blackwell Scientific Publications Ltd for their considerable help in producing this book.

C. A. Seymour, London
A. P. Weetman, Sheffield
February 1994

PART 1
LECTURES

Visions of the brain: imaging the mind in action

R. S. J. FRACKOWIAK

One of the more interesting challenges to clinical science is to understand how the human brain works. What is it in the way the brain is structured and organized that permits the generation of percepts, action, communication through language and feelings? An understanding of how the human brain works is a programme that needs to be tackled at many levels, from the genetic, molecular and neurochemical through to the study of brain systems, maps and networks of neurones. Clinical neurologists have a long tradition of inferring function from the minute observation of disturbed behaviour and correlation of such clinical findings with a description of the extent of anatomical brain damage. Advances in basic animal neurophysiology and anatomy have enlarged that perspective in recent years. The advent of non-invasive imaging and monitoring techniques applicable to the human brain in life indicates a way forward for the direct investigation of the functional organization of the human brain in a more accurate, sensitive and controlled fashion than previously possible. The theme of this lecture is to describe experiments that have aimed to investigate the human visual system with such modern, non-invasive techniques, and to communicate the excitement in such a clinical scientific endeavour.

INTRODUCTION TO FUNCTIONAL MAPPING OF THE BRAIN

Knowledge of the functions of a biological system almost invariably depends on a precise knowledge of the anatomy of that system [1]. The study of the functional anatomy of the human brain is a long one, dating from the speculations of the phrenologists, to the anatomical observations of clinicians such as Broca [2], Fritsch and Hitzig as well as others in this century who capitalized on the effects of penetrating missile injuries [3], or neurosurgical operations, on behaviour. Following these studies, neurosurgeons attempted to define cortical areas associated with aspects of brain function by intra-operative cortical stimulation studies in patients who could report the effects of such stimulation on their behaviour or perceptions [4]. Unfortunately, all of these pioneers, of necessity, dealt with brains that were damaged, or at least potentially damaged to a greater or lesser extent by disease or epilepsy. In any event, the efforts of these workers resulted in a number of powerful ideas which, like the homuncular map of the human sensorimotor cortex, were seductive and useful enough in clinical practice to remain viable even today, despite often being profoundly flawed as explanations for how sensory or motor functions are actually embodied in the structure of the brain [5].

A considerable impetus has been provided to the investigation of brain function by two methodological advances. The first has been the explosion of knowledge occasioned by advances in neuroanatomical tracing methods and also by the technical possibility of recording from focal sites in the awake behaving monkey's brain during the performance of specific tasks or learned behaviours.

The second has been the development of non-invasive techniques for imaging the structure and function of the human brain *in vivo*. The former studies have demonstrated, in the monkey, anatomical connections within and between distant cortical areas and evidence for basic principles of brain organization such as functional specialization [6], modularity [7,8] and parallelism [9] in the cortex, which have led to novel theories of brain function. The latter have opened the way to an analysis of the functional architecture of the human brain.

Non-invasive imaging of the brain has had its greatest impact on diagnostics, with the introduction of computerized tomography (CT) scanning in 1974 and magnetic resonance imaging (MRI) scanning in the early 1980s. Abnormalities of brain structure associated with disease have become readily recognizable and the images have had an immense and immediate impact on clinical practice. MRI scans are a powerful way of studying the normal anatomy of the human brain in life, free of the artefacts of shrinkage, fixation and compression. Volumetric images can now be obtained in less than 15 minutes, with T_1 weighting to enhance grey to white matter contrast, and with a resolution of 1 mm in each of the three orthogonal planes. The images can be viewed, using readily available software, as rendered images of the surface anatomy of the cortex, or axially through any desired plane, or segmented into constituent components, such as grey matter and cerebrospinal fluid (CSF). It is arguable that the normal gross anatomy of the brain is now more easily examined in the living human than postmortem. To date, this degree of anatomical description has been largely under-used because of the absence of corresponding functional information. However, over the last decade new functional scanning techniques have been introduced that now make analysis of structure–function relationships possible in the human brain.

One of these techniques is called positron emission tomography (PET). This is a very sensitive radiotracer based method, which depends on recording the distribution of a perfusion tracer in the brain during the performance of brain work [10]. Perfusion is intimately linked to energy metabolism and hence to glucose consumption, and is easy to measure with the use of water, labelled in trace quantities with oxygen-15, the short-lived positron-emitting isotope of oxygen ($H_2{}^{15}O$). The majority of the energy consumed by neural tissue during activity is consumed at the synaptic nerve endings and not in the cell body region. The changes of perfusion associated with a particular brain task, therefore, map the distribution of the projection sites of the brain areas engaged by the task [11]. Measurements of the distribution of perfusion in the brain can be carried out in 45–90 seconds, the resulting scans representing the integrated activity in the brain, as indexed by blood flow, over a physiological event or period of stimulation of 30–45 seconds. The images of neural activity, indexed by the PET scans, have a resolution of about $6 \times 5 \times 5$ mm with present day commercial equipment, with a theoretical limitation of approximately $2 \times 2 \times 2$ mm.

Another functional technique that has begun to be developed is functional MRI (fMRI) [12]. A number of methods have been proposed, but the most interesting is one that depends on an uncoupling of oxygen consumption from the focal increases in blood flow that accompany cerebral activation [13]. This uncoupling results in an increase in local venous oxyhaemoglobin which, unlike deoxyhaemoglobin, is not paramagnetic and therefore does not degrade the local MRI signal as does deoxy-haemoglobin. This means that neuronal activity can produce a local increase in MRI signal which can then be recorded. There are many aspects of this new method that require development and, indeed, the sensitivity of MRI may be such that the small local changes in blood flow that accompany certain types of brain activity, often in the association cortices, may be below the limits of detectability by the method. Nevertheless, the possibility of obtaining functional information without any need for ionizing radiation, by using the same scanning instrument that provides concurrent anatomical information, is very attractive.

THE VISUAL SYSTEM: BASIC PRINCIPLES

The visual system has proved a very fruitful field for the study of the functional organization of the brain. Notions about the function of the calcarine cortex, the primary cortical receiving area for visual signals from the retina, which viewed it as an area onto which visual 'information' was faithfully impressed, were apparently supported by demonstrations by Henschen, Holmes and others of the retinotopic organization of that cortex – similar points in visual space lay side by side in cortical space [14,15]. These notions, elaborated by neurologists at the turn of the century, have given way to more sophisticated ideas about the way the visual world is generated by the brain. The visual cortex is no longer regarded as a biological 'film', but as a structure that selectively recognizes invariant aspects of the visual world to generate meaningful percepts that predict how that world is likely to behave and hence how the individual should respond within it.

The work of Hubel and Wiesel [8] established the modular organization of primary visual cortex (area V1), and its arrangement into functionally specialized columns. Subsequently, cytochrome oxidase rich patches (blobs), stripes and other specialized components have been demonstrated in this area and in the immediately surrounding cortex (area V2) [16,17]. Zeki [9] has shown that subspecialized regions in area V1 are anatomically and physiologically connected to specialized regions in V2, and that there are also parallel connections to other extrastriate areas, which themselves exhibit specific and diverse functional attributes [6,16]. Maps of the macaque visual cortex now comprise some 32 separate specialized areas with around 310 connections between them, each connection invariably associated with a reverse reciprocal connection [18]. Some of these areas, those most closely connected to striate cortex, are associated with elemental aspects of visual function such as the perception of colour, of visual motion, of depth and of form. The integration of signals from these specialized areas to produce the unified, spatially and temporally congruent visual image that we normally perceive has only just become an object of study.

A critical assumption in the interpretation of such work in relation to the functional architecture of the human brain has been that the human brain is organized along analogous lines to the brain of the macaque monkey. This is an assumption that is not without danger, given that major changes in cortical anatomy, especially in the association cortices, distinguish these primate species. It is therefore as important to confirm in the human brain those principles of functional brain organization that have been deduced from highly controlled experiments in monkey, as it is to explore the new and additional functions that flow from the particularities of the organization of the human brain *per se*.

Disease in the visual system has been, often in retrospect, very informative about the functional organization of the human visual cortex. Patients with hemi-achromatopsia were described as early as 1888 [19,20]. In this condition, all aspects of the visual scene, except for colour, are perceived normally in the appropriate hemifield. A patient with akinetopsia was described in 1983 [21,22], who retains normal visual function except for the fact that she has immense difficulties perceiving objects in motion. These specific abnormalities of visual perception have been associated with lesions in distinct and different parts of the prestriate visual cortex (see below). However, the relationship of these lesions to the areas normally associated with the different aspects of visual function that have been lost or distorted has not, until recently, been defined. The work that I shall describe in the remainder of this lecture explores these aspects of human brain function. The results of this work are an example of the new information about the human brain that we can expect from non-invasive brain scanning techniques. The eventual aim of such work is a clearer understanding of the disturbances of brain function that underlie abnormal human behaviour. Such behaviour often has no obvious structural counterpart, e.g. the visual and auditory hallucinations of psychotic patients, the difficulties that dyslexic people experience when attempting to read, and the psychomotor retardation that characterizes depression and some frontal lobe disorders.

EARLY PET STUDIES OF THE VISUAL SYSTEM OF HUMANS

The earliest functional imaging studies of the human visual system were carried out with deoxyglucose labelled with fluorine-18 (^{18}FDG) [23]. This is a tracer of glucose consumption, which changes in parallel with blood flow under conditions of focal brain activation. The local rate of glucose consumption was found to increase in the occipital cortex as the visual stimuli presented to the subjects became increasingly complex. Unfortunately, the half-life of ^{18}F (110 minutes) precludes its repeated use to make multiple sequential measurements of brain function in individuals. Repetitive measurements in subjects at different visual stimulus rates were made possible by use of the short-lived ^{15}O-labelled water, because ^{15}O has a half-life of 2.1 minutes. Thus, $H_2{}^{15}O$ can be administered comfortably up to 12 times in a single scanning session. Such studies showed that regional perfusion in the striate cortex is dependent on the presentation rate of a flashing visual stimulus [24]. A similar result has been obtained recently with fMRI by J.W. Belliveau *et al.* (personal communication). In fact, the relationship between stimulus frequency and striate perfusion is approximately linear up to 7.8 Hz at which rate it peaks before declining progressively at stimulation rates of 15.5, 33.1 and 61 Hz.

Use of an optimized flash stimulus, with presentation of the visual stimulus in one or other hemifield at various eccentricities, has permitted a mapping of the retinotopic representation of visual space in the striate cortex [25]. Changes in stimulus location from macular to perimacular to peripheral, in upper and lower quadrants, caused reliable changes in blood flow response sites in the striate cortex. The response locus with each stimulus was plotted into a standard stereotactic brain space and distances between response loci were correlated with the retinal eccentricity of the stimuli. This experimental design permitted calculation of the magnification factor, i.e. the linear extent of striate cortex to which each degree of the retinal visual field projects. Thus, at the macula, every degree of retinal representation is mapped onto 3.4 mm of cortex, and from the perimacular region to the periphery, every degree is mapped onto 0.9 mm of cortex. These values were calculated without compensation for cortical infolding or curvature of the calcarine fissure and are therefore underestimates, but nevertheless, estimates obtained non-invasively in life. It is of interest that these early reports, and some early reviews [26], indicated that a number of extrastriate areas were also activated, in addition to striate visual cortex, by a flashing annular stimulus, but they do not specify which areas, or their functional significance, further.

FUNCTIONAL SPECIALIZATION: COLOUR VISION

Our own work, carried out in collaboration with Semir Zeki, has focused on two organizational principles, about which there were already data from the macaque visual cortex. We asked whether functional specialization and parallelism were equally important organizational principles in the brain of humans. Indeed, we used the monkey data to guide our experiments. Colour vision was the first visual attribute we investigated because of the clear demonstration of the response characteristics of the visual area associated with this attribute (area V4) in the monkey [27]. The visual world is represented in area V4 comparatively coarsely with little of the precise retinotopic organization characteristic of striate cortex (area V1). The cells are almost all sensitive to the colour or wavelength composition of the presented stimuli. The area is directly and reciprocally connected to area V1 and to a second visual area (V2) which surrounds V1 and receives massive projections from it.

Our experiment set out to identify the functional homologue of V4 in humans [28]. We did this by making measurements of relative blood flow distribution in a group of normal subjects whilst they viewed a Mondriaan, which is an abstract collage of 12 rectangles, rendered in different colours. This blood flow distribution was compared to the distribution recorded during viewing of precisely the same collage, except that it was rendered in shades of grey, with care taken to equate the luminance from each equivalent rectangle in the two montages (Plate 1, facing p. 18). The result was the identification of significant activation (increase in blood flow) in an area lying in the inferior part of the occipital lobe, in the caudal part of the fusiform gyrus (Plate 2), that was associated with the presence of colour. This observation confirms that an area in the extrastriate cortex of man is functionally specialized for a particular attribute of vision, namely colour perception, and that the area is homologous behaviourally to area V4 defined electrophysiologically in the monkey.

The question of anatomical as well as functional homology is worth discussing. The assumption that the anatomical disposition of functionally specialized visual areas is similar in monkey and humans may be invalid. A critical piece of evidence is the published anatomical MRI scan of the vascular lesion suffered by a patient who, as a result, acquired hemi-achromatopsia (Fig. 1) [29]. This image clearly shows an infarct in the same site in the brain, lying inferiorally in the occipital cortex in the

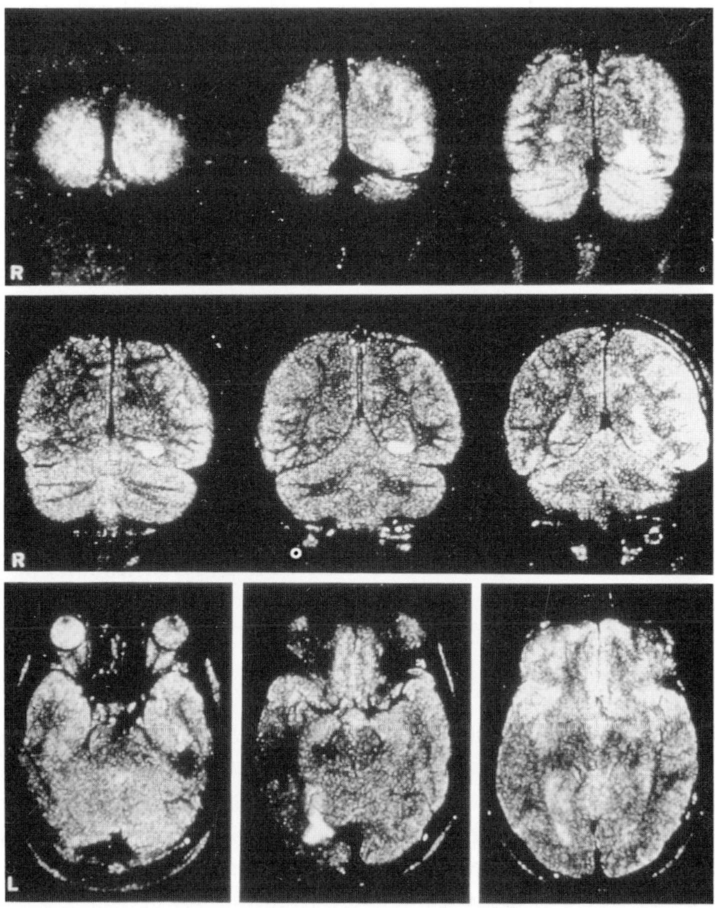

Fig. 1 The MRI scan with coronal views of the occipital pole in the top two rows, and transaxial views through approximately the same planes as in Plate 2 in the bottom row (R, right; L, left) of the patient of Kölmel with right hemiachromatopsia. The lesion lies in the fusiform gyrus. The correspondence between the region associated with colour perception in normal subjects and the loss of colour vision in a lesioned patient is obvious (By permission from Kölmel [29].)

region of the lingual and fusiform gyri on the side opposite to the field with disturbed colour perception, that we have demonstrated by PET to be associated with colour perception in normal subjects. This convergent evidence is very persuasive and has led us to identify the area of the human brain activated by coloured visual stimuli as the human homologue of monkey area V4 [30]. This area lies more ventrally in the brain of humans than it does in the monkey, in which it lies on the lateral surface of the cortical convexity. However, the parietal cortex of humans is much more highly developed than in the monkey. In addition, the relative disposition of visually specialized areas in this part of the extrastriate cortex seems to be relatively conserved in humans, as will be described below. It is therefore possible that the apparent lack of anatomical congruity between V4 in the brain of the monkey and that of humans is brought about by a selective development of the human parietal cortex, resulting in a more ventral localization for V4 and other visual extrastriate areas in humans than in the monkey.

There is a further area that has been shown by PET to activate when normal subjects attend to the colours of visual objects, but in this case they were discrete small objects of different shapes and colours and moving in different directions [31]. This area lies on the convexity of the brain at the parieto-occipital junction some 10–30 mm above the intercommissural plane. It is important not to equate this area with V4 simply because of the apparent identity of anatomical sites between monkey V4 and this human visual area. The cognitive aspects of attending to one of a number of visual attributes are not the same as the controlled situation in which colour is the only aspect of the visual world that is changed, and for which no major demand on attention is made for it to be perceived. The additional area may well be a higher order area associated specifically with the attribution of attentional resources to different aspects of visual perception.

PARALLELISM: VISUAL MOTION

The notion that visual signals are processed in parallel arose initially from anatomical studies in the macaque, which clearly demonstrated independent connections between area V1 and all the adjacent functionally specialized areas lying in prestriate cortex [9]. This evidence spoke against serial processing of visual signals in a caudal/rostral direction, which had been at the centre of thinking about the formation of 'cortical images' and their subsequent interpretation by comparison with previously experienced 'percepts' stored in association cortex. We therefore decided to demonstrate parallelism formally by showing the presence of a second functionally specialized visual area. For this, we chose the area concerned with the perception of visual motion, known as area V5. Basic experiments had shown that in the monkey, brain cells in area V5 are interested in large part, if not exclusively, with moving objects in the visual field [32]. This area, which in the macaque lies at the junction of the occipital and mid-temporal lobes, is characterized by heavy cortical and subcortical myelination [33]. It receives signals from V1 and V2 and also has a relatively coarse retinotopic organization.

Our experiment consisted of measuring the distribution of relative blood flow with PET whilst subjects viewed a static image of numerous, randomly distributed black and white squares, each subtending 1° of visual space [30]. The recorded blood flow distribution was compared to that found when the image was viewed moving *en bloc* in one of each of the four cardinal directions or the four diagonals, changing direction randomly every 6 seconds. The average blood flow map obtained when viewing the moving as opposed to the stationary versions of the image differed in that there was highly significant activation (blood flow increase) in two areas, lying in the right and left hemisphere over the convexity of the brain, at the junction of the occipital and temporal lobes just above the intercommissural plane (Plate 3). This region was clearly quite different from that demonstrated with the colour experiment. In each experiment, the control and experimental stimuli differed from each other by only one visual attribute. The experimental and control stimuli were closely matched in the colour experiment as indicated by no net difference in activity in the primary visual area. In the motion experiment, the matching was less perfect, as one stimulus contained moving edges and therefore a possible additional stimulation of orientation sensitive areas, which may not have been activated by the stationary control.

As in the case of defective colour vision, there is evidence from pathology in humans to substantiate the conclusion that the area identified in a group of normal subjects is indeed the human homologue of area V5 in the monkey. A patient with akinetopsia, the inability to perceive

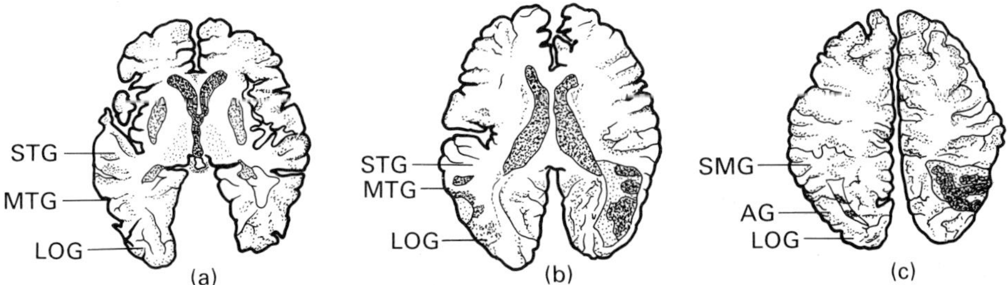

Fig. 2 A diagram of the lesions drawn from CT scans of the patient of Zihl *et al.* with cerebral akinetopsia. The lesions, consequent on venous infarction, are extensive but encompass the area demonstrated in normal volunteers to be associated with visual motion perception (Plate 3). STG, Superior temporal gyrus; MTG, middle temporal gyrus; LOG, lower occipital gyrus; AG, angular gyrus. (Data from Zihl *et al.* [21], by permission of Oxford University Press.)

visual motion with preservation of other visual modalities, has been described in the literature, as noted above [22]. This patient suffered a superior sagittal sinus thrombosis which resulted in bilateral parieto-temporo-occipital infarctions of the brain and the abnormality of a greatly degraded perception of visual motion. The lesions are shown in Fig. 2 which demonstrates that, though large, they encompass the regions that become active with the perception of visual motion in normal humans. Once again, the convergence of results from recordings in normal subjects and from clinicopathological correlations is persuasive evidence supporting the designation of the activated region in human brain as human V5 – the homologue of monkey V5.

VISUAL MOTION AREA: STRUCTURE–FUNCTION RELATIONSHIPS

Recent technical advances in the design of PET scanners have increased the sensitivity for the detection of radioactivity five-fold, thus permitting meaningful studies in single individuals. The results described above were obtained by averaging data from groups of individuals, which necessitated reformatting all the scans into a common, standard, anatomical space. Studies in individuals provide the very considerable advantage of permitting direct correlation of functional maps with the anatomy of the same individual recorded with MRI. The brains of normal subjects differ considerably in size and shape. There are also differences in the orientation, disposition and sometimes number of sulci in different brains. Functionally specialized areas may lie at different places in a sulcus depending on the developmental history of the brain in question. Some areas of the brain are hypervariable in terms of gross anatomical features such as those described above, and the occipital cortex is one of the most hypervariable areas of the human brain. We have asked ourselves whether there is any relationship between particular functionally defined areas and any anatomical landmarks, to see whether there are anatomical or developmental rules which govern what the function of a particular brain area will be. To answer this question we studied 12 normal individuals with the visual motion paradigm described above [34]. We were able to carry out six recordings in each condition and by averaging them were able to obtain maps of significantly changed blood flow associated with the perception of visual motion in each of them. These were then coregistered with the T_1-weighted MRI scans from the same individuals using an algorithm developed especially for the purpose.

Our results indicated that in 16 of the 24 available hemispheres for which we had collected data, and in all of which we had identified area V5, it was possible to show a constant anatomical relationship of area V5 to two variable cortical sulci. These sulci, the ascending limb of the inferior temporal sulcus (ALITS) and the inferior or lower occipital sulcus, define the anterior and upper limits of V5. This observation establishes a link between anatomy and function (Plate 4). Our experiments have indicated a further link to development. The myelo-architectonic studies of Flechsig [35] at the beginning of the century described the maturation of the human brain in terms of the progressive pattern of myelination of cortical areas. Flechsig described an area (Feld 16) which was the sixteenth most myelinated area in the infant brain that lies in exactly the same location as area V5 described with PET in the human adult [34]. Early myelination is associated with the primary cortices – visual, auditory, sensorimotor, olfactory and limbic. It is therefore of interest that the area of the human brain associated with the perception of visual motion, so crucial to establishing fixation in the newborn, is also heavily myelinated at birth. The presumed implication is that function of the area is determined prenatally and hence in the absence of visual stimulation. This indicates that there must be a major genetic component to the determination of its anatomical locus, despite the apparent individual variability of the anatomy of this area. An indication of the variability is given by the fact that area V5 differed in location by up to 20 to 30 mm in this cohort of 12 subjects.

VISUAL INTEGRATION

The parallel distribution of visual signals from the primary visual cortex to other specialized prestriate regions, each of which is associated with a restricted number of visual attributes, begs the question of how the brain synthesizes the signals back into the visual scene that we experience, which is a unitary experience that is congruent in space and time for all its component attributes. To explore this issue further we have performed two experiments using visual stimuli chosen to highlight the integrative functions of the visual cortex. In the first experiment we capitalized on the fact that one can display moving sheets of random dots on a monitor in such a way that they appear as such, or alternatively so that an illusion of form is generated. In common experience this effect is found with a badly adjusted TV set on which one can see horizontal stationary or moving lines. Our experimental setup involved moving sheets of dots in a side-to-side direction thus setting up the illusion of standing columns of variable width from the moving stimuli. As control stimuli we used the random motion setup and also a static form that mimicked the illusory form in the size, width and disposition of the columns, but which did not use motion to generate them.

Thus, we were able, by contrasting the perfusion map associated with form-from-motion with the aggregate of that produced by the static form stimulus and the random motion stimulus, to ask whether there were areas in the brain in which there was more activity in the illusory stimulus than in the other two stimuli, which served to control as far as possible for the individual components of the experimental stimulus. One prediction might be that areas in the association cortex distal to the prestriate areas would be responsible for the integration of cortical signals necessary to generate the form-from-motion percept. Another, favoured by us, was that the excess activity would be found in the striate cortex itself reflecting signals that are fed back, by a process of re-entry [36], from specialized areas for visual motion and orientation, to modulate new signals as they arrive from the retina. Our result unequivocally indicated that area V1 showed greater activity with form-from-motion than with random motion alone or with the aggregate of random motion and static form. This is clear evidence that the integration of visual signals necessary to generate the percept of form-from-motion requires re-entry of signals to the primary visual cortex.

The second experiment used another illusion which is that of motion-from-form [37]. In this case the experimental visual stimulus and the control stimulus were virtually identical. The stimulus consists of a geometrical pattern, a painting by I. Leviant that hangs in the Palais de la Decouverte in Paris. The pattern consists of concentric rings on a background of radially arranged, regular spokes. The painting is coloured but we rendered it in black and white to avoid contaminating the cerebral signals. If the picture is viewed by fixation of the centre, very soon the majority of observers become aware of apparent motion in the concentric rings that is in opposite directions in adjacent rings and that can reverse direction at random intervals. On the other hand if, as in the control version, the spokes run through the rings rather than between them, no apparent motion is perceived. The perfusion maps were compared and the sites of activation on the convexity of the brain in the parieto-occipital and temporo-occipital regions were compared with those elicited in the same subjects with the standard visual motion experimental paradigm described above. We found that with the conscious perception of visual motion, even though no physical motion was present in the stimulus, there was activation of a region of prestriate cortex that overlapped at least in part with area V5, the visual motion area. This leads to the rather startling conclusion that the activation of a cortical area is sufficient to generate a percept without the usual physical stimulus that normally elicits that percept being necessarily present.

CONCLUSION

The presence of lesions in the human visual brain can lead to various deficits of function. Some of these, such as the problems of residual vision and 'blindsight' [38], may provide opportunities for the study of the functional anatomy of consciousness itself, through the investigation of patients with these disorders. Equally, there are diseases, both degenerative and of uncertain aetiology, that lead to theoretically interesting visual misperceptions or hallucinations. A better understanding of the functional significance of other areas of the human visual cortex than those with already defined functions will increase our understanding of the organization of the visual cortex and of the mechanisms underlying the symptoms of visual dysfunction. Recovery from cortical visual deficits is not understood but is in certain circumstances a well recognized phenomenon. In the motor system we have shown that the adult human brain is capable of considerable plastic reorganization [39–41], which suggests that an improved understanding of the reorganization that underlies the recovery from visual deficits may suggest new ways for rehabilitating patients with selective cortical visual pathology.

More generally, the non-invasive imaging techniques are providing new information about the functioning of the human brain, capitalizing on the simultaneous acquisition of functional information from the whole brain at once. New methods of image analysis are becoming available which allow the exploration of functional connectivity as well as the description of functional localization. Such techniques combined with new information about other levels of cerebral organization present us with challenges and opportunities for a deeper understanding of human vision and the unique capacities and capabilities of the human brain in general.

ACKNOWLEDGEMENTS

I wish to acknowledge my collaborators Dr John Watson of University College London and the MRC Cyclotron Unit, and currently of the University of Sydney, and Professor Semir Zeki of University College London.

REFERENCES

1 Zeki SM. *A Vision of the Brain*. Oxford: Blackwell Scientific Publications, 1993.
2 Broca PP. Perte de la parole, ramollisement chronique et destruction partielle du lobe antérieure gauche du cerveau. *Bull Soc Anthropol* 1861;2:235–238.
3 Holmes G. A contribution to the cortical representation of vision. *Brain* 1931;54:470–479.
4 Penfield W, Boldrey E. Somatic motor and sensory representation in the cerebral cortex of man as studied by electrical stimulation. *Brain* 1937;60:389–443.
5 Schott GD. Penfield's homunculus: a note on cerebral cartography. *J Neurol Neurosurg Psychiatry* 1993;56:329–333.
6 Zeki SM. Functional specialisation in the visual cortex of the *rhesus* monkey. *Nature* 1978;274:423–428.

7 Hubel DH, Wiesel TN. Receptive fields and functional architecture in two non striate visual areas (18 and 19) of the cat. *J Neurophysiol* 1965;28:279–298.
8 Hubel DH, Wiesel TN. *The Ferrier Lecture*: functional architecture of macaque monkey visual cortex. *Proc R Soc Lond B* 1977;198:1–59.
9 Zeki SM. The functional organisation of projections from striate to prestriate visual cortex in the *rhesus* monkey. *Cold Spring Harb Symp Quant Biol* 1975;40:591–600.
10 Phelps ME, Mazziotta JC. Positron emission tomography: human brain function and biochemistry. *Science* 1985;228:799–809.
11 Mata H, Fink DG, Gainer H, *et al.* Activity dependent energy metabolism in rat posterior pituitary primarily reflects sodium pump activity. *J Neurochem* 1980;34:213–215.
12 Belliveau JW, Kennedy DN, McKinstry D, *et al.* Functional mapping of the human visual cortex by magnetic resonance imaging. *Science* 1991;254:716–719.
13 Kwong KK, Belliveau JW, Chesler DA, *et al.* Dynamic magnetic resonance imaging of human brain activity during primary sensory stimulation. *Proc Natl Acad Sci USA* 1992;89:5675–5679.
14 Daniel PM, Whitteridge D. The representation of the visual field on the cerebral cortex in monkeys. *J Physiol (Lond)* 1961;159:203–221.
15 Talbot SA, Marshall WH. Physiological studies of neural mechanisms of visual localisation and discrimination. *Am J Ophthalmol* 1941;24:1255–1264.
16 Livingstone MS, Hubel DH. Thalamic inputs into cytochrome-rich regions in monkey visual cortex. *Proc Natl Acad Sci USA* 1982;79:6098–6101.
17 Horton JC. Cytochrome oxidase patches: a new cytoarchitectonic feature of monkey visual cortex. *Phil Trans R Soc Lond B* 1984;304:199–253.
18 Felleman DJ, Van Essen DC. Distributed hierarchical processing in the primate cerebral cortex. *Cerebral Cortex* 1991;1:1–47.
19 Verrey L. Hémiachromatopsie droite absolue. *Arch Ophthalmol (Paris)* 1888;8:289–301.
20 Zeki S. A century of cerebral achromatopsia. *Brain* 1990;113:1721–1777.
21 Zihl J, von Cramon D, Mai N. Selective disturbance of movement vision after bilateral brain damage. *Brain* 1983;106:313–340.
22 Zeki S. Cerebral akinetopsia (cerebral visual motion blindness). *Brain* 1991;114:811–824.
23 Phelps ME, Kuhl DE, Mazziotta JC. Metabolic mapping of the brain's response to visual stimulation: studies in humans. *Science* 1981;211:1445–1448.
24 Fox PT, Raichle ME. Stimulus rate dependance of regional cerebral blood flow in human striate cortex demonstrated by positron emission tomography. *J Neurophysiol* 1984;51:1109–1120.
25 Fox PT, Miezin FM, Allman JM, *et al.* Retinotopic organisation of human visual cortex mapped with positron emission tomography. *J Neurosci* 1987;7:913–922.
26 Mora BN, Carman GJ, Allman JM. *In vivo* functional localisation of the human visual cortex using positron emission tomography and magnetic resonance imaging. *Trends Neurosci* 1989;12:282–285.
27 Zeki SM. Colour coding in *rhesus* monkey prestriate cortex. *Brain Res* 1973;53:422–427.
28 Lueck CJ, Zeki S, Friston KJ, *et al.* The colour centre in the cerebral cortex of man. *Nature* 1989;340:386–389.
29 Kölmel HW. Pure homonymous hemiachromatopsia: findings with neuroophthalmologic examination and imaging procedures. *Eur Arch Psychiatr Neurol Sci* 1988; 237:237–243.
30 Zeki S, Watson JDG, Lueck CJ, *et al.* A direct demonstration of functional specialization in human visual cortex. *J Neurosci* 1991;11:641–649.
31 Corbetta M, Miezin FM, Dobmeyer S, *et al.* Selective and divided attention during visual discriminations of shape, color, and speed: functional anatomy by positron emission tomography. *J Neurosci* 1991;11:2383–2402.
32 Wurtz RH, Yamasaki DS, Duffy CJ, Roy JP. Functional specialisation for visual motion processing in primate cerebral cortex. *Cold Spring Harb Symp Quant Biol* 1991;55:717–727.

33 Clarke S, Miklossy J. Occipital cortex in man: organisation of callosal connections, related myelo- and cytoarchitecture, and putative boundaries of functional visual areas. *J Comp Neurol* 1990;298:188–214.
34 Watson JDG, Myers R, Frackowiak RSJ, *et al.* Area V5 of the human brain: a combined study using positron emission tomography and magnetic resonance imaging. *Cerebral Cortex* 1993;3:79–94.
35 Flechsig P. Developmental (myelogenetic) localisation of the cerebral cortex in the human subject. *Lancet* 1901;ii:1027–1029.
36 Edelman G. *Neural Darwinism.* Oxford: Oxford University Press, 1989.
37 Zeki S, Watson JDG, Frackowiak RSJ. Going beyond the information given: the relation of illusory visual motion to brain activity. *Proc R Soc Lond B* 1993;252:215–222.
38 Weiskrantz L. *Blindsight.* Oxford: Clarendon Press, 1986.
39 Chollet F, DiPiero V, Wise RJS, *et al.* The functional anatomy of motor recovery after ischaemic stroke in man. *Ann Neurol* 1991;29:63–71.
40 Weiller C, Chollet F, Friston KJ, *et al.* Functional reorganisation of the brain in recovery from striatocapsular infarction in man. *Ann Neurol* 1992;31:463–472.
41 Weiller C, Ramsay SC, Wise RSJ, *et al.* Individual patterns of functional reorganisation in the human cerbral cortex after capsular infarction. *Ann Neurol* 1993;33:181–189.

Distribution of nitric oxide synthase in human and experimental animal tissues: involvement in disease

D. R. SPRINGALL, L. D. K. BUTTERY & J. M. POLAK

Nitric oxide (NO) is an important regulatory molecule, acting both as a second messenger and neurotransmitter, and is involved in a diverse range of physiological functions. Recognition of this has stemmed from several lines of research, including the search for nitrate-producing cells in mammals [1], the phenomenon of endothelium-mediated relaxation of smooth muscle [2] and the identity of mediators of non-adrenergic non-cholinergic (NANC) neurotransmission [3].

Numerous mammalian cell types and tissues synthesize NO, including vascular endothelium [4], platelets [5], macrophages [6], vascular smooth muscle [7], neutrophils [8], hepatocytes [9], Kupffer cells [10], and central and peripheral nervous tissues [11]. The principal action of NO is on target cells, close to its site of synthesis, where it activates soluble guanylate cyclase by binding to the haem moiety of the enzyme, forming a transient NO–haem complex [12]. NO-activated guanylate cyclase elevates intracellular cyclic guanosine monophosphate (cGMP) levels and cGMP acts as an intracellular messenger to initiate cellular functions such as relaxation of vascular smooth muscle and inhibition of platelet aggregation [12]. When present in sufficient quantities NO is also a cellular cytotoxic agent inhibiting mitochondrial respiration and DNA synthesis as part of the cell-mediated immune response [13].

The physico-chemical properties of NO are well suited to its role as a local transcellular messenger. It has a small molecular size, lipophilic nature and short half-life, making it unnecessary to have membrane transporters and enzyme systems for initiating or terminating its action.

Endogenous NO is derived from the oxidation of one or more guanidino nitrogen atoms of L-arginine, via the catalytic action of the enzyme NO synthase, yielding NO and L-citrulline (reviewed in Moncada *et al.* [14]). This reaction is specific since a number of analogues of L-arginine, including its D-enantiomer, are not substrates. Furthermore, the analogues N^G-monomethyl-L-arginine (L-NMMA) and N^G-nitro-L-arginine (L-NNA) reversibly inhibit synthesis. What has now become known as the L-arginine–NO pathway has been demonstrated in a wide,

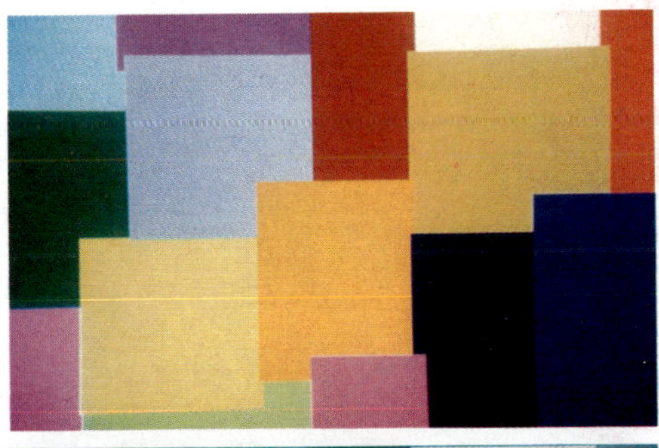

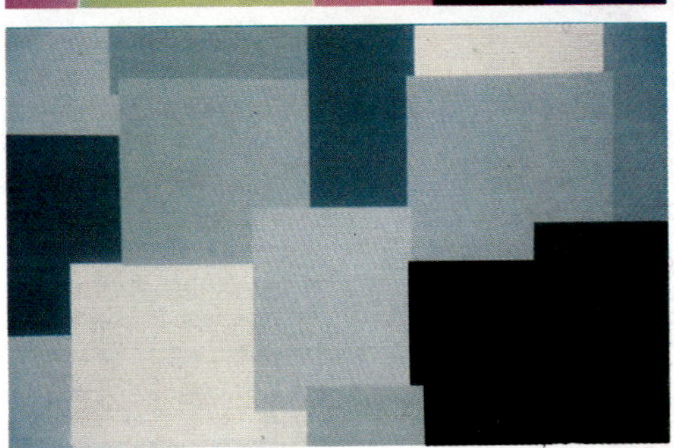

Plate 1 The stimuli used to excite the visual system during recordings of the distribution of cerebral blood flow in a group of normal human subjects. The abstract collages (Mondrians) differ only by the presence (above) or absence (below) of colour in the images.
The comparison of blood flow distributions resulted in the identification of human visual area V4 – see Plate 2.

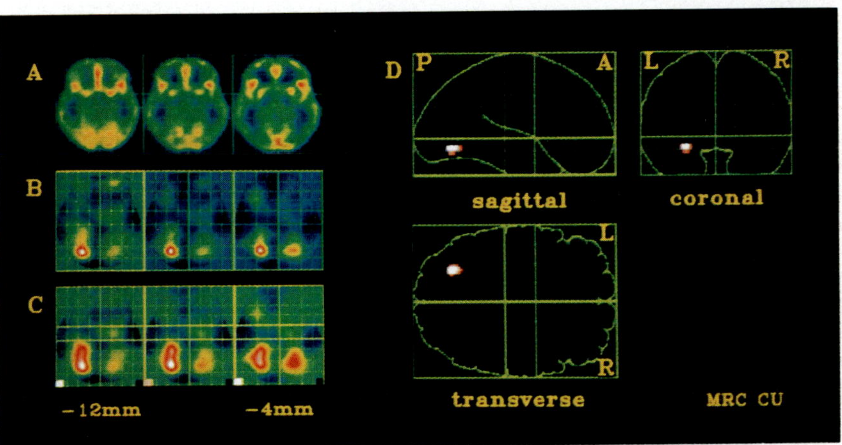

Plate 2 The result of a comparison of perfusion maps obtained with the stimuli shown in Plate 1. (A) denotes the average blood flow maps at −12, −8 and −4 mm below the intercommissural line. The grid superimposed on the maps is the reference proportional anatomical space of Talairach and Tournoux (*A Stereotactic Coplanar Atlas of the Human Brain*. Stuttgart, Thieme, 1989). A similar configuration is used for the rCBF difference maps (B) and for the statistical parametric maps (C) which show significant changes in cerebral blood flow associated with the difference in the brain states corresponding to the two viewing conditions. A bilaterally homologous region is seen to lie in the inferior occipital cortex in the region of the fusiform gyrus. The point of most significant change is demonstrated on the projections (D) in which the data from the whole volume of brain can be inspected from the sagittal, posterior coronal and superior transaxial views. The most significant area in this experiment lay in the left fusiform gyrus. (By permission from Watson *et al.* [34].)

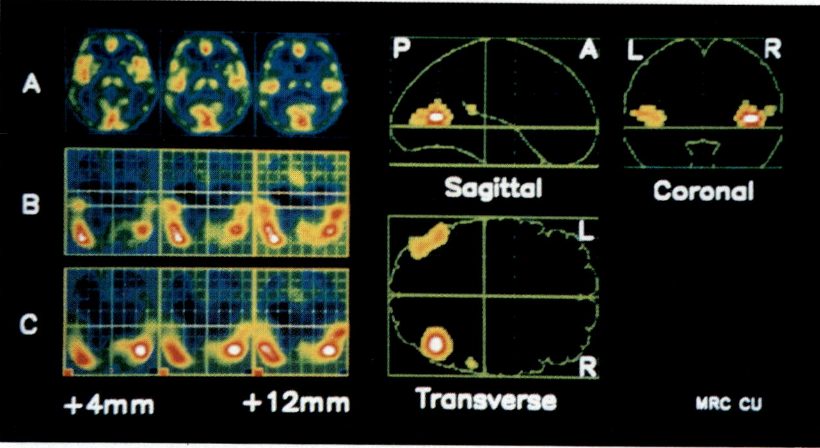

Plate 3 The result of an experiment designed to highlight areas associated with the perception of visual motion in a group of normal subjects. The layout of the figure is identical to the description in the legend to Plate 2. The transaxial images now lie from 4 to 12 mm above the intercommissural plane and the sites of significant activation are located on the convexities of the hemispheres at the junction of the occipital and temporal lobes. (By permission from Zeki *et al.* [30].)

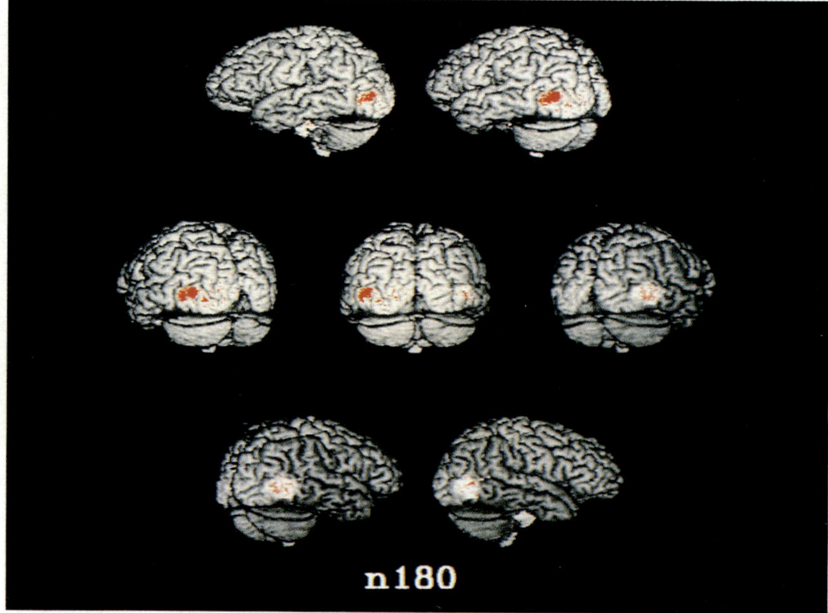

Plate 4 The surface of a single subject's brain (n180) rendered from a volumetric T_1-weighted MRI data set with the areas associated with visual motion perception (V5) coregistered onto the surface in red and white to demonstrate their relationship to the sulcal anatomy. The image in the middle is the posterior view and those around the periphery show 30° rotations, with the lateral view at the top left of the figure and the right lateral view at the bottom right. Area V5 lies in the angle formed by the ascending limb of the inferior temporal sulcus and the inferior occipital sulcus.

and ever increasing, variety of different cells and tissues, and contributes to a diverse range of physiological and pathophysiological processes.

Based on pharmacological and biochemical differences of synthesis [4–11] and from isolation and purification of NO synthase there is clear evidence of multiple forms of the enzyme [14,15]. Three distinct isoforms have been described to date: the neuronal (constitutive) NO synthase, the endothelial (constitutive) NO synthase and the macrophage (inducible) NO synthase. The constitutive enzymes are absolutely dependent on calcium ions (Ca^{2+})/calmodulin for activity and are responsible for the rapid and continuous release of low levels of NO following activation of cell-surface receptors or in response to physical stimuli. Constitutive NO synthesis is involved in functions as varied as regulation of basal vascular tone [16], neurotransmission in the central and peripheral nervous system [14] and penile erection [17]. In contrast, activation of the inducible NO synthase occurs over several hours in response to specific cytokine stimuli and is largely independent of Ca^{2+}/calmodulin. Once synthesized, the enzyme produces high levels of NO for prolonged periods. Inducible NO synthesis is mainly involved in cell-mediated immunity effecting cytotoxicity/cytostasis in invading organisms and in tumour cells [14]. Both constitutive and inducible enzymes additionally require certain redox cofactors such as the reduced form of nicotinamide-adenine-dinucleotide phosphate (NADPH) for activity [18] and also tetrahydrobiopterin [15] which is essential for synthesis of the inducible enzyme [19,20].

More recently, the deduced protein sequences of molecular clones of the constitutive rat and human brain NO synthase [21,22], the constitutive bovine and human endothelial NO synthase [23,24] and the inducible murine macrophage [25], rat smooth muscle [26] and rat liver NO synthase [27] have shown that there are substantial sequence differences between these three enzyme isoforms suggesting that they may be the products of distinct genes. Indeed, the structure and chromosomal localization of the human constitutive neural [28] and endothelial [29] NO synthase has now been described and will undoubtedly provide more information on the function of the NO synthase gene family. However, in spite of the differing biochemical, pharmacological and molecular profiles, all three enzyme isoforms do contain several highly conserved regions with consensus sequences for binding several redox cofactors. In addition, all of the NO synthase isoforms characterized thus far catalyze the same reaction, producing NO and L-citrulline from L-arginine. It is therefore likely that all enzymes will have similar substrate binding sites, although as yet the active site has not been described in any of the enzyme isoforms.

Interestingly, the NO synthases also share significant sequence homology with cytochrome P450 reductase and also have similar properties, both being oxidative enzymes that have recognition sites for two flavins and NADPH [21]. Hence it has been postulated that cytochrome P450 reductase and NO synthase are closely related in evolution. NO synthase is also of ancient evolutionary origin and is present in the starfish [30] and the horseshoe crab [31], which dates back at least 500 million years. Taken together these data strongly suggest that the NO synthase gene family had a common ancestor which has been manipulated by a variety of different cell types to effect a diverse range of physiological functions.

MEASUREMENT AND DETECTION OF THE L-ARGININE–NO PATHWAY

There are many methods of investigating the L-arginine–NO pathway. Direct measurement of NO is difficult since the molecule is highly reactive, has a short half-life and is present in small amounts. However, several methods of NO assay have been developed (reviewed in Archer [32]), the most commonly used being: (i) chemiluminescence, which relies on the generation of light in the reaction between NO and ozone that is directly proportional to NO levels; (ii) 'trapping' of NO by reduced haemoglobin or nitroso compounds which can then be detected by electron paramagnetic resonance; and (iii) oxidation of reduced haemoglobin by NO to methaemoglobin which is detected by dual wavelength spectrophotometry. While these methods are the most sensitive, they do, for the most part, require specialized equipment. Hence other methods of measuring NO activity have been developed which do not require specialized equipment, although these are less sensitive and more indirect. Direct methods include spectrophotometric monitoring of nitrite production, which is indicative of NO oxidation. Indirect methods of determining NO activity include: (i) accumulation of cGMP (measured by radio-immunoassay or enzyme-linked immunoadsorbent assay), which assesses the effect of NO on guanylate cyclase activation in a reporter cell; (ii) the use of inhibitors of NO synthesis such L-NMMA or L-NNA, which can be used to monitor the effect of blocking NO release by recording changes in a number of physiological parameters such as blood flow or blood pressure; and (iii) measurement of citrulline, the coproduct of NO synthesis. While providing information on the relative activity of NO synthase at different levels of the L-arginine–NO pathway, none of these methods necessarily provides an accurate account of which cell type is synthesizing NO.

LOCALIZATION OF NO SYNTHASE

The isolation and purification of the enzyme isoforms and the molecular cloning of the NO synthase genes has permitted the development of highly specific probes. Using immunocytochemical and *in situ* hybridization techniques, this has allowed the detailed morphological localization and mapping of NO synthase isoforms in numerous tissues and species as well as providing a quantitative assessment of the amount of stored enzyme. More recently, radiolabelled L-arginine and L-arginine analogues have been used to detect enzyme binding sites [33], and to provide information on morphological localization of the enzyme by autoradiography, and on enzyme activity by competitive inhibition studies.

DISTRIBUTION OF NO SYNTHASE

Constitutive neural NO synthase

This enzyme has been shown to be expressed in distinct neural populations within both the central nervous system and peripheral nervous system [34–36], in a variety of different animal species. On Western blots the neural enzyme has been shown to have a molecular weight of 160 kDa [14,15]. Molecular cloning of the enzyme reveals high interspecies sequence conservation, with almost identical enzymes present in rat, pig, cow and human.

In the brain the enzyme has been localized immunocytochemically to discrete neuronal populations, being present in the molecular and granular layers of cerebellum (Fig. 1), medium-sized neurones of caudate (Fig. 2), and multipolar neurones of claustrum pallidus, olfactory tubercle, hypothalamus and tegmentum [34–36].

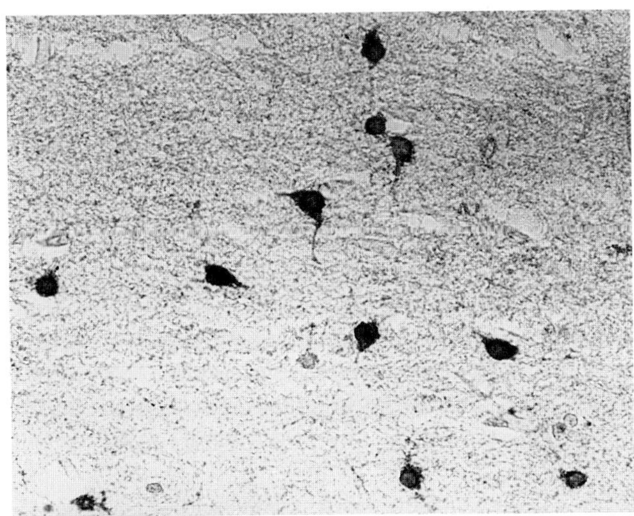

Fig. 1 Human brain immunostained with antiserum to neural NO synthase. Strong staining is evident in numerous bipolar neurones in cerebellum. Indirect immunoperoxidase. (Original magnification ×360.)

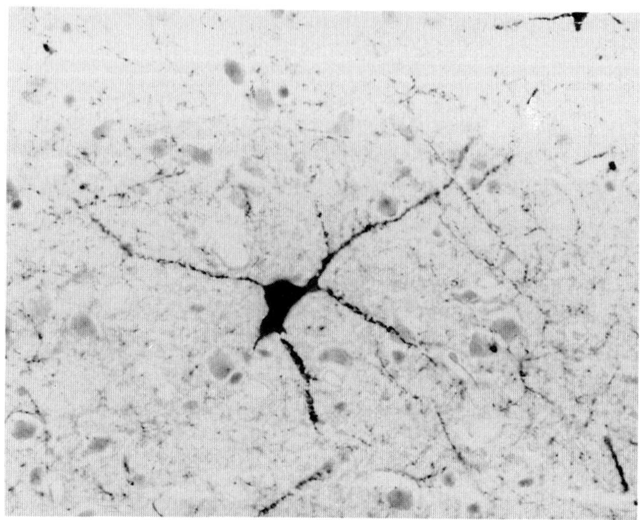

Fig. 2 Human brain immunostained with antiserum to neural NO synthase. Strong staining is evident in a medium-sized multipolar neurone in cerebral cortex. Indirect immunoperoxidase. (Original magnification ×360.)

Prior to the discovery of NO synthase it was known that selected neuronal populations within the brain could be identified histochemically through the reduction of a dye salt nitro-blue-tetrazolium in the presence of NADPH [37]. Subsequently, some studies have demonstrated that the localization of NO synthase has absolute coincidence with the staining observed using the NADPH-diaphorase technique, implying that they are the same enzyme [35]. Furthermore, there are now numerous reports which have utilized the NADPH-diaphorase technique as a marker for neuronal NO synthase. However, doubt has recently been cast on the use of the NADPH-diaphorase technique as an absolute marker of NO synthase [38,39], with increasing evidence for some differences in the localization of some neuronal populations using the separate histochemical and immunocytochemical techniques. The disparity may be due to a number of reasons. It has been shown that much of the NADPH-diaphorase activity can be inactivated if tissue is preserved in fixative, so that caution is required if comparing the distribution of staining when different tissue processing regimes may have been used. More recently, further molecular characterization of the enzyme has indicated that there may in fact be two separate isoforms of neural NO synthase [40]. The two forms appear to be the product of alternative splicing of the NO synthase gene, with resulting expression of two distinct enzymes which may have differing activities. As well as having major implications for the function of neural NO synthase, the expression of two neural isoforms may also help to explain the anomalies of NADPH-diaphorase and NO synthase staining.

The release of NO in the central nervous system is mediated through elevations of intracellular Ca^{2+} following stimulation of *N*-methyl-D-aspartate (NMDA) receptors [41]. Once released it can serve as an agent of classical anterograde neuronal signalling, but NO also has unique properties as a retrograde signalling agent, thereby strengthening the association between the neurone transmitting and the neurone receiving the signal [42]. This has led to the suggestion that NO may promote synaptic plasticity, and may therefore be involved in longterm potentiation which is believed to be one mechanism contributing to the development of memory and the learning process [42]. It has been observed that NO synthase-containing neurones appear particularly refractile to neural damage (reviewed in Bredt and Snyder [43]), which occurs following an insult such as stroke or as a result of neurodegenerative diseases such as Huntington's chorea. Interestingly, when present at high levels, NO is neurotoxic. Hence, it has been suggested that increased NO production, possibly through overstimulation of NMDA receptors, may directly contribute to neural damage. This may also explain why in areas of brain damage NO synthase-containing neurones are often spared.

In the spinal cord NO synthase has a differential distribution which is consistent in a number of different species [44]. Staining is present in neural cell bodies and processes in the superficial dorsal horn, intermediolateral cell column of thoracic and sacral levels and lamina X. Scattered positive cells are also present in the deeper dorsal horn, ventral horn and white matter [44]. While most workers agree on this localization, there is contention regarding localization in motor neurones with some reports indicating that NO synthase is localized to this site [45] (Fig. 3), while others suggest that it is not [46]. In addition it has been shown that spinal motor neurones express NO synthase following some methods of experimentally induced traumatic neural injury, such as ventral root avulsion, but not after ventral root transection [47]. Early expression of NO synthase in the motor neurones seems to be associated with axonal sprouting and growth. However, it is interesting that the neurones expressing lesion-induced NO synthase ultimately die, although it is not known whether expression of NO synthase is related to their death. NO synthase is also present in dorsal root ganglia (Fig. 4), being most abundant in the lower thoracic to first lumbar/sacral ganglia, and it has been suggested that here NO may act as a messenger between neurones and satellite cells in sensory ganglia [48]. Following spinal nerve ligation or transection of the sciatic nerve, there is an increase in the number of cells expressing NO synthase in the dorsal root ganglia. Several lines of research have indicated that increased NO production may be involved in nociceptive processing following a neural

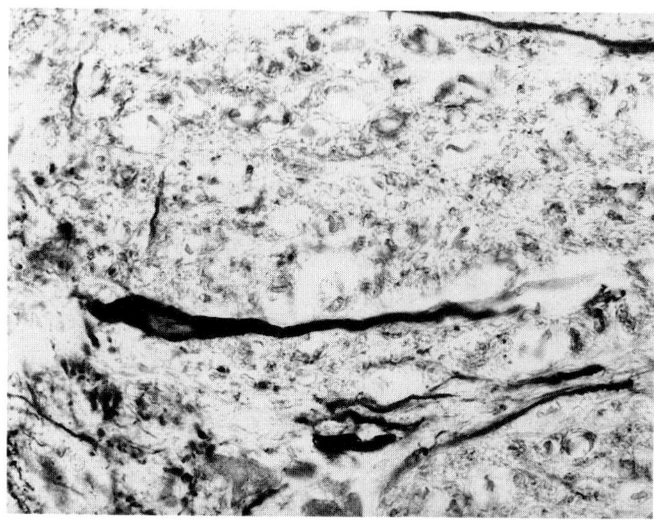

Fig. 3 Human spinal cord immunostained with antiserum to neural NO synthase. Strong staining is seen in a motor neurone in ventral horn of lumbar spinal cord. Indirect immunoperoxidase. (Original magnification ×360.)

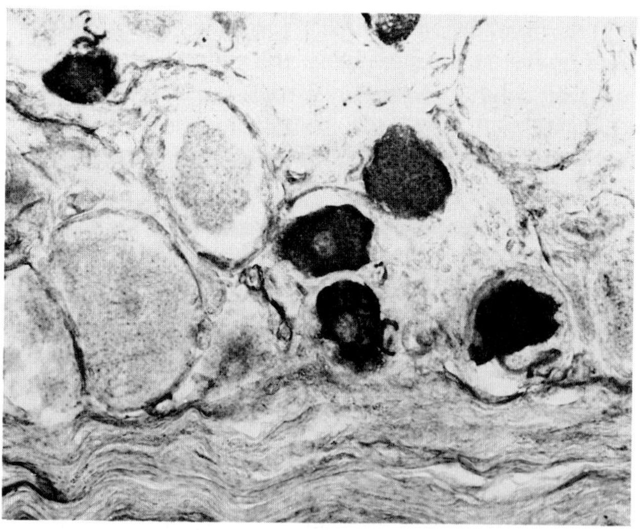

Fig. 4 Human dorsal root ganglia immunostained with antiserum to neural NO synthase. Strong staining is seen in small/medium-sized primary sensory neurones. Indirect immunoperoxidase. (Original magnification ×360.)

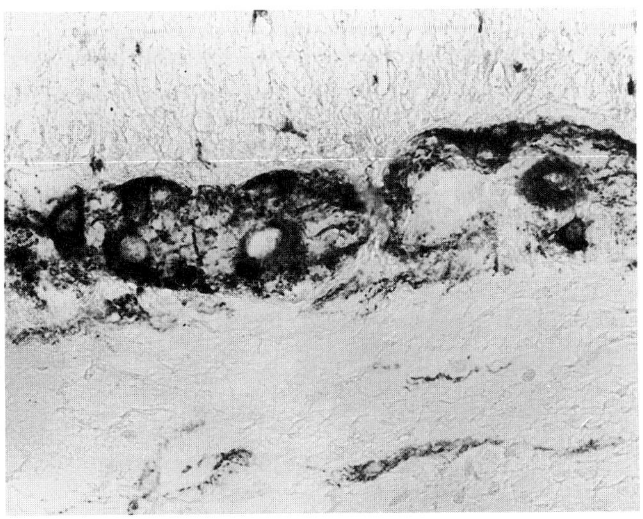

Fig. 5 Human colon stained with antiserum to neural NO synthase. Strong staining is present in ganglion cells and fibres of myenteric plexus. Indirect immunoperoxidase. (Original magnification ×360.)

insult (reviewed in Meller and Gebhart [49]) and this is substantiated by the antinociceptive effects of administration of inhibitors of NO synthase [50].

In addition to the central nervous system, NO synthase-containing nerves are abundantly distributed in the peripheral nervous system [35,36]. Inhibitory NANC nerves are an important population of nerves in peripheral tissues, and it is increasingly apparent that NO is one of the major agents involved in the signalling of this system. These so-called nitroxidergic nerves have previously been most studied in rat anococcygeus muscle [51] and bovine retractor penis muscle [52], but examples of these nerves are found in almost every area of the periphery. In normal gut from many different species, including rat and human, NO synthase immunostaining is localized mainly in fibres and ganglion cells of myenteric plexus (Fig. 5) and muscularis externa, and to a lesser extent in the submucosa and mucosa [35,36]. This distribution is consistent at various levels of the gut. So far, there is little or no evidence of colocalization of NO synthase and any neuropeptide in humans [53]. However, NO synthase is almost always colocalized with vasoactive intestinal peptide (VIP) in the rat, and it has been suggested that both substances are cotransmitters of the enteric inhibitory NANC system [54]. Electrical stimulation of the myenteric neural plexus evokes relaxation of the gut smooth muscle, which can be blocked by inhibitors of NO synthase, thus indicating that NO serves as a neurotransmitter in the gut contributing to the modulation of gut smooth muscle tone [55]. Furthermore, an assessment of the relative contribution of NO and VIP in mediating relaxation of guinea-pig stomach following vagal nerve stimulation indicates that NO is the principal agent of NANC inhibitory neurotransmission in the gut [56].

The neuronal NO synthase may have a role in gut pathology. A study of inflammatory bowel disease in humans revealed that the distribution of NO synthase immunoreactivity is comparable to that seen in uninvolved areas of gut, and hence there is no apparent involvement of NO synthase immunoreactive nerves in the neuromatous hyperplasia of inflammatory bowel disease. This may be due to the fact that NO synthase-containing nerves originate in the myenteric rather than the submucous plexus [53]. However, there is evidence that the levels of NO are increased in this condition but the exact site or sites of synthesis have yet to be firmly established. It has been shown that in a mouse model of opioid-induced constipation, administration of L-arginine can reverse the constipation, indicating that NO may have an important role in the neurogenic control of gut motility, which when compromised contributes to gut pathophysiology [57].

Nitroxidergic nerves also supply blood vessels in a number of vascular beds, including cerebral, mesenteric and pulmonary arteries [58] and have a prominent role in mediating neurogenic vasodilatation [59], and may thus complement endothelium-dependent NO-mediated mechanisms of vasodilatation. Similarly, NO synthase-containing nerves have been localized to the corpora cavernosum and to neuronal plexuses in the adventitia of penile arteries, and also to the endothelium of penile blood vessels. Corpus cavernosum tissue is known to relax both after administration of acetylcholine and by electrical stimulation of penile NANC nerves. Hence, both sources of NO may be involved in the processes leading to dilatation of cavernosal sinusoids and erection. Administration of inhibitors of NO synthesis completely blocks erection produced by electrical stimulation of cavernous nerves, as does de-endothelialization of penile blood vessels, indicating that NO is central to the process of penile erection. Thus, defects in NO-mediated mechanisms in the penis may be involved in some forms of impotence [17].

In the rat, guinea pig, pig and human lung, staining for NO synthase is mainly evident in fibres associated with tracheobronchial and pulmonary smooth muscle with some staining also present in intrinsic ganglia. In guinea-pig airways, NO synthase is reported to be principally colocalized with VIP, but with no evidence of localization in sensory or adrenergic fibres [60]. In human normal lung, we have found NO synthase to be present in airway smooth muscle, around seromucous glands, in the submucosa and, to a lesser degree, around blood vessels but not in the airway epithelium. In airway smooth muscle, the immunoreactive nerves comprised about 30% of total nerves, compared with 40% immunoreactive for VIP, and therefore a partial colocalization of the two is possible (Figs 6 and 7). The relative importance of VIP and NO as neurotransmitters in the NANC innervation is not clear. However, it has recently been shown that in the human lung NO is the principal agent of NANC neurotransmission, with VIP only having a minor contribution [61], although in other species such as guinea pig the role of NO may be less prominent [62].

Because NO is a potent mediator of vaso- and bronchodilatation it has been suggested that it may play a role in the postnatal adaptation of the lung, which essentially changes from a vasoconstricted to a vasodilated state at birth. Support for this hypothesis has come from observations in the developing pig lung. We have found that NO synthase immunoreactive fibres supplying airways and blood vessels decrease significantly with age, from the newborn up to 10 days postpartum, and remain at similar levels in the adult. Thus, the expression of the enzyme may have a prominent role in the physiological adaptation to extrauterine life [63].

Endothelial NO synthase

Endothelial NO synthase has been described in the endothelium of a number of different vascular beds in a range of animal species, where it has a prominent role in the regulation of vascular tone. This enzyme is distinct from the neural enzyme, having a molecular weight of 135 kDa. Cloning of the bovine and human endothelial enzymes reveals that they share 94% sequence homology and suggests that in human and cow, at least, there is very high interspecies conservation [18,19].

The endothelial enzyme is ubiquitously distributed, being evident in macrovascular and microvascular endothelium of arterial and venous circulations in a wide range of vascular beds, including heart, lung (Fig. 8), kidney and brain (Fig. 9) [64], although it has been suggested that the localization of NO synthase is more prominent in larger vessels [34]. Detailed immunochemical investigation reveals that the enzyme may, in fact, have variable levels of expression both in different vascular beds and also within the same vascular bed. For example, in the placenta endothelial NO synthase immunoreactivity is evident in umbilical (Figs 10 and 11) and chorionic vessels, but as the size of vessels decreases, staining disappears and is totally absent from the smallest vessels of the placental villous tree. Interestingly, staining is also detected in the syncytiotrophoblast (Fig. 12) of the placental villous tree – one of the few instances, to date, of a cell type other than the endothelial cell expressing the endothelial enzyme. It is highly probable that syncytiotrophoblast-derived NO contributes to control of the smaller vessels, where the

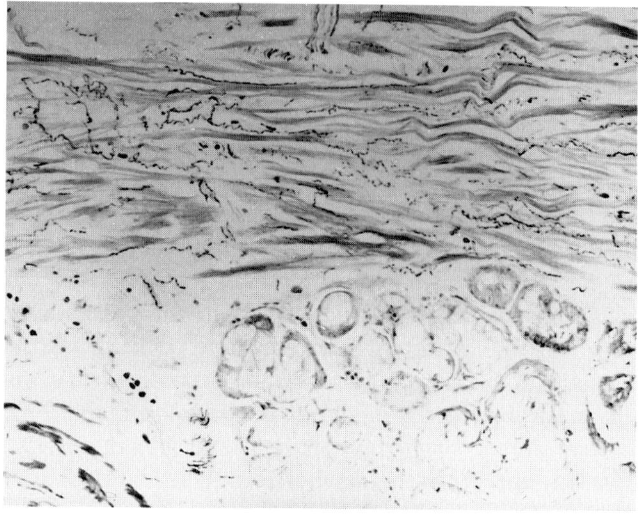

Fig. 6 Serial sections of human trachea stained with antisera to neural NO synthase. Staining is seen in similar populations of fibres in Fig. 7, associated with tracheal smooth muscle. Indirect immunoperoxidase. (Original magnification ×230.)

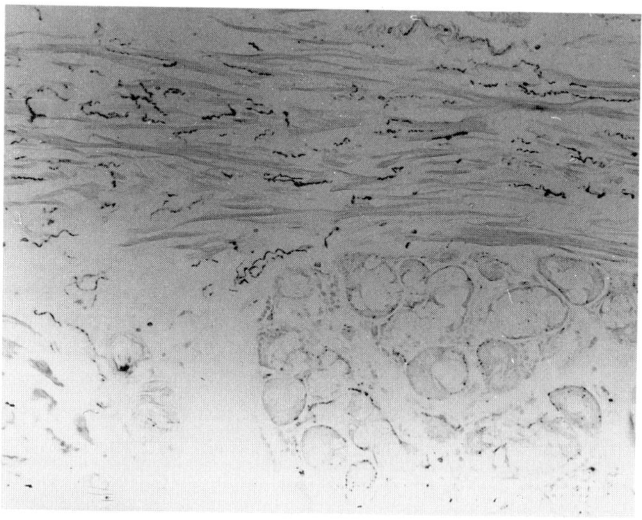

Fig. 7 Serial sections of human trachea stained with antisera to VIP. Staining is seen in similar populations of fibres in Fig. 6, associated with tracheal smooth muscle. Indirect immunoperoxidase. (Original magnification ×230.)

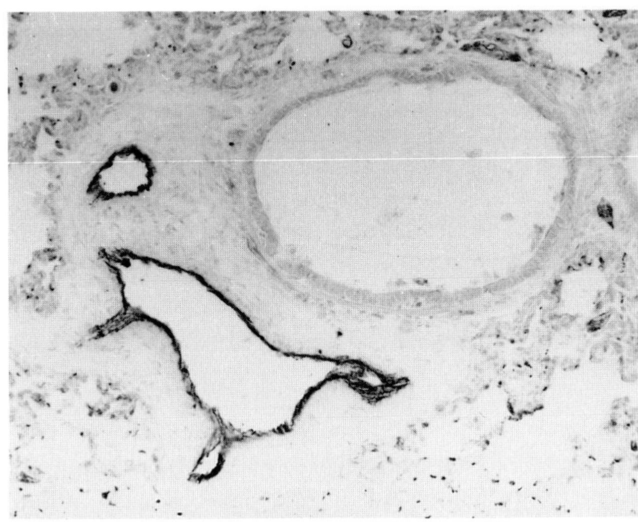

Fig. 8 Pig lung immunostained with antiserum to endothelial NO synthase. Strong staining is seen in endothelia of pulmonary artery and vein. Indirect immunoperoxidase. (Original magnification ×360.)

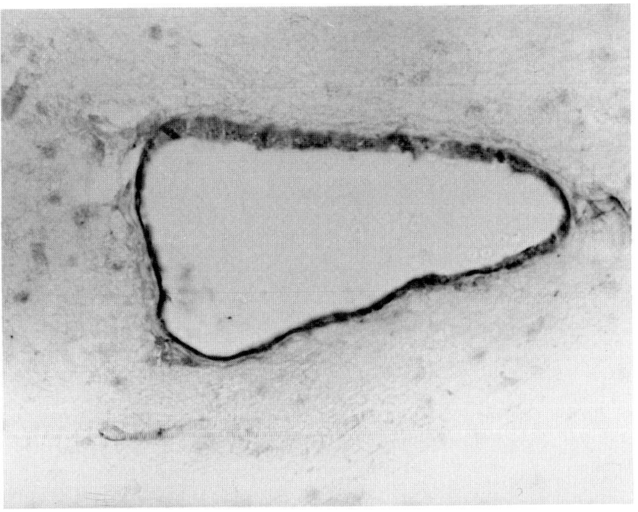

Fig. 9 Sheep brain immunostained with antiserum to endothelial NO synthase. Staining is seen in the endothelium of a cerebral vessel. Indirect immunoperoxidase. (Original magnification ×500.)

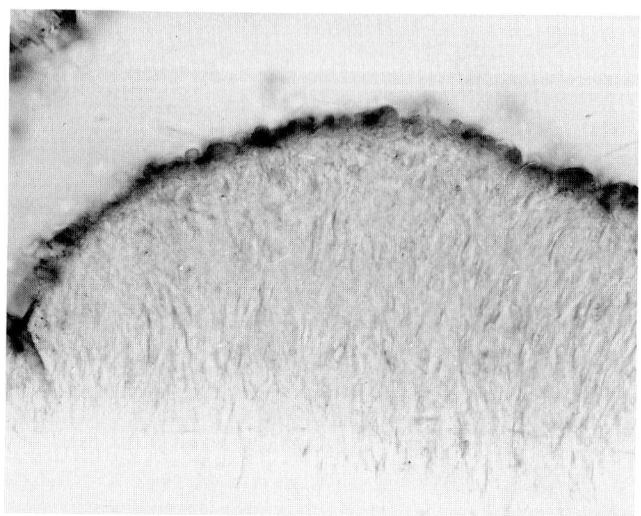

Fig. 10 Human umbilical cord immunostained with antiserum to endothelial NO synthase. Strong staining is seen in the endothelia of umbilical artery. Indirect immunoperoxidase. (Original magnification ×500.)

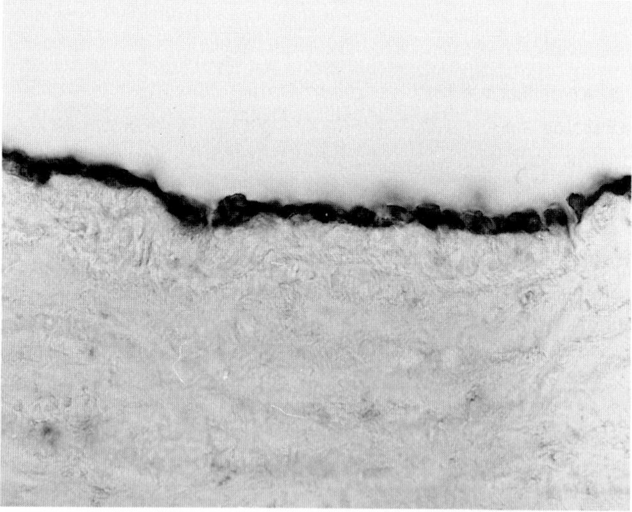

Fig. 11 Human umbilical cord immunostained with antiserum to endothelial NO synthase. Strong staining is seen in the umbilical vein. Indirect immunoperoxidase. (Original magnification ×500.)

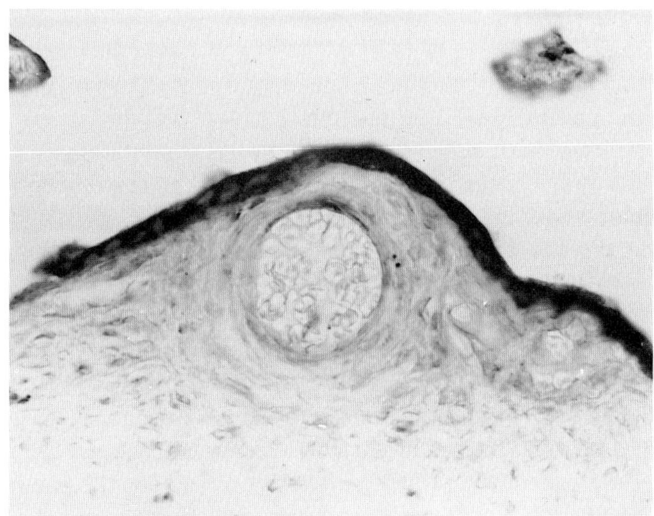

Fig. 12 Human placenta immunostained with antiserum to endothelial NO synthase. In the placenta staining is evident in syncytiotrophoblast layer of placental villus, but is apparently absent from the foetal blood vessel. Indirect immunostaining. (Original magnification ×500.)

enzyme is apparently not expressed and, perhaps more importantly, inhibits platelet aggregation in the intervillous space. This differential distribution of endothelial NO synthase in the placenta strongly suggests that NO derived from this enzyme has a pivotal role in the regulation of placental perfusion and also illustrates that the variable expression of the enzyme might well be intimately related to physiological function [65].

In the pig lung, endothelial NO synthase, like the neuronal form, shows an age-related variation in the level of expression and distribution in pulmonary blood vessels during the first few days after birth. From newborn to 3 days postpartum, the level of enzyme expression increases significantly, and then gradually decreases again 1–2 weeks postpartum and then remains at similar levels in the adult [66]. This suggests that the high levels of enzyme may play a role in reversing the essentially hypertensive state of the newborn, but that as lung function normalizes, the level of enzyme regresses to a level which is sufficient to maintain normal perfusion. The similar age-related changes in the level of neuronal enzyme expression, as reported above, illustrate that physiological function and adaptation of certain organ systems may be the result of contributions from both endothelium-dependent and endothelium-independent NO-mediated mechanisms.

NO is the most potent vasorelaxant known and is one of the principal agents in the control of vascular tone and basal blood pressure [16].

Endothelium-derived NO is released in response to physical stimuli, such as shear stress due to local variations in blood flow, and chemical stimuli, including acetylcholine, adenosine triphosphate (ATP), substance P and bradykinin [14]. Endothelium-derived NO has been shown to form complexes with small proteins, forming stable adducts such as *S*-nitrosothiol [67]. These NO-adducts may prevent scavenging of NO by haemoglobin, and may also help to deliver NO to specific sites, thus extending the life and potentiating the actions of NO. The release of NO-adducts has subsequently been demonstrated in other cell types, such as macrophages [68], and their formation may add a new dimension to ascertaining the physiological and pathophysiological function, and possible cellular trafficking of NO.

Unlike other isoforms, the endothelial enzyme is *N*-terminally myristoylated. This is important in determining the subcellular localization of the enzyme. It is predominantly associated with the particulate fraction (i.e. membranes) of the cell and this may be important for substrate binding. However, activity is also dependent on phosphorylation of the enzyme, which may subsequently be translocated from the particulate to the cytosolic fraction of the cell, thus illustrating that the activity of this enzyme is highly regulated [69,70].

Altered function of the enzyme may have a significant contribution to the pathogenesis of vascular diseases, such as pulmonary hypertension and atherosclerosis. At present, it is not clear how important a factor NO is or where exactly it fits into the time-course of disease progression. Decreased synthesis of NO could be the result of decreased enzyme activity, which may be a consequence of substrate availability or blockade of the enzyme by endogenous inhibitors [71]. Similarly, decreased synthesis of NO may be due to the lack of agonist-induced activation of the enzyme. In addition, oxidized low density lipoproteins are potent inhibitors of the L-arginine–NO pathway [72], possibly affecting L-arginine mobilization, since an excess of exogenous L-arginine can normalize or improve impaired endothelium-dependent relaxation. It is important to note that the constitutive enzymes are highly regulated, requiring multiple cofactors and possibly protein phosphorylation for full activity. The endothelial enzyme may also be subject to subcellular trafficking. Decreased enzyme expression may be significant, inferring that abnormal function lies at the level of the gene.

However, in spite of the lack of detailed information on the mechanisms involved, there is certainly good evidence that reduced availability of NO does contribute to some diseases, since controlled inhalation of authentic NO is effective in alleviating symptoms of the adult respiratory distress syndrome (ARDS) and also partially reverses pulmonary hypertension [73]. Similarly, administration of the enzyme substrate L-arginine has been shown to be an effective therapeutic agent for Raynaud's phenomenon [74] and restores acetylcholine-induced vasoconstriction in atheromatous human coronary arteries [75]. Immunocytochemical evidence suggests that in some diseases such as pre-eclampsia, where decreased NO has been postulated to be important in contributing to the disease, the level of enzyme appears similar to that in normal healthy subjects. However, in coronary vessels obstructed by atheromatous plaques and also in vessel grafts obstructed by neo-intima, the expression of the enzyme is often greatly reduced when compared to the normal healthy native vessel, suggesting that the loss of patency seen in these vessels may ultimately be due to a decrease or a total loss of expressed enzyme.

Inducible NO synthase

The inducible enzyme is distinct from all other known forms of NO synthase in that it is generally absent from normal healthy tissues. The enzyme is only expressed following exposure to immunological stimuli, which can induce the *de novo* synthesis of the enzyme in an extensive range of tissues [14]. The conditions necessary for induction vary between cell types, but endotoxin, interferon γ, tumour necrosis factor α and interleukin 1, either alone or particularly in combination, lead to induction in most cells. The inducible enzyme has a molecular weight of 130 kDa which is similar to the endothelial enzyme. However, cloning reveals that the inducible enzyme only shares about 50% homology with both the neural and endothelial enzymes and thus (like the two constitutive enzymes) [24] is the product of a distinct gene. Inducible NO synthase has now been purified to homogeneity and cloned from a variety of cells including murine macrophages, rat smooth muscle and rat liver [25–27]. These studies indicate that the enzyme(s) are virtually identical thus implying that, in rodents at least, there is only one isoform of inducible NO synthase.

Investigation of the induction and tissue distribution of NO synthase has primarily focused on easily manipulated models such as endotoxin-treated rat and human or animal cells in culture (Figs 13 and 14). *In vitro* and *in vivo* induction of NO synthase by endotoxin and or combinations of cytokines has been demonstrated in numerous cells including macrophages [6], vascular smooth muscle [7], hepatocytes [8], Kupffer cells [9], mesangial cells [76], myocytes [77] and chondrocytes [78]. In fact, induction of this enzyme has been demonstrated in virtually every cell type and has prompted the suggestion that induction of NO synthase represents a primitive and comparatively rapid immune effector system [79].

Interestingly, some cells appear to have different requirements for induction of the enzyme. For example, endotoxin alone does not appear

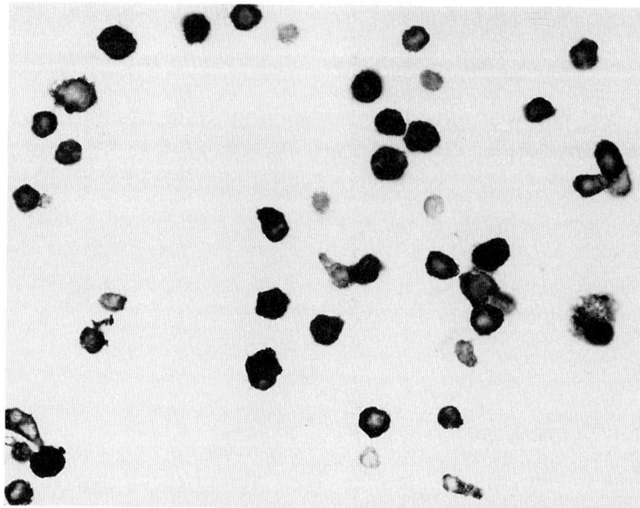

Fig. 13 Murine RAW 264 macrophages immunostained with antiserum to inducible NO synthase. Strong staining is seen in endotoxin-stimulated cells. Indirect immunoperoxidase. (Original magnification ×360.)

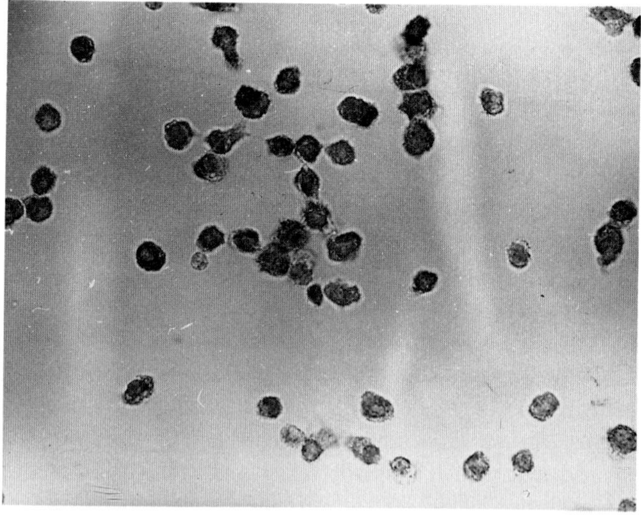

Fig. 14 Murine RAW 264 macrophages immunostained with antiserum to inducible NO synthase. No staining is present in unstimulated cells. Indirect immunoperoxidase. (Original magnification ×360.)

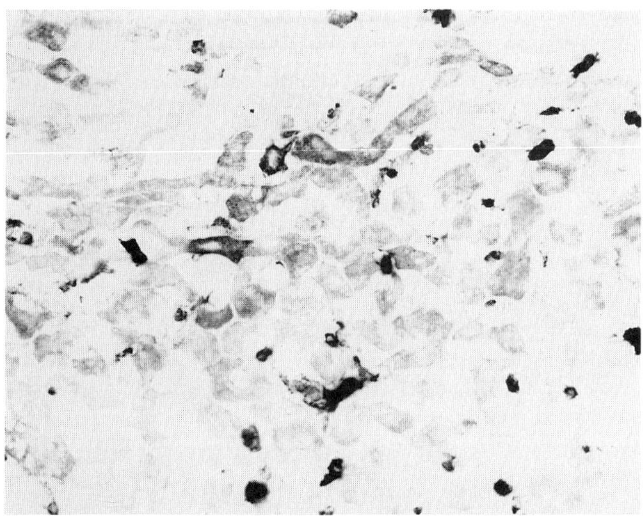

Fig. 15 Endotoxin-treated rat liver immunostained with antiserum to inducible NO synthase. Strong staining is evident in numerous macrophages and also a few hepatocytes. Indirect immunoperoxidase. (Original magnification ×360.)

to be a particularly potent stimulus for induction in hepatocytes [80] (Fig. 15), whereas robust expression can be detected in macrophages [81] (Fig. 15). This may be due to different thresholds of induction in different cells and probably relates to cellular function; the macrophage is one of the principal cells involved in cell-mediated immunity, and hence even a mild stimulus may be effective in inducing high levels of the enzyme. In addition, the macrophage for the most part is freely circulating; for NO to be effective, it may be necessary to generate very high levels of NO, hence the need for high expression of the enzyme. As suggested above, the efficacy of macrophage-derived NO may be increased by the formation of NO-adducts, which could have a significant contribution in directing NO to a specific site such as the blood vessel wall. In contrast, some tissues such as vascular smooth muscle or cardiac myocytes may express levels of the enzyme that are sufficient to exert profound physiological effects, such as hypotension [14] and abnormal myocardial contraction [77], but at levels below the limits of detection of some investigative techniques such as immunocytochemistry.

The induction of NO synthase has been demonstrated in some human tumour cell-lines [82] and has also been shown to regulate tumour blood flow in an experimental murine tumour model [83] (Fig. 16). Further investigation of this model has revealed that the enzyme is primarily expressed in the tumour neovasculature and is induced several days after introduction of the tumour cells. The induction of this enzyme in

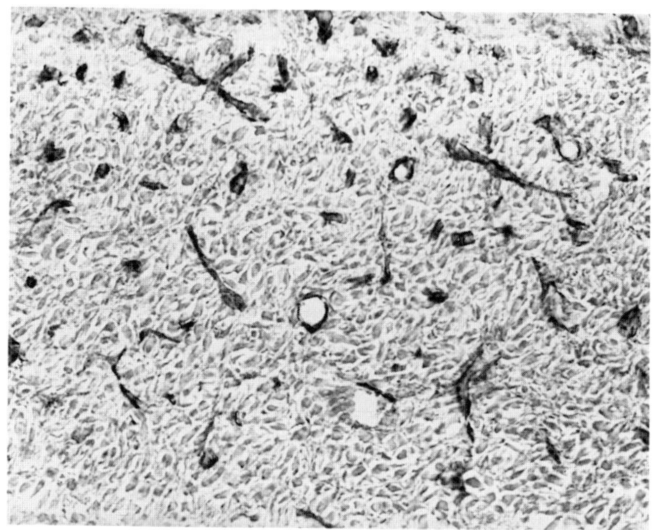

Fig. 16 Experimental murine tumour (adenocarcinoma) immunostained with antiserum to inducible NO synthase. Strong straining is seen in the endothelium of tumour neovasculature. Indirect immunoperoxidase. (Original magnification ×360.)

tumours is a somewhat surprising finding, since NO is both cytotoxic and cytostatic when present at sufficient levels. This may be partially explained from the observation that some cells have different sensitivities to NO [14], hence the tumour cells may be less susceptible to NO toxicity. In addition, it is possible that the role of inducible NO synthesis in regulating tumour blood flow, thereby maintaining perfusion and sustaining tumour growth, may outweigh the tumouricidal actions. It is interesting that many solid tumours have necrotic cores, which may well be the direct result of NO-mediated cell damage. Furthermore, the inducible NO synthase immunoreactive vessels appear more prominent at the periphery of the tumour which is the most active site of tumour growth.

Induction of NO synthesis has also been demonstrated in bone tissue following administration of endotoxin. Immunostaining for inducible NO synthase was observed in a variety of bone cells including growth plate chondroblasts, differentiating peri-epiphyseal chondroblastic cells, osteoclasts and articular chondrocytic cells. The significance of inducible NO synthesis on bone tissue function is complex and not fully understood, although it has been suggested that increased NO production inhibits osteoclast activity thereby affecting bone resorption [84].

In humans there is little or no evidence to suggest that inducible NO synthase is present in macrophages, unlike in other animals where macrophages are a prominent source of inducible NO synthesis. Recently, an inducible NO synthase from human hepatocytes has been purified to homogeneity and cloned. The human enzyme may be a distinctive form of NO synthase sharing approximately 80% homology with the rodent inducible enzyme [79]. However, antisera to rodent enzymes have successfully been shown to crossreact with human tissues. For example, in a study of bronchial biopsies from asthmatic subjects, inducible NO synthase immunoreactivity was localized to the airway epithelium in 90% of subjects. This strongly suggests that increased NO production is a feature in the process of asthma, possibly reflecting the inflammatory nature of the disease, and could mediate local bronchodilatation and also contribute to epithelial cell damage and stripping [85].

The role of inducible NO synthesis is multifactorial. Once activated, the inducible NO synthase is unregulated, generating high (nanomolar) levels of NO with actions which are cytotoxic/cytostatic and mediating prolonged vasodilatation, contributing to the profound hypotension seen in some conditions such as sepsis. Inhibition of NO synthesis by arginine analogues such as L-NMMA has been used successfully to alleviate life-threatening hypotension in two human subjects with sepsis, thus illustrating the profound physiological effects of this enzyme. However, caution should be made in drawing conclusions, since inhibition of the enzyme in some organs such as lung, liver and kidney may actually potentiate cellular injury, thus indicating that the inducible enzyme may also exert protective effects [86,87].

CONCLUSIONS

In the short time since the discovery of NO, this small, labile, soluble gas has become established as a versatile, tissue- and species-diverse messenger molecule. The synthesis and control of NO is exquisitely manipulated by a family of enzymes, the NO synthases, all of which catalyze the same reaction but, according to their tissue localization and the level of NO produced, effect a wide range of profound physiological and pathophysiological actions. Although the mechanisms involved in regulation of these enzymes are only just beginning to be unravelled, the cloning of the NO synthase gene family will clarify the full role of these enzymes (and possibly, as yet undiscovered NO synthase isoforms) in both health and disease.

REFERENCES

1 Tannenbaum SR, Fett D, Young UR, *et al.* Nitrite and nitrate are formed by endogenous synthesis in the human intestine. *Science* 1978;200:1487–1488.

2 Furchgott RF, Zawadzki JV. The obligatory role of endothelial cells in relaxation of arterial smooth muscle by acetylcholine. *Nature* 1980;288:373–376.

3 Gillespie JS. The rat anococcygeus muscle and its response to nerve stimulation and to some drugs. *Br J Pharmacol* 1972;45:404–416.
4 Palmer R, Moncada S. A novel citrulline forming enzyme implicated in the formation of nitric oxide by vascular endothelial cells. *Biochem Biophys Res Commun* 1989;158: 348–352.
5 Radomski MW, Palmer RMJ, Monacada S. An L-arginine:nitric oxide pathway in human platelets regulates aggregation. *Proc Natl Acad Sci USA* 1990;87:5193–5197.
6 Marletta MA, Yoons PS, Iyenga R, *et al.* Macrophage oxidation of L-arginine to nitrite and nitrate: nitric oxide as an intermediate. *Biochemistry* 1988;27:8706–8711.
7 Rees DD, Celleck S, Palmer RMJ, Moncada S. Dexamethasone prevents the induction by endotoxin of nitric oxide synthase and associated effects on vascular tone. An insight into endotoxin shock. *Biochem Biophy Res Commun* 1990;173:541–547.
8 Schmidt HHHW, Seifart R, Bohme E. Formation and release of nitric oxide from human neutrophils and HL-6 cells induced by chemotactic peptide, platelet activating factor and leukotriene B_4. *FEBS Lett* 1989;244:357–360.
9 Curran RD, Billiar TR, Stuehr DJ, *et al.* Hepatocytes produce nitrogen oxides from L-arginine in response to inflammatory products from Kupffer cells. *J Exp Med* 1989;170: 1769–1774.
10 Billiar TR, Curran RD, Stuehr DJ, *et al.* An L-arginine-dependent mechanism mediates Kupffer cell inhibition of hepatocyte protein synthesis *in vitro*. *J Exp Med* 1989;169: 1467–1472.
11 Knowles RG, Palacios M, Palmer RMJ, Moncada S. Formation of nitric oxide from L-arginine in the central nervous system: a transduction mechanism for stimulation of soluble guanylate cyclase. *Proc Natl Acad Sci USA* 1989;86:5159–5162.
12 Ignarro LJ. Haem-dependent activation of guanylate cyclase by nitric oxide: a novel signal transduction mechanism. *Blood Vessels* 1991;28:67–73.
13 Hibbs JB, Taintor RR, Vavrin Z, Rachlin EM. Nitric oxide: a cytotoxic activated macrophage effector molecule. *Biochem Biophys Res Commun* 1988;157:87–94.
14 Moncada S, Palmer RMJ, Higgs EA. Nitric oxide: physiology, pathophysiology and pharmacology. *Pharmacol Rev* 1991;43:109–142.
15 Fosterman U, Schmidt HHHW, Pollock JS, *et al.* Isoforms of nitric oxide synthase. *Biochem Pharmacol* 1991;42:1849–1857.
16 Vallance P, Collier J, Moncada S. Effects of endothelium-derived relaxing factor on peripheral arterial tone in man. *Lancet* 1989;ii:997–1000.
17 Burnnett AL, Lowenstein CJ, Bredt DS, *et al.* Nitric oxide: a physiological mediator of penile erection. *Science* 1992;257:401–403.
18 Knowles RG, Palacois M, Palmer RMJ, Moncada S. Kinetic characteristics of nitric oxide synthase from rat brain. *Biochem J* 1990;269:207–210.
19 Kwon NS, Nathan CF, Steuhr DJ. Reduced biopterin as a co-factor in the generation of nitrogen oxides by murine macrophages. *J Biol Chem* 1989;264:20496–20501.
20 Tayeh MA, Marletta MA. Macrophage oxidation of L-arginine to nitric oxide, nitrite and nitrate. Tetrahydrobiopterin is required as a co-factor. *J Biol Chem* 1989;264: 19654–19658.
21 Bredt DS, Hwang PM, Glatt CE, *et al.* Cloned and expressed nitric oxide synthase structurally resembles cytochrome P-450 reductase. *Nature* 1991;351:714–718.
22 Nakane M, Schmidt HHHW, Pollock JS, *et al.* Cloned human brain nitric oxide synthase is highly expressed in skeletal muscle. *FEBS Lett* 1993;316:175–180.
23 Lamas S, Marsden PA, Gordon KL, *et al.* Endothelial nitric oxide synthase: molecular cloning and characterization of a distinct constitutive isoform. *Proc Natl Acad Sci USA* 1992;89:6348–6352.
24 Marsden PA, Schappert KT, Chen Hai S, *et al.* Molecular cloning and characterization of human endothelial nitric oxide synthase. *FEBS Lett* 1992;307:287–293.
25 Xie Q-W, Cho HJ, Calaycay J, *et al.* Cloning and characterisation of inducible nitric oxide synthesis from mouse macrophages. *Science* 1992;256:225–228.
26 Nunokawa Y, Ishida N, Tanaka S. Cloning of inducible nitric oxide synthase in rat vascular smooth muscle cells. *Biochem Biophys Res Commun* 1993;191:89–94.
27 Wood ER, Berger H Jr, Sherman PA, Lapetina EG. Hepatocytes and macrophages express an identical inducible nitric oxide synthase gene. *Biochem Biophys Res Commun* 1993;191:767–774.

28 Kishimoto J, Spurr N, Liao M, *et al.* Localization of brain nitric oxide synthase to human chromosome 12. *Genomics* 1992;14:802–804.

29 Marsden PA, Heng HH, Scherer SW, *et al.* Structure and chromosomal localization of the human constitutive endothelial nitric oxide synthase gene. *J Biol Chem* 1990;268: 17478–17488.

30 Martinez A, Riveros-Moreno V, Polak JM, *et al.* Nitric oxide synthase-immunoreactivity in the starfish *Marthasterias glacialis. Cell Tissue Res* 1994 (in press).

31 Radomski MW, Martin JF, Moncada S. Synthesis of nitric oxide by the heamocytes of the American horseshoe crab (*Limulus polyphemus*). *Phil Trans R Soc Lond B* 1991;334: 129–133.

32 Archer S. Measurement of nitric oxide in biological models. *FASEB J* 1993;7:349–360.

33 Wharton J, Springall DR, Rutherford RAD, *et al.* Placental nitric oxide synthase visualized by *in vitro* autoradiography and immunocytochemistry. *Placenta* 1993;14:A82.

34 Bredt DS, Hwang PM, Snyder S. Localisation of nitric oxide synthase indicating a neural role for nitric oxide. *Nature* 1990;347:768–770.

35 Bredt DS, Glatt CE, Hwang PM, *et al.* Nitric oxide synthase protein and mRNA are discretely localized in neuronal populations of mammalian CNS together with NADPH diaphorase. *Neuron* 1991;7:615–624.

36 Springall DR, Riveros-Moreno V, Buttery LDK, *et al.* Immunological detection of nitric oxide synthase(s) in human tissues using heterologous antibodies suggesting different isoforms. *Histochemistry* 1992;98:259–266.

37 Thomas E, Pearse AGE. The solitary active cells. Histochemical demonstration of damage-resistant nerve cells with a TPN-diaphorase reaction. *Acta Neuropathol* 1964;3: 238–249.

38 Michel T. Nitric oxide synthesis in infantile hypertrophic pyloric stenosis. *N Engl J Med* 1992;327:1690–1691.

39 Schmidt HHHW, Gagne GD, Nakane M, *et al.* Mapping of neural nitric oxide synthase in the rat suggests frequent co-localization with NADPH diaphorase but not with soluble guanylyl cyclase, and novel paraneural functions for nitrinergic signal transduction. *J Histochem Cytochem* 1992;40:1439–1456.

40 Ogura T, Yokoyama T, Fujisawa H, *et al.* Structural diversity of neuronal nitric oxide synthase mRNA in the nervous system. *Biochem Biophys Res Commun* 1993;193:1014–1022.

41 Garthwaite J, Garthwaite G, Palmer RMJ, Moncada S. NMDA receptor activation induces nitric oxide synthesis from L-arginine in rat brain slices. *Eur J Pharmacol* 1989;172:413–416.

42 Baringa M. Is nitric oxide the 'retrograde messenger'. *Science* 1992;254:1296–1297.

43 Bredt DS, Synder S. Nitric oxide as a neuronal messenger. *TIPS* 1991;12:125–128.

44 Dun NJ, Dun SL, Wu SY, *et al.* Nitric oxide synthase immunoreactivity in the rat, mouse, cat and squirrel monkey spinal cord. *Neuroscience* 1993;54:845–857.

45 Terenghi G, Riveros-Moreno V, Hudson L, *et al.* Immunohistochemistry of nitric oxide synthase demonstrates immunoreactive nuerons in spinal cord and dorsal root ganglia of man and rat. *J Neurol Sci* 1993;118:34–37.

46 Dun NL, Dun SL, Forsterman U, Tseng LF. Nitric oxide synthase immunoreactivity in rat spinal cord. *Neurosci Lett* 1992;147:217–220.

47 Wu W. Expression of nitric oxide synthase (NOS) in injured CNS neurons as shown by NADPH diaphorase histochemistry. *Exp Neurol* 1993;120:153–159.

48 Morris R, Southam E, Braid DJ, Garthwaite J. Nitric oxide may act as a messenger between dorsal root ganglion neurones and their satellite cells. *Neurosci Lett* 1992;137: 29–32.

49 Meller ST, Gebhart GF. Nitric oxide and nociceptive processing in the spinal cord. *Pain* 1993;52:127–136.

50 Przewlocki R, Machelska H, Przewlocka B. Inhibition of nitric oxide synthase enhances morphine antinociception in the rat spinal cord. *Life Sci* 1993;53:1–5.

51 Li CG, Rand MJ. Evidence for a role of nitric oxide in the neurotransmitter system mediating relaxation of the anococcygeus muscle. *Clin Exp Pharmacol Physiol* 1989; 16:933–938.

52 Gillespie JS, Sheng H. A comparison of haemoglobin and erythrocytes as inhibitors of

smooth muscle relaxation by the NANC transmitter in the BRP and rat anococcygeus and by EDRF in the rabbit aortic strip. *Br J Pharmacol* 1989;98:445–450.
53 Bishop AE, Dodoo A, Riveros-Moreno V, *et al.* Morphological evidence for nitric oxide production by the human enteric nervous system. *Regul Peptides* 1993;47:97.
54 Aimi Y, Kiumura H, Kinoshita T, *et al.* Histochemical localization of nitric oxide synthase in rat enteric nervous system. *Neuroscience* 1993;514:553–560.
55 Sanders KM, Ward SM. Nitric oxide as a mediator of non-adrenergic non-cholinergic neurotransmission. *Am J Physiol* 1992;262:G379–392.
56 Desai KM, Warner TD, Bishop AE, *et al.* Nitric oxide, and not VIP, is the main neuotransmitter of vagally induced relaxation of the guinea pig stomach. *Br J Pharmacol* 1994 (in press).
57 Calignano A, Moncada S, Di Rosa M. Endogenous NO modulates morphine-induced constipation. *Biochem Biophys Res Commun* 1991;181:889–893.
58 Toda N, Okamura T. Regulation by nitroxidergic nerve of arterial tone. *NIPS* 1992; 7:148–152.
59 Toda N, Okamura T. Mechanism underlying the response to vasodilator nerve stimulation in isolated dog and monkey cerebral arteries. *Am J Physiol* 1991;261:H1511–H1517.
60 Kummer W, Fischer A, Mundel P, *et al.* Nitric oxide synthase in VIP-containing vasodilator nerve fibres in the guinea pig. *Neuroreport* 1992;3:653–657.
61 Belvisi MG, Stretton CD, Miura M, *et al.* Inhibitory NANC nerves in human tracheal smooth muscle: a quest for the neurotransmitter. *J Appl Physiol* 1992;73:2505–2510.
62 Belvisi MG, Miura M, Stretton CD, Barnes PJ. Endogenous vasoactive peptide and nitric oxide modulate cholinergic neurotransmission in guinea pig trachea. *Eur J Pharmacol* 1993;231:97–102.
63 Springall DR, Buttery LDK, Hislop AA, *et al.* Nitric oxide synthase immunoreactive nerves in pig lung decrease during postnatal development. *Am Rev Respir Dis* 1993; 147:A939.
64 Pollock JS, Nakane M, Buttery LDK, *et al.* Characterization and localization of endothelial nitric oxide synthase using specific monoclonal antibodies. *Am J Physiol* 1993;C1379–C1387.
65 Buttery LDK, McCarthy A, Springall DR, *et al.* Placental NO synthase: a possible regulator of the feto-maternal interface. *Placenta* 1994 (in press).
66 Hislop AA, Buttery LDK, Springall DR, *et al.* Postnatal changes in localisation of endothelial nitric oxide synthase in the porcine pulmonary vasculature. *Am Rev Respir Dis* 1993;147:A224.
67 Stamler JS, Simon DI, Osborne JA, *et al.* S-Nitrosylation of proteins with nitric oxide: synthesis of and characterization of biologically active compounds. *Proc Natl Acad Sci USA* 1992;89:444–448.
68 Uchizumi H, Hattori R, Sase K, *et al.* A stable L-arginine-dependent relaxing factor released from cytotoxic-activated macrophages. *Am J Physiol* 1993;264:H1472–H1477.
69 Busconi L, Michel T. Endothelial nitric oxide synthase: N-terminal myristoylation determines subcellular localization. *J Biol Chem* 1992;268:8410–8413.
70 Michel T, Li KG, Busconi L. Phosphorylation and subcellular translocation of endothelial nitric oxide synthase. *Proc Natl Acad Sci USA* 1993;90:6252–6256.
71 Vallance P, Leone A, Calver A, *et al.* Accumulation of an endogenous inhibitor of nitric oxide synthesis in chronic renal failure. *Lancet* 1992;389:572–575.
72 Tanner FC, Noll G, Boulanger CM, Luscher TF. Oxidized low density lipoproteins inhibit relaxations of porcine coronary arteries. Role of scavenger receptor and endothelium-derived nitric oxide. *Circulation* 1991;83:2012–2020.
73 Faule KJ, Rossaint R, Keitel M, *et al.* *Successful Treatment of Severe Adult Respiratory Distress Syndrome With Nitric Oxide: The First Three Patients.* Presented at Second International Meeting on the Biology of Nitric Oxide, London, October, 1991.
74 Agostoni A, Marasini B, Biondi ML, *et al.* L-arginine therapy in Raynaud's phenomenon. *Int J Clin Lab Res* 1991;31:202–203.
75 Dubois JL, Zelinsky R, Roudot F, *et al.* Effects of infusion of L-arginine into the left anterior descending coronary artery on acetylcholine-induced vasoconstriction of human atheromatous coronary arteries. *Am J Cardiol* 1992;70:1269–1275.

76 Pfeilschifter J, Rob P, Mulsch A, *et al.* Interleukin-1-β and tumour necrosis factor-α induce a macrophage-type of nitric oxide synthase in rat renal mesangial cells. *Eur J Biochem* 1992;203:251–255.
77 Brady AJB, Poole-Wilson PA, Harding SE, Warren JB. Nitric oxide production within cardiac myocytes reduces their contractility in endotoxaemia. *Am J Physiol* 1992; 263:H1963–H1966.
78 Palmer RMJ, Andrews T, Foxwell NA, Moncada S. Glucocorticoids do not affect the induction of a novel calcium-dependent nitric oxide synthase in rabbit chondrocytes. *Biochem Biophys Res Commun* 1992;188:209–215.
79 Geller DA, Lowenstein CJ, Shapiro RA, *et al.* Molecular cloning and expression of inducible nitric oxide synthase from human heptocytes. *Proc Natl Acad Sci USA* 1993;90:3491–3495.
80 Geller DA, Nussler AK, Di Silvio M, *et al.* Cytokines, endotoxin and glucocorticoids regulate the expression of inducible nitric oxide synthase in hepatocytes. *Proc Natl Acad Sci USA* 1993;90:522–526.
81 Buttery LDK, Evans TJ, Springall DR, *et al.* Distinct localization of inducible nitric oxide synthase in endotoxin-treated rats. *Endothelium* 1993;1:S27.
82 Radomski MW, Jenkins DC, Holmes L, Moncada S. Human colorectal adenocarcinoma cells: differential nitric oxide synthesis determines their ability to aggregate platelets. *Cancer Res* 1991;51:6073–6078.
83 Buttery LDK, Springall DR, Andrade S, *et al.* Induction of nitric oxide synthase in the neo-vasculature of experimental murine tumours. *J Pathol* 1993;171:311–319.
84 Umeda T, Gross SS, Cudd A, *et al.* Osteoclasts contain both inducible and constitutive NOS isoforms: a key role in bone resorption? *Endothelium* 1993;1:S47.
85 Schultz P, Raij L. Inhibition of nitric oxide (NO) synthesis in vivo potentiates endotoxin (LPS) induced renal injury. *J Am Soc Nephrol* 1991;3:563.
86 Billiar TR, Curran RD, Harbrect BG, *et al.* Modulation of nitrogen oxide synthesis in vivo: NG-monomethyl-L-arginine inhibits endotoxin-induced nitrite/nitrate biosynthesis while promoting hepatic damage. *J Leuk Biol* 1990;48:565–569.

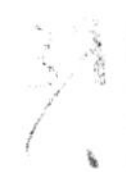

Is asthma a disease of affluence?

A. J. WOOLCOCK

INTRODUCTION AND DEFINITIONS

The prevalence of asthma in children is increasing in many countries. This paper draws attention to the fact that asthma is now a major problem in affluent countries and presents evidence that the house-dust mite is the link between increasing asthma and increasing affluence.

Asthma is an inflammatory disease of the airways that makes them prone to narrow too easily and too much in response to many different provoking stimuli.

Airway hyperresponsiveness (AHR) is the increased narrowing of the airways which occurs in response to a provoking stimulus. Both AHR and symptoms of wheeze and chest tightness are thought to result from a combination of factors, including thickening of the airway wall, increased bulk of the smooth muscle, uncoupling of the local elastic recoil, loss of epithelium, an alteration in the contractility of the smooth muscle and, perhaps, exposure of the sensory nerves. A normal person has a dose–response curve to inhaled methacholine as shown by curve F in Fig. 1 while the curves of asthmatic subjects are shifted to the left. It appears that many allergic people who do not have symptoms of asthma have abnormal dose – response curves [1] and many have some inflammation of the airways [2].

Current asthma is defined in epidemiological studies as the presence of AHR plus symptoms of asthma (usually wheeze or chest tightness) in the last year.

EPIDEMIOLOGY OF CHILDHOOD ASTHMA IN AUSTRALIA

Australia is a dry continent but is humid near the sea and most of the population lives in the areas where it is humid at all times. Table 1 shows the prevalence of current asthma (symptoms plus AHR) in a number of populations of children in different countries. The bronchial provocation tests used to define AHR were different but it is now possible to compare

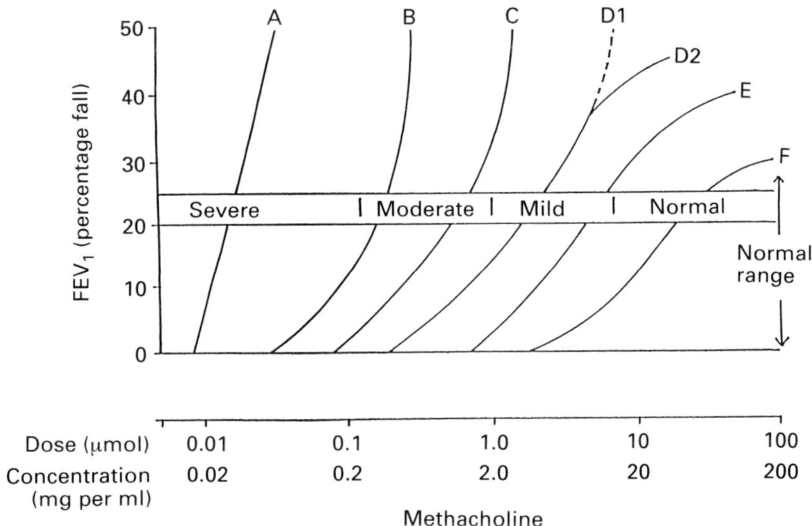

Fig. 1 Cumulative dose–concentration response curves to methacholine. The curve marked F is from a normal person, E is abnormal and found in some asymptomatic atopic people, D indicates mild AHR – curves in this position may or may not have a measurable plateau. The curves C, B, A represent increasing severity of AHR and are found in symptomatic asthma.

Table 1 Prevalence of current asthma, diagnosed asthma, wheeze and airway hyperresponsiveness (AHR) in populations of children

Country	Study year	Number	Age	Current asthma (%)	Diagnosed asthma (%)	Wheeze ever (%)	AHR (%)	References
Australia	82	1487	8–10	5.4	11.0	21.7	10.1 (H)	[8]
	86	1217	8–11	6.7	17.3	26.5	10.0 (H)	[36]
	91	1339	8–11	11.0	23.5	33.4	17.2 (H)	[37]
New Zealand	81	813	9	11.1†	27.0		22 (M)	[40]
	88	1084	6–11	9.1	14.2	27.2	20 (H)	[39]
	89	873	12	8.1†	16.8	26.6	12 (E)	[38]
England	80	1613	7	8.0†		14.8*	? (H)	[42]
Wales	89	965	12	5.3†	12	22.3	8 (E)	[38]
Germany	90	5768	9–11	4.2†	7.9		? (C)	[43]
Denmark	87	527	7–16	5.3			16 (H)	[41]
Indonesia	81	406	7–15	1.2	2.3	14.5	2.2 (H)	[14]
China	88	3067	11–17	1.9	2.4	6.3	4.1 (H)	[16]
Papua New Guinea	85	257	6–20	0	0	1.7	1.0 (H)	[15]
Kenya	91	402	9–12	3.3	11.4		10.7 (E)	[44]
Australia indig.	91	215	7–12	0.1	0	1.4	2.8 (H)	[11]

* Since starting school.
† Indicates a figure calculated from published data.
Current asthma, AHR + wheeze in last 12 months; H, histamine; M, methacholine; E, exercise; C, cold air hyperventilation; ?, test done, data not reported in paper; Australia indig., Aborigines.

the figures for current asthma with some confidence. In Australia and New Zealand the prevalence of childhood asthma is increasing and the figures for 'asthma ever diagnosed' are now the highest in the world (in some populations more than 25% of children have been diagnosed at some time as having asthma [3,4]). Furthermore, deaths in 5–34-year-olds were 1.14 per 100 000 in 1990, which was higher than New Zealand (0.80) in this age group. Clearly Australia and New Zealand have a problem with childhood asthma that needs to be addressed.

In order to identify the risk factors for asthma, we started epidemiological studies about 12 years ago with the aim of comparing different populations. In these continuing studies we select schools randomly and study the 8–10-year-olds. A questionnaire is sent home to the parents which contains a consent form and the questionnaire is checked with the child; height and weight are measured and skin tests to 14 common aero-allergens are performed [5].

Spirometric function is carried out, followed by a histamine inhalation test [6], except when the lung function is abnormal. Dust is collected from the beds and homes using a specially designed portable vacuum cleaner [7]. The methods have been described in a number of our publications [8,9].

The results are expressed as shown in Fig. 2. The area of the outside box represents the total number of children; the relationship between children with wheeze in the previous 12 months, AHR (a 20% fall in the forced expiratory volume in 1 second (FEV_1) after less than 4.0 μmol of histamine) and atopy (one or more skin-test wheals of 3 mm or greater) are shown. The children with both symptoms and AHR are defined as having 'current asthma'. We have shown that these children have more frequent symptoms, are more atopic, use more medications and have more variability of peak flow readings than children with symptoms

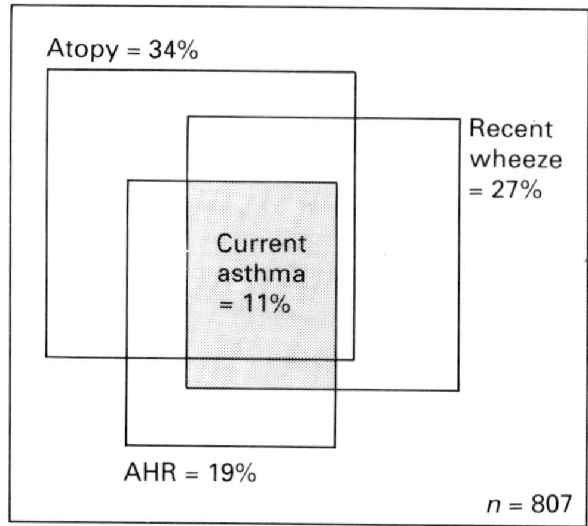

Fig. 2 The relationship between wheeze in the previous 12 months, AHR and atopy in children aged 8–10 years living in Lismore, New South Wales in 1991. The children with wheeze and AHR are considered to have 'current asthma'.

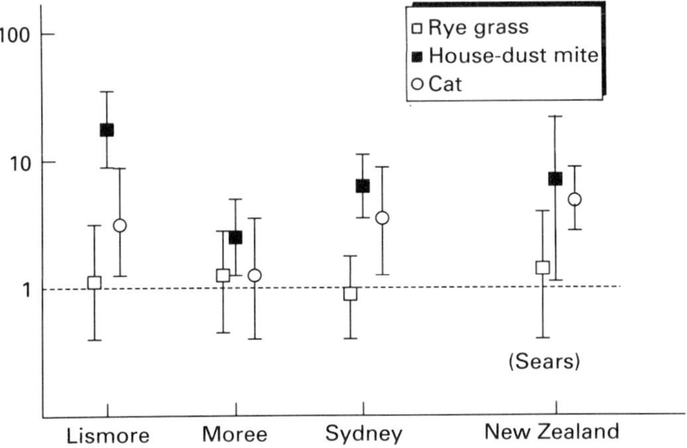

Fig. 3 Adjusted odds ratios for current asthma with different allergens in three Australian and one New Zealand population [12].

alone or children with AHR alone [10]. These data are from the town of Lismore which has a humid climate. In Table 1 the three populations shown for Australia are all from coastal Australia. We have shown that the prevalence has been increasing in children since 1982 and the increase is occurring only in children who are allergic. On the other hand, as can be seen from Table 1, there is little asthma in Australian Aboriginal children living in rural areas of Australia [11].

In epidemiological studies in Caucasian populations we have found that atopy is the greatest risk factor for asthma in all populations and, when the risk of being allergic to individual allergens is calculated using adjusted odds ratios, mites are the only allergens that are consistently a risk, as shown in Fig. 3 for three Australian towns and for Dunedin in New Zealand [12]. Furthermore, in children who are allergic to mites, those living in towns where the most mite allergen is found have the most symptoms [13].

EPIDEMIOLOGY OF ASTHMA IN THE WORLD

As can be seen from Table 1, childhood asthma is common in New Zealand and England but uncommon in a number of less affluent populations including Indonesia [14], Papua New Guinea (0%) [15] and China (1.9%) [16]. In Europe there have been studies that show that asthma is less common in the Alps than near the coast of France [17].

Table 2 shows prevalence figures from a number of countries where the same methods have been used on two separate occasions in populations under the age of 20 years. It clearly demonstrates that increases are occurring as well as an astonishing difference between New Zealand

Table 2 Changes in prevalence of asthma or symptoms in same population studied with same method on two occasions

Country	Study year	Number	Age	Current asthma	Diagnosed asthma	References
Australia	82	769	8–11	6.5	12.9	[8]
	92	795	8–11	12.9	19.3	[45]
New Zealand	75		12–18		26.2*	[46]
	89		12–18		34.0*	[46]
Wales	73	?	12		6.0	[47]
	88	965	12		12.0	[48]
USA	71–74	large	6–11		4.8	[49]
	76–80	27 275	6–11		7.6	[49]
Finland	61	38 000	19	0.1		[50]
	89	38 000	19	1.8		[50]
France	68	8 140	21		3.3	[51]
	82	10 559	21		5.4	[51]
Tahiti	79	3 870	16		11.5	[51]
	84	6 731	13		14.3	[52]

* Cumulative prevalence of asthma and/or wheeze.

and Finland. The figures for Finland are for 'current asthma', rather than for 'diagnosed asthma' but nevertheless are extremely low. Unfortunately there are insufficient data to correlate levels of mite allergen and the prevalence of childhood asthma in all populations studied because allergen levels and asthma prevalence have been measured at the same time only in France and Australia. However, in Australia, there is more asthma in the towns where it is humid than in dry areas and the same was found in France. Figure 4 shows the relationship between size of skin-test wheals and the prevalence of symptoms in children in Australia.

EVIDENCE FOR A CAUSAL RELATIONSHIP BETWEEN ASTHMA AND MITES

The causal relationship between exposure to mite allergen and asthma can be examined by asking about several important aspects of the relationship as suggested by Bradford Hill in 1965 [18] when he demonstrated the causal relationship between cigarette smoking and lung cancer.

First, is the association both strong and consistent? The strength is shown in Figs 3 and 4 and indirectly in Fig. 2. Tables 1 and 2 also show that asthma is uncommon in Scandinavia where there appear to be fewer mites than in England where it is more humid and mite counts are consistently high. In some populations there is a relationship between the severity of asthma and the degree of exposure [19,20]. It must be stressed that these data are for Caucasian populations who, on the whole, are affluent and sleep on mattresses and in houses that tend to be humid. In non-affluent populations, such as in China, it is not clear if the lower

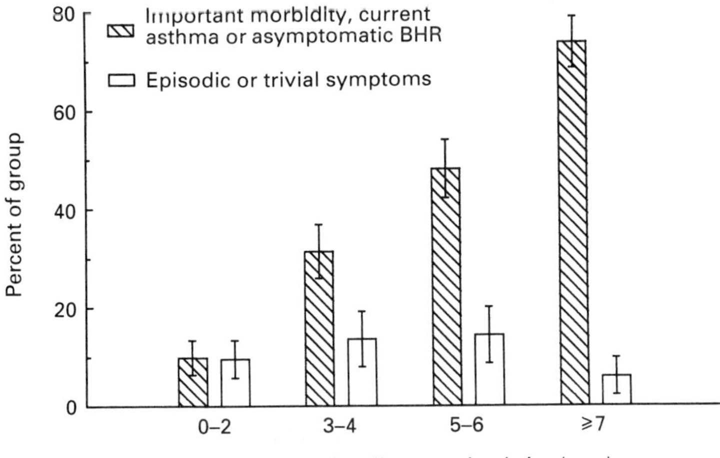

Fig. 4 The relationship between wheal size and prevalence of measurements of asthma in an Australian population of children.

prevalence is related to less exposure to mite allergen or if other protective factors are operating. It is of interest that within non-affluent populations in Africa, the prevalence of AHR, as measured by exercise, varies with the local level of affluence [21,22]. In these African relatively humid environments, affluence may well be associated with increasing levels of mites.

Second, is the temporality correct? If asthma is linked to house-dust mites and is increasing, is there evidence that mites are increasing? There are few data about changes in mite numbers or allergen with time in any population. However, there is evidence from Australia [23], as shown in Fig. 2, and indirectly from studies of specific immunoglobulin E in children living in the same environment in Switzerland [24] as well as other evidence from studies of numbers of skin-test reactions to mites in Australia [25]. In the absence of predators, house-dust mites will multiply when there is sufficient humidity and a source of food (skin scales). It seems likely that conditions favouring their growth, particularly in beds, are increasing throughout much of the world.

Third, is there a biological gradient? Evidence for this comes from studies showing the higher the concentration of mite or mite allergen, the greater the skin test positivity [26], the greater the risk of AHR and symptoms of asthma [20]. In addition, the prevalence of skin-test positivity is higher in humid than in dry climates [8,17,27]. Moreover, experiments where people are placed in low mite allergen environments consistently show that improvement in asthma using different measures occurs [28–30]. These experiments have included a stay of 6 months in hospital, periods in the Alps and rigid treatment of homes. Not all studies of home treatment have been shown to be effective but where there has been failure, the authors have not shown a consistent fall in mite allergen levels.

Fourth, is the relationship plausible? The airway inflammation of asthma is characterized by eosinophils, mast cells and thickening of the airway walls. This inflammation results in symptoms and in abnormal airway function which is best characterized by measurements of AHR. This inflammation appears to be the result of repeated challenge of the airways by the allergen to which the individual is sensitized. Mite allergens, most of which appear to be enzymes [31], are a particularly potent cause of atopy and of airway inflammation. There are relatively few animal models in which mite allergen has been used. But it is known that mites can cause allergic inflammation, typical of that seen in asthma in guinea pig [32] and mouse and rat [33].

Finally, are there other causes of asthma which are similar to mite allergen? The occupational sensitizers, western red cedar dust (plicatic acid) and toluene diisocyanate cause sensitization and workers who develop wheezing have a disease that is not different in pathology, clinical format or response to treatment from allergic asthma in the general population. In fact we learn from the occupational model that only some people get sensitized, that removal from the sensitizing agent is the only effective way to treat the disease, and if exposure continues for long enough the disease becomes persistent, even after complete removal from the allergen.

CONCLUSIONS

The data show that asthma, its symptoms and AHR are increasing in children in many affluent countries and that the association with mites is becoming more and more evident. Thus, it appears that asthma is a disease of affluence and countries that are not yet affluent may be at risk for having increased asthma in their children.

Since low mite environments are associated with less asthma [17,34] and high mite environments are associated with asthma, it seems reasonable to try to reduce the mite allergen in homes, particularly in the beds of infants and young children, as has been suggested in a recent editorial in *Thorax* [35].

REFERENCES

1 Boonsawat W, Salome CM, Woolcock AJ. Effect of allergen inhalation on the maximal response plateau of the dose-response curve to methacholine. *Am Rev Respir Dis* 1992;146:565–569.

2 Djukanovic R, Lai CKW, Wilson JW, *et al*. Bronchial mucosal manifestations of atopy: a comparison of markers of inflammation between atopic asthmatics, atopic nonasthmatics and healthy controls. *Eur Respir J* 1992;5:538–544.

3 Robertson CF, Heycock E, Bishop J, *et al.* Prevalence of asthma in Melbourne schoolchildren: changes over 26 years. *Br Med J* 1991;302:1116–1118.
4 Henry RL, Abramson R, Adler JA, *et al.* Asthma in the vicinity of power stations: 1. A prevalence study. *Pediatr Pulmonol* 1991;11:127–133.
5 Pepys J. Skin testing. *Br J Hosp Med* 1975;14:412–417.
6 Yan K, Salome C, Woolcock AJ. Rapid method for measurement of bronchial responsiveness. *Thorax* 1983;38:760–765.
7 Tovey ER, Marks GB, Matthews M, Woolcock AJ. Changes in mite allergen Der p 1 in house dust following spraying with a tannic acid/acaracide solutuion. *Clin Exp Allergy* 1992;22:67–74.
8 Britton WJ, Woolcock AJ, Peat JK, *et al.* Prevalence of bronchial hyperresponsiveness in children: the relationship between asthma and skin reactivity to allergens. *Int J Epidemiol* 1986;15:202–209.
9 Peat JK, Salome CM, Woolcock AJ. Factors associated with bronchial hyperresponsiveness in Australian adults and children. *Eur Respir J* 1992;5:921–929.
10 Toelle BG, Peat JK, Salome CM, *et al.* Towards a definition of asthma for epidemiology. *Am Rev Respir Dis* 1992;146:633–637.
11 Veale A, Peat JK, Salome CM, Woolcock AJ. Low prevalence of asthma and atopy in aboriginal children. *Proc Thoracic Soc Aust NZ* 1992;02.
12 Sears MR, Herbison GP, Holdaway MD, *et al.* The relative risks of sensitivity to grass pollen, house dust mite and cat dander in the development of childhood asthma. *Clin Exp Allergy* 1989;19:419–424.
13 Peat JK, Mellis CM, Tovey E, *et al.* Further evidence for the importance of house dust mite atopy in childhood asthma. *Proc Thoracic Soc Aus NZ* 1992;069.
14 Woolcock AJ, Konthen PG, Sedgwick CJ. Allergic status of children in an Indonesian village. *Asian Pac J Allergy Immunol* 1984;2:7–12.
15 Turner KJ, Dowse GK, Stewart GA, Alpers MP. Studies on bronchial hyperreactivity, allergic responsiveness, and asthma in rural and urban children of the highlands of Papua New Guinea. *J Allergy Clin Immunol* 1986;77:558–566.
16 Zhong NS, Chen RC, O-yang M, *et al.* Bronchial hyperresponsiveness in young students of southern China: relation to respiratory symptoms, diagnosed asthma, and risk factors. *Thorax* 1990;45:860–865.
17 Charpin D, Birnbaum J, Haddi E, *et al.* Altitude and allergy to house-dust mites. *Am Rev Respir Dis* 1991;143:983–986.
18 Bradford Hill A. The environment and disease: association or causation? *Proc Roy Soc Med* 1965;58:295–300.
19 Sporik R, Holgate ST, Platts MT, Cogswell JJ. Exposure to house-dust mite allergen (Der p I) and the development of asthma in childhood. A prospective study. *N Engl J Med* 1990;323:502–507.
20 Marks G, Tovey E, Woolcock A. In subjects with asthma the concentration of Der P 1 in beds correlates with the severity of bronchial hyperresponsiveness and symptoms. *Am Rev Respir Dis* 1993;147:A458.
21 Van Niekerk CH, Weinberg EG, Shore SC, *et al.* Prevalence of asthma: a comparative study of urban and rural Xhosa children. *Clin Allergy* 1979;9:319–324.
22 Keeley DJ, Neill P, Gallivan S. Comparison of the prevalence of reversible airways obstruction in rural and urban Zimbabwean children. *Thorax* 1991;46:549–553.
23 Green W, Tolle B, Woolcock A. House dust mite increase in Wagga Wagga houses. *Aust NZ J Med* 1993;23:409.
24 Gassner M, Wuthrich B. Prevalence of inhalative sensitizations in schoolchildren in a rural area. *Schweitz med Wschr* 1991;121(Suppl 40/1):41.
25 Peat JK, van den Berg RH, Mellis CM, *et al.* Changes in the prevalence of asthma and allergy in Australian children 1982–1992. *Am Rev Respir Dis* 1993;147:A800.
26 Lau S, Falkenhorst G, Weber A, *et al.* High mite-allergen exposure increases the risk of sensitization in atopic children and young adults. *J Allergy Clin Immunol* 1989;84: 718–725.
27 Murray AB, Ferguson AC, Morrison BJ. Sensitisation to house dust mites in different climatic areas. *J Allergy Clin Immunol* 1985;76:106–112.
28 Ehnert B, Lau-Schadendorf S, Weber A, *et al.* Reducing domestic exposure to dust

mite allergen reduces bronchial hyperreactivity in sensitive children with asthma. *J Allergy Clin Immunol* 1992;90:135–138.

29 Murray AB, Ferguson AC. Dust-free bedrooms in the treatment of asthmatic children with house dust or house dust mite allergy: a controlled trial. *Pediatrics* 1983;71: 418–422.

30 Platts-Mills TAE, Tovey ER, Mitchell EB, *et al.* Reduction of bronchial hyperreactivity during prolonged allergen avoidance. *Lancet* 1982;ii:675–678.

31 Stewart GA, Bird CH, Thompson PJ. Do the group II dust mite allergens correspond to lysozyme? *J Allergy Clin Immunol* 1992;90:141–142.

32 Ishii A, Ito K, Ino Y, Miyamoto T. Experimental asthma in guinea pigs sensitized with mites (*Dermatophagoides farinae*). *Int Arch Allergy Appl Immunol* 1989;89:400–403.

33 Stewart GA, Holt PG. Immunogenicity and tolerogenicity of a major house dust mite allergen, Der p 1 from Dermatophagoides pteronyssinus, in mice and rats. *Int Arch Allergy Appl Immunol* 1987;83:44–51.

34 Bonet AL, Nicro E, Antonioni J, *et al.* Pulmonary function and bronchial hyperreactivity in asthmatic children with house dust mite allergy during prolonged stay in the Italian Alps. *Ann Allergy* 1985;54:42–45.

35 Feather IH, Warner JA, Holgate ST, *et al.* Cohabiting with domestic mites. *Thorax* 1993;48:5–9.

36 Hurry VM, Peat JK, Woolcock AJ. Prevalence of respiratory symptoms, bronchial hyperresponsiveness and atopy in schoolchildren living in the Villawood area of Sydney. *Aust NZ J Med* 1988;18:745–752.

37 Peat J, Gray E, Mellis C, Woolcock A. *Asthma and Allergy in Primary Schoolchildren Living Close to Incinerators Operated by the Waterboard of New South Wales.* Summary report for the waterboard of New South Wales, 1992.

38 Barry DMJ, Burr ML, Limb ES. Prevalence of asthma among 12 year old children in New Zealand and South Wales: a comparative survey. *Thorax* 1991;46:405–409.

39 Pattemore PK, Asher MI, Harrison AC, *et al.* Ethnic differences in prevalence of asthma symptoms and bronchial hyperresponsiveness in New Zealand schoolchildren. *Thorax* 1989;44:168–176.

40 Sears MR, Jones DT, Holdaway MD, *et al.* Prevalence of bronchial reactivity to inhaled methacholine in New Zealand children. *Thorax* 1986;41:283–289.

41 Backer V, Bach MN, Dirkson A. Prevalence and predictors of bronchial hyperresponsiveness in children aged 7–16 years. *Allergy* 1989;44:214–219.

42 Lee DA, Winslow NR, Speight AN, Hey EN. Prevalence and spectrum of asthma in childhood. *Br Med J* 1983;286:1256–1258.

43 Nicolai T, Mutius EV, Reitmeir P, Wjst M. Reactivity to cold air hyperventilation in normal and asthmatic children in a survey of 5697 school chlldren in Southern Bavaria. *Am Rev Respir Dis* 1993;147(3):565–572.

44 Ng'ang'a LW, Odhiambo JA, Gicheha CG, *et al.* The prevalence of bronchial asthma in primary school children in Nairobi. *Am Rev Respir Dis* 1992;145:A537.

45 Peat JK, van den Berg RH, Mellis CM, Leeder SR. Evidence for an increase in the prevalence of asthma in Australian children. *Br Med J* 1994 (in press).

46 Shaw RA, Crane J, O'Donnell TV, Porleous LE, Coleman ED. Increasing asthma prevalence in a rural New Zealand adolescent population: 1975–1989. *Arch Dis Child* 1990;65:1319–1323.

47 Barry DMJ, Burr ML, Limb ES. Prevalence of asthma among 12 year old children in New Zealand and South Wales: a comparative survey. *Thorax* 1991;46:405–409.

48 Burr ML, Butland BK, King S, Vaughan WE. Changes in asthma prevalence: two surveys 15 years apart. *Arch Dis Child* 1989;64:1452–1456.

49 Cergen PJ, Mullally DI, Evans R. National survey of prevalence of asthma among children in the United States, 1976 to 1980. *Pedlatrics* 1988;81:1–7.

50 Haahtela T, Lindohlm H, Bjorksten F, *et al.* Prevalence of asthma in Finnish young men. *Br Med J* 1990;301:266–268.

51 Laird R, Chansin R, Neukirch F, *et al.* Prevalence of asthma among teenagers attending school in Tahiti. *J Epidemiol Comm Health* 1988;2:149–151.

52 Perdrizet S, Neukirch F, Cooreman J, Liard R. Effects of long-term inhaled salbutamol therapy on the provocation of asthma by histamine. *Chest* 1987;6:104S–106S.

PART 2
CLINICAL PHARMACOLOGY AND THERAPEUTICS

Drug chirality and its clinical relevance

M. S. LENNARD

Many doctors are probably unaware that a large number of the medicines they prescribe are mixtures containing only 50% of the active drug, the rest being an impurity that is inactive or even toxic. The reason for this is that many drugs have a molecular structure that lacks symmetry and as a consequence exist in 'left-' and 'right-handed' *isomeric** forms called *enantiomers*. (The terms 'enantiomer' and 'isomer' are often used indiscriminately.) Mixtures of drug enantiomers of 50:50 are called *racemates*. The phenomenon is known as *chirality* from the Greek word 'cheir' meaning 'a hand'. Indeed, like our own hands, drug enantiomers are non-superimposable, mirror images of each other (e.g. warfarin, Fig. 1).

Approximately 40% of synthetic drugs are chiral and because it has usually been easier to produce mixtures of enantiomers than the pure forms themselves, about 90% of chiral drugs have been marketed as racemates.

PHARMACOLOGICAL SIGNIFICANCE OF CHIRALITY

Why should chirality influence drug action? Although enantiomers have identical physical properties, except for the rotation of plane polarized light, they interact differently with pharmacological receptors which themselves are composed of chiral constituents (e.g. amino acids). Because of this, in many instances only one enantiomer will occupy the receptor and produce a significant pharmacological effect. Thus, the active enantiomer (eutomer) alone will be responsible for the therapeutic and also the unwanted effects. However, for some drugs the so-called

* *Isomers* are compounds having the same number and kind of atoms. Isomers having different spatial arrangements of their chemical groups are referred to as *stereoisomers*. Chirality is dependent on the presence of a centre of asymmetry in the chemical structure. Usually this centre is a carbon atom with four different atoms or groups attached to it. The nomenclature used by chemists to describe enantiomers can be confusing. The universally accepted classification system is based on the spatial arrangement of the atoms and chemical groups around the chiral atom and enantiomers are referred to as '*R*' (right, from the Latin 'rectus') or '*S*' (left, meaning 'sinister'). However, older systems of naming enantiomers, namely as (−) or (+), (*l*) or (*d*), and (L) or (D) are still used.

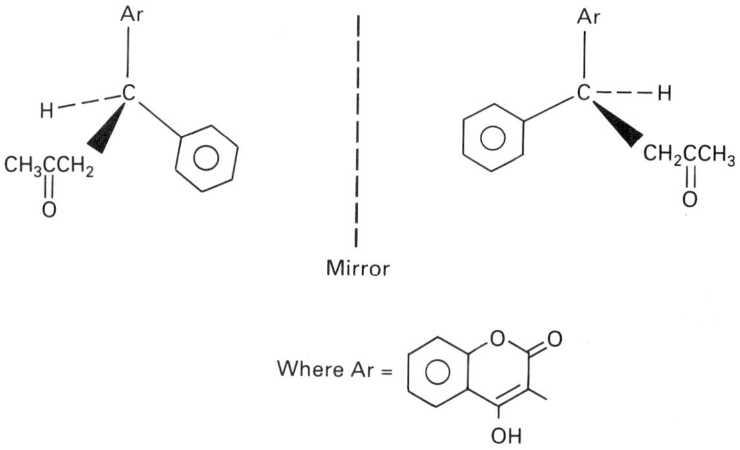

Fig. 1 The chemical structures of warfarin enantiomers, which are non-superimposable mirror images of each other. (By permission from Drayer [11].)

inactive enantiomer (distomer) does have significant pharmacological activity but is less potent than the eutomer. Furthermore, there is an increasing number of examples of enantiomers that are inactive with respect to one pharmacological action but have comparable activity to the other enantiomer when another pharmacological effect is considered. However, the possibility that the inactive enantiomer may actually be toxic has been of greatest concern and questions regarding the safety of racemates began to be raised about 10 years ago. The case of thalidomide has frequently been used to highlight the dangers of racemates and to promote the case for the development and use of pure enantiomers. Several authors have implied in rather emotive terms that the teratogenic effects of this racemic drug could have been avoided if the *R*-enantiomer had been used as a hypnosedative. However, the evidence that only *S*-thalidomide is teratogenic is inconclusive [1]. Furthermore, the possibility that racemization occurs rapidly *in vitro* and *in vivo* may make it difficult to attribute unequivocally any biological effect of thalidomide to one of its enantiomers.

Rapid progress in analytical methodology has allowed much information to be gathered on the biological fate of enantiomers following administration of the racemate, and many examples of stereoselectivity in the processes of drug absorption, distribution, metabolism and excretion have been documented (Fig. 2). It is clear from these and other clinical pharmacological studies that the therapeutic use of pure enantiomers has potential advantages. These are a less complex and more selective pharmacological profile, a greater therapeutic index, less complex pharmacokinetics, less complex drug interactions and less complex plasma

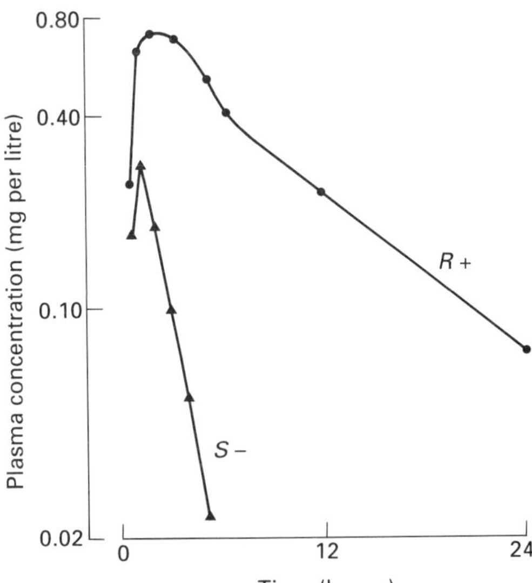

Fig. 2 The plasma concentration time profile of *S*(−)-nicoumalone (▲) and *R*(+)-nicoumalone (●) in one subject following a single oral 20 mg dose of the racemic drug. The *S*-isomer is more pharmacologically active yet it makes a negligible contribution to anticoagulant effect because of a much more rapid elimination. (By permission from Gill *et al.* [12].)

concentration–response relationships. Although the consensus is now clearly in favour of the clinical use of enantiomerically pure drugs, the implications of this both for the development of new chiral drugs and for those that are in current therapeutic use deserve further consideration. The key question in any discussion of the clinical relevance of drug chirality must be whether or not the therapeutic index of the single enantiomer differs from that of its racemate.

IMPLICATIONS OF CHIRALITY FOR NEW DRUGS

Development of enantiomers from existing racemates

To date two drugs, dexfenfluramine [2] and dilevalol [3], have reached the clinic as enantiomers having been developed to replace the existing racemates, fenfluramine and labetalol, respectively. The anorectic effect of racemic fenfluramine is due to the action of dexfenfluramine (D-fenfluramine), which increases presynaptic output and decreases postsynaptic uptake of 5-hydroxytryptamine. Through its action on catecholamines, L-fenfluramine may cause many of the adverse effects of the racemate. Thus, there appears to be some advantage in the use of dexfenfluramine as an adjunct to dietary restriction in obesity.

Unlike labetalol, dilevalol (the *R*,*R*-enantiomer) is a partial β_2-adrenoceptor agonist with peripheral vasodilating activity, but it is without α_1-adrenoceptor blocking action. Dilevalol was launched in Japan and Portugal in 1990 and was due to be marketed in the UK in the same year. However, it was withdrawn because of a low but significant number of cases of reversible hepatitis. Although there have been a few reports of liver abnormalities with labetalol, enantiomeric dilevalol appears to be more hepatotoxic than racemic labetalol.

These examples are likely to be the first of many enantiomers to be developed from existing racemates. In the USA about 40 use-patents have been filed for single isomer drugs including *S*-terfenadine (allergy), *R*-salbutamol, *R*-salmeterol, *R,R*-famoterol (asthma), *S*-ketoprofen, (periodontal disease), *R*-ketoprofen (analgesia), *S*-fluoxetine (depression), *S*-ondansetron (emesis) and *S*-amlodipine (hypertension). Similar developments are also occurring in the UK and other countries. Single isomers that are at an advanced stage of clinical testing include *S*-atenolol (hypertension) and *S*-ofloxacin (infection).

Development of new chemical entities

Guidelines from national regulatory bodies on chiral drug development are imminent and it is expected that the pharmaceutical industry will be asked to justify the use of new racemates. This regulatory pressure is already being felt and the industry is clearly moving away from racemates and even, perhaps unfortunately, chiral drugs. To support this Campbell [4] quotes registration statistics for 1986–87, which indicate that 66% of the new chiral compounds being dealt with by the UK Committee of the Safety of Medicines were single enantiomers, whereas there was a 40% decrease from the previous year in the number of chiral drugs being considered for a product licence. By the year 2000, a drug brought to the market as a racemate may be a rarity.

IMPLICATIONS OF CHIRALITY FOR DRUGS ALREADY IN USE

A few synthetic drugs, including some very old ones, are given as a single isomer and there are compelling reasons to do so. These include L-dopa, which is less toxic than D-dopa, and L-methotrexate and L-thyroxine, which are more active than their corresponding D-enantiomers. Interestingly, D-thyroxine has been used as a hypocholesterolaemic agent on the basis that it has about the same potency as L-thyroxine in lowering the concentration of blood cholesterol, but has only one-quarter the potency to increase overall metabolic rate.

Dextropropoxyphene is an analgesic whereas its enantiomeric twin, levopropoxyphene, is an antitussive and the brand names Darvon and Novrad, which are used respectively in the USA, are mirror images.

D-penicillamine is less toxic that L-penicillamine in the treatment of Wilson's disease. For this reason the D-isomer was adopted for the treatment of rheumatoid arthritis. However, although the doses used are generally much lower for this indication, the relative therapeutic indices of the isomers have not been compared in this condition.

Quinidine and quinine are diastereoisomers, that is stereoisomers but not mirror images. Quinidine has greater antiarrhythmic and antimalarial activity than quinine, but the latter is preferred for the treatment of malaria because it is much less cardiodepressant than quinidine. Quinine is also widely used for the treatment of muscle cramps.

Tamoxifen is not chiral but exists as two *geometrical* isomers. *Trans*-tamoxifen is an antagonist at oestrogen receptors and is used clinically to treat breast cancer. In contrast, *cis*-tamoxifen is oestrogenic. There is some evidence that *trans*-4-hydroxytamoxifen, a metabolite of *trans*-tamoxifen and also a potent antioestrogen, can be converted *in vivo* to *cis*-4-hydroxytamoxifen which, like its *cis*-parent, is oestrogenic [5]. If substantiated, these findings may help to explain why many patients are or become resistant to tamoxifen and could have important implications with respect to the debate on the long-term safety of prophylactic tamoxifen in women at familial risk of breast cancer.

For some drugs given as racemates there is a case for one of the enantiomers to be made available clinically because of the greater toxicity of the other enantiomer. One such example is the intravenous anaesthetic ketamine, the use of which is limited by the occurrence of psychotic emergence reactions. The results of limited clinical studies have indicated that *S*-ketamine is three times as potent an anaesthetic but causes significantly fewer psychotic episodes than the *R*-enantiomer.

Both enantiomers of sotalol have significant class III antiarrhythmic activity and the racemate is used clinically for this purpose. However, *l*-sotalol also has β-blocking activity, which may be undesirable in certain patients, especially those with heart failure. Thus, *d*-sotalol, which is not a β-blocker, may offer a clinical advantage over the racemate as an antiarrhythmic agent and is now being evaluated as such.

Similarly, patients being treated with racemic disopyramide for arrhythmias may gain more benefit from the use of the (+)-enantiomer, since the less potent (−)-disopyramide is thought to be mostly responsible for the heart failure precipitated by the racemate through its marked negative inotropic effect.

Another cardiovascular drug whose therapeutic index might be improved by using a single enantiomer is verapamil. Its (+)-enantiomer has little of the negative chronotropic, dromotropic or inotropic effect of the (−)-form and, thus may be a safer antianginal drug than the racemate. A potential new indication for verapamil is its ability to reverse multiple drug resistance to cytotoxic agents during cancer chemotherapy (Fig. 3) [6]. However, the high doses of the racemate needed to do this are associated with unacceptable cardiotoxicity. Early trials suggest that this

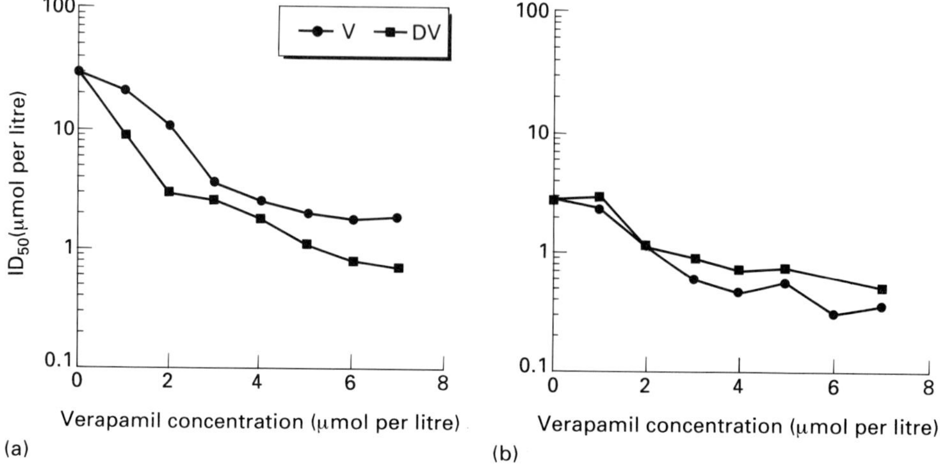

Fig. 3 The sensitivity of drug resistant cell lines 2780AD (a) and H69LX10 (b) to adriamycin in the presence of racemic verapamil (V) or D-(+)-verapamil (DV). The ID_{50} is the drug concentration required to kill 50% of the cells. (Reprinted from Plumb *et al.* [6], with permission from Pergamon Press Ltd, Oxford.)

problem might be overcome by using the less cardiotoxic (+)-enantiomer, which has a similar potency to (−)-verapamil as a modulator of multiple drug resistance.

Severe, sometimes fatal cardiotoxicity, which is sudden in onset, has occurred following administration of the local anaesthetic bupivacaine. This drug is given as a racemate and data from non-human species indicate that the *R*-enantiomer has the greater myocardial toxicity [7]. Since the local anaesthetic potencies of the two isomers of bupivacaine are similar, the use of *S*-bupivacaine may be safer than the racemate. The *S*-enantiomer of ropivacaine, a chemical analogue of bupivacaine, is now being developed for clinical use.

As well as being an effective oral therapy for hypertension, *S*-timolol is widely used in eyedrops for the treatment of open-angle glaucoma. However, there have been numerous reports of systemic toxicity associated with its topical use including some fatal asthmatic attacks. Based on studies in rabbit and healthy volunteers it has been suggested that *R*-timolol might be a safer alternative, since it is about 50 times less potent as an antagonist at β_2-adrenoceptors but only four times less potent at lowering intraocular pressure than the *S*-enantiomer. However, in asthmatic patients *R*-timolol has been found to cause bronchoconstriction at a dose only four times higher than that of *S*-timolol [8]. Thus, the margin between the therapeutic and adverse effects of *R*-timolol may not be as great as previously thought.

For many existing and well established chiral drugs there is no proven advantage in replacing the racemate with the active enantiomer. Most of the β-adrenoceptor antagonists are administered as racemates for the treatment of hypertension and angina. For the majority of these drugs almost all of the β-adrenoceptor blocking activity and their adverse effects reside in the (−)-enantiomers. Thus, although 50% of a dose is of no clinical value, it seems unlikely that this therapeutically inactive portion contributes significantly to adverse effects.

Although *S*-warfarin is about three to five times more potent than *R*-warfarin, the therapeutic indices of the isomers are similar. Thus, the only gain in replacing racemic warfarin by its *S*-enantiomer would seem to be a lower dose requirement. On the other hand changing to a single enantiomer would theoretically decrease the range of the drug interactions involving warfarin, since such reactions are specific to one or other isomer. For example, metronidazole, amiodarone, co-trimoxazole and sulphinpyrazone specifically inhibit the metabolism of *S*-warfarin, whereas cimetidine and enoxacin inhibit that of the less active *R*-form. However, these potential advantages are outweighed by the accumulated clinical experience with the racemate and by the increased cost of producing enantiomers.

The issue of whether the single enantiomers of non-steroidal anti-inflammatory drugs (NSAIDs) have additional benefits over their racemates is becoming increasingly complex. The property of inhibition of prostaglandin cyclooxygenase resides almost exclusively in the *S*-enantiomers of these compounds and, until very recently, it was thought that all of the anti-inflammatory and analgesic effects of the NSAIDs were mediated through this mechanism. Thus, replacement of the racemate with the active *S*-form has been suggested. However, the case for this is somewhat weakened by the fact that the *R*-enantiomers of many NSAIDs are converted *in vivo* to their *S*-counterparts (chiral inversion). Furthermore, many of the adverse effects of these drugs are attributed to the *S*-enantiomer through its action on prostaglandin synthesis and it has even been suggested that the *R*-form should be used as a prodrug to avoid the gastrointestinal ulceration caused by NSAIDs. However, since the side-effects of these drugs are thought to be produced systemically as well as locally, this approach must be questioned. On the other hand concern has been expressed that, because it can be incorporated into triacylglycerols, the *R*-enantiomer of ibuprofen is more toxic than *S*-ibuprofen. However, a direct link between the formation of these 'hybrid' triglycerides, which have been postulated to interfere with normal lipid metabolism, and toxicity, has not been established. It is now becoming evident that perhaps the 'inactive' *R*-forms of several NSAIDs possess intrinsic analgesic activity. For example, *R*-flurbiprofen, which is only inverted chirally to a small extent in humans, has been shown to exert significant analgesic activity in different animal models of pain and

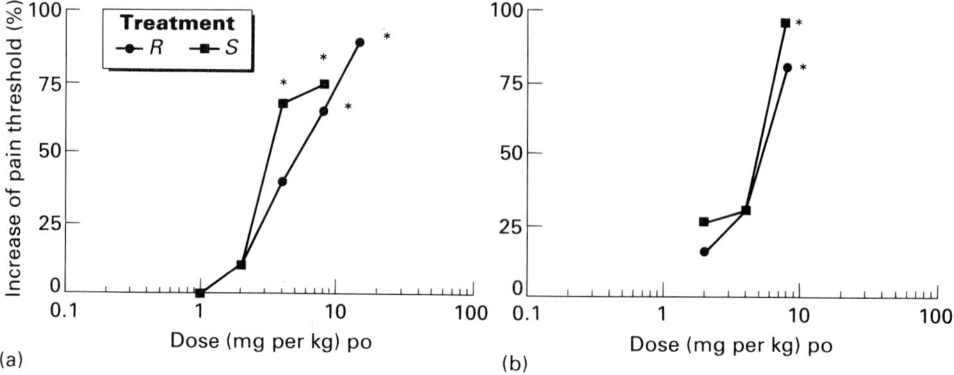

Fig. 4 The antinociceptive effects of *S*-flurbiprofen and *R*-flurbiprofen in the rat Randall-Selitto assay following injection of baker's yeast (a) and of interleukin 1 (b). $^{*}P < 0.05$ for the comparison of the pain threshold of the inflamed paw between treated and control animals. (By permission from Brune *et al.* [9].)

nociception (Fig. 4) [9], although it is practically devoid of effects on prostaglandin synthesis and, therefore, should not cause gastrointestinal side-effects. Thus, in addition to the racemate, both single enantiomers of NSAIDs may have a role to play in the drug therapy of pain and inflammatory disorders. In this context each of the enantiomers of ibuprofen and ketoprofen is being developed for clinical use.

The safety and effectiveness of long-term treatment with β_2-adrenoceptor agonists in asthma have recently been called into question. Salbutamol and other β_2-adrenoceptor agonists are given as racemates, but only *R*-salbutamol causes relaxation of airways smooth muscle. Recent work in guinea pig has suggested that repeated dosing with the 'inactive' *S*-enantiomer causes hyperreactivity to allergens leading to bronchoconstriction [10]. Based on these findings it has been postulated that *S*-salbutamol may be responsible for the deleterious effects, but the case for single enantiomer development is not yet convincing.

WHAT DOES THE PRESCRIBER NEED TO KNOW ABOUT DRUG CHIRALITY?

It is quite difficult for the ordinary prescriber to find out whether a drug is chiral and, if so, whether it is available as a racemate or a single enantiomer. The most readily accessible sources of drug information, such as the *British National Formulary*, the Data Sheet Compendium, and even most of the standard texts on clinical pharmacology, do not define the chirality of a drug except in a minority of cases. This is beginning to change and, with respect to nomenclature, if each isomer and racemate were given a different Approved Name, it would be apparent whether a medicine contained a single isomer or a mixture. From a practical standpoint it is probably unimportant for the clinician to know whether the great majority of the drugs they prescribe are single isomers or racemates. There is a strong argument for the issue of drug chirality to be resolved among clinical pharmacologists, the regulatory authorities and the pharmaceutical industry so that the final product is the best available to the clinician. Because fewer new compounds are now being developed as racemates, drug therapy should be simplified. However, one area of confusion may still lie in the increasing number of drugs for which a single enantiomer is being developed to replace a racemate. As discussed earlier this was done for dexfenfluramine yet both the new enantiomer and the old racemate are available. It seems reasonable that in such cases products are clearly marked as racemates or pure isomers and that sufficient information on their pharmacological and therapeutic properties is provided to encourage the rational prescribing of these drugs. In conclusion, some awareness of 'looking glass' drugs by the doctor might benefit the patient.

ACKNOWLEDGEMENT

Professor G.T. Tucker is thanked for his comments on the manuscript.

REFERENCES

1 Winter W, Frankus E. Thalidomide enantiomers. *Lancet* 1992;339:365.
2 Anonymous. Dexfenfluramine. *Lancet* 1991;337:1315–1316.
3 Lennard MS. Clinical pharmacology through the looking glass: reflections on the racemate vs enantiomer debate. *Br J Clin Pharmacol* 1991;31:623–625.
4 Campbell DB. Stereoselectivity in clinical pharmacokinetics and drug development. *Eur J Drug Metab Pharmacokin* 1990;15:109–125.
5 Osborne CK, Coronado E, Allred DC, *et al.* Acquired tamoxifen resistance: correlation with reduced breast tumor levels and isomerization of trans-4-hydroxytamoxifen. *J Natl Cancer Inst* 1991;83:1477–1482.
6 Plumb JA, Milroy R, Kaye SB. The activity of verapamil as a resistance modifier *in vitro* in drug resistant human tumour cell lines is not stereospecific. *Biochem Pharmacol* 1990;39:787–792.
7 Aberg G. Toxicological and local anaesthetic effects of optically active isomers of two local anaesthetic compounds. *Acta Pharmacol Toxicol* 1972;31:273–286.
8 Richards R, Tattersfield AE. Comparison of airways response to eye drops of timolol and its isomer L-714,465 in asthmatic subjects. *Br J Clin Pharmacol* 1987;24:485–492.
9 Brune K, Geisslinger G, Menzel-Soglowek S. Pure enantiomers of 2-arylpropionic acids: tools in pain research and improved drugs in rheumatology. *J Clin Pharmacol* 1992;32:944–952.
10 Morley J, Chapman ID, Foster A, *et al.* Effects of (+) and racemic salbutamol on airway responses in the guinea pig. *Br J Pharmacol* 1991;104:295P.
11 Drayer DE. Pharmacodynamic and pharmacokinetic differences between drug enantiomers in humans: an overview. *Clin Pharmacol Ther* 1986;40:125–133.
12 Gill TS, Hopkins KJ, Rowland M. Stereospecific assay of nicoumalone: application to pharmacokinetics studies in man. *Br J Clin Pharmacol* 1988;25:591–598.

Further reading

Smith DF. *Handbook of Stereoisomers: Therapeutic Drugs*. Boca Rouge: CRC Press, 1989.
Tucker GT. The clinical relevance of chirality. *Prescriber's J* 1991;31:189–197.
Tucker GT, Lennard MS. Enantiomer specific pharmacokinetics. *Pharmacol Ther* 1990; 45:309–329.
Williams KM. Enantiomers in arthritic disorders. *Pharmacol Ther* 1990;46:273–295.

Diurctic-induced cardiotoxicity: malign influence or myth?

G. T. McINNES

SUMMARY

Long-term treatment with thiazide diuretics reduces serum potassium and may reduce serum magnesium, but an important reduction in total body potassium or magnesium does not follow. Thiazide treatment also causes a rise in serum urate, occasionally precipitates diabetes mellitus, and may elevate serum total cholesterol slightly. It is often suggested that diuretics have a malign cardiotoxic influence, i.e. thiazide-induced potassium or magnesium disturbances are arrhythmogenic, and that thiazide-related changes in lipids, glucose tolerance or urate may be atherogenic. Much of the evidence that thiazide treatment may predispose to myocardial infarction or sudden death is flawed, or is based on unproven hypotheses. The results of large prospective controlled outcome trials in hypertensive patients employing thiazide diuretics do not support the hypothesis that the thiazides are cardiotoxic even when they are used at high dosage. When considered collectively these trials provide strong evidence for the safety, efficacy, tolerability and convenience of these inexpensive drugs. Furthermore, unwanted biochemical effects of thiazides can be minimized or in some instances avoided entirely by using the low doses which should now be standard therapy in hypertension. In clinical practice possible contraindications to the use of thiazides (diabetes, gout) and potential adverse drug interactions (with lithium, digoxin, and drugs which prolong the QT interval) must be considered. Except in this minority of patients the thiazide diuretics remain eminently suitable drugs for use as first-line therapy in hypertension and in other conditions.

INTRODUCTION

Diuretics have made a major contribution to the management of heart failure and hypertension over many years. These drugs are effective, well tolerated, and widespread long-term experience supports their safety. Why then should there be concern about their cardiotoxic potential?

Diuretics formed the basis of the therapeutic regimens in all the major long-term prospective outcome trials which established the value of treating hypertension. However, while diuretic-based therapy achieved the anticipated benefit in reducing cerebrovascular events, this treatment appeared to have less than the expected impact in preventing myocardial infarction and sudden death. Although these findings have several possible explanations independent of the drugs employed, attention has been focused on postulated malign cardiotoxic influences of thiazides [1–3]. The most persistently advanced hypothesis proposes that diuretic-induced disturbances in potassium and magnesium metabolism cause serious cardiac arrhythmias while hyperlipidaemia, carbohydrate intolerance and hyperuricaemia secondary to diuretics are assumed to be atherogenic and predispose to myocardial infarction.

The case against thiazide diuretics has been prosecuted almost entirely outside the columns of the legitimate medical press. Much of it has been sponsored by pharmaceutical companies with a vested interest in displacing thiazides from their important role in the management of hypertension. Studies of dubious quality have been published repeatedly without ever appearing in a refereed journal and have eventually been cited in independent review articles, some of which have expressed doubt about the safety of diuretics. Replacement of generic thiazide by the much more expensive newer branded drugs would add greatly to the drug bill. The purpose of this article is to review the evidence for and against a malign cardiotoxic influence of diuretics.

DIURETIC-INDUCED METABOLIC DISTURBANCES

Potassium

Diuretics cause variable reductions in plasma potassium concentration [4]. Falls are greater with thiazides than with loop diuretics and levels tend to be lower in hypertension than in heart failure. At higher doses (e.g. bendrofluazide 10 mg daily), about 50% of hypertensive patients develop hypokalaemia (serum potassium less than 3.5 mmol/l) although values below 3.0 mmol/l are unusual.

The evidence that diuretics cause potassium *deficiency* (reduction in total body potassium) is weak. In heart failure, findings are inconsistent [5,6] with the few adequately controlled studies showing little or no change in total body potassium. Reduced tissue potassium of a magnitude similar to that seen after diuretics has been reported in untreated heart failure and does not correlate with the duration of diuretic treatment [7,8]. Thus, the potassium deficit appears to be due primarily to alterations associated with heart failure. During treatment of hypertension with thiazides, tissue potassium loss amounts to less than 5% [9], a change of little physiologic significance.

Magnesium

Diuretics increase urine magnesium excretion acutely [10] but adequate studies suggest at most modest falls in plasma magnesium (0.02–0.05 mmol/l) within the reference range [11–14]. On the basis of poorly controlled observations, it has been suggested that the elderly are particularly at risk of diuretic-induced hypomagnesaemia [15,16]. In neither of these studies can low serum magnesium be attributed with confidence to diuretic treatment. The evidence in favour of diuretic-induced magnesium *depletion* in heart failure has been derived from inappropriate interpretation of the data often from inadequately designed studies [5,15,17]. Limited information in hypertension indicates negligible changes [18]. Falls are unlikely to exceed 4%.

The hypothesis that hypomagnesaemia contributes to refractory potassium depletion [15] stems from observations that severe magnesium deficiency in animals causes depletion of muscle potassium [19] which persists despite a large intake of potassium. In the most frequently cited study in humans [20], magnesium sulphate infusion appeared to increase muscle potassium by 8%, or about 240 mmol in diuretic treated subjects over 12 hours while potassium chloride infusion had no effect. The extracellular space contains only 48 mmol potassium, however, and could not support a shift of potassium into cells of this magnitude in only 12 hours. The magnesium infusion seemed to conjure up potassium which did not exist.

Lipids

Trials with sufficient sample size demonstrate that, in the short-term, thiazide diuretics raise total cholesterol, low-density lipoprotein cholesterol, very low-density lipoproteins, cholesterol and triglycerides [21]. In seven trials with more than 25 subjects, the mean increase in total cholesterol was 5%. Long-term findings are less clear. In the large prospective intervention trials, changes in total cholesterol following thiazides were in the order of 1% [22] although there were small differences from concurrent control groups in several trials (mean 0.1 mmol/l) and thiazides may blunt a reduction in total cholesterol due to dietary intervention [23]. Long-term changes in cholesterol subfractions and triglycerides are variable and modest [22].

Carbohydrate

Thiazide-induced impairment of carbohydrate metabolism has been amply confirmed by numerous short- and long-term studies [24]. Some of the changes in blood sugar may be due to regression effects since larger increases tend to be seen in those at the lower end of the blood sugar distribution. Therefore, the risks of developing frank hyperglycaemia appear to be small. In the large outcome trial only about 0.5–1% of subjects treated with a thiazide developed hyperglycaemia and/or diabetes mellitus [25]. Alterations are reversible on discontinuation of thiazides [26].

It has been widely assumed that diuretic-induced carbohydrate intolerance is a direct consequence of altered potassium homeostasis [27] but it remains to be demonstrated that diuretic regimens which maintain a normal potassium status are superior with respect to glucose tolerance during long-term treatment. Some studies have suggested alterations in pancreatic insulin secretion [28] and recent work provides some evidence that diuretics may decrease tissue sensitivity to insulin [29], i.e. reduced glucose uptake leading to persistent hyperglycaemia and hyperinsulinaemia. While diabetes mellitus undoubtedly predisposes to coronary heart disease, the available evidence suggests that hyperglycaemia and elevated insulin levels are independent risk factors only at the upper extremities of their distribution [30,31]. Therefore, only those few thiazide-treated patients who develop diabetes mellitus are likely to have an increased risk of coronary heart disease over and above that related to hypertension.

Uric acid

Thiazides tend to increase blood levels of uric acid and hyperuricaemia has been suggested as an independent risk factor for coronary heart disease and sudden death [32]. However, this association ignores important confounding influences and a subsequent analysis has cast considerable doubt on the causality of the relationship [33].

DIURETICS AND CARDIAC ARRHYTHMIAS

Diuretics reduce plasma potassium concentrations and extreme hypokalaemia is associated with cardiac arrhythmias. Thus, it is hypothesized that diuretics are responsible for serious cardiac arrhythmias and sudden death.

An early study in uncomplicated hypertension [34] has been cited widely in support of thiazide-induced arrhythmogenicity but more recent work [35–39] has not supported this observation. A representative sample of prospective studies employing ambulatory electrocardiogram (ECG) monitoring is shown in Table 1.

A substudy of a large Medical Research Council trial of treatment of mild to moderate hypertension [38] reported an association between thiazide treatment and ventricular ectopic activity during 24-hour ambulatory monitoring. Ventricular ectopic activity correlated with the

Table 1 Hypokalaemia and ventricular ectopy in hypertension

Reference	Number of patients	Plasma K		Hours of ECG	Arrhythmic change
		Basal	Diuretic		
[34]	7	4.0	3.0	24	Increase
	14	3.9	3.0	24	No change
[35]	27	4.0	3.0	48	No change
	17	4.2	3.8	48	No change
[36]	13	4.0	3.0	48	No change
[37]	20	4.4	3.0	24	No change
[38]	16	4.2	3.6	24	No change
[39]	45	4.2	3.6	48	No change

degree of hypokalaemia and could be complex with multifocal beats, bigeminy, couplets and the R on T phenomenon. The substudy had three components.

1 In a cross-sectional study in 155 patients, ventricular ectopy, including complex arrhythmias, was significantly more frequent in bendrofluazide-treated subjects after 2 years but there was no correlation with serum potassium, which was reduced by 0.5 mmol/l after the diuretic. Importantly, 24-hour monitoring was not conducted before treatment in this group.

2 Sixteen patients preselected because of severe hypokalaemia on bendrofluazide were randomized to continue diuretic alone or to receive additional potassium chloride (48 mmol daily) for 5 days; despite a major difference in serum potassium (0.7 mmol/l), there was no difference in ectopic activity between the groups.

3 In patients randomly assigned to bendrofluazide, the frequency of ventricular ectopy was not increased despite a mean fall in serum potassium of 0.6 mmol/l (Table 1).

Although pooled data from the three studies showed a highly significant overall correlation between the frequency of ventricular ectopic beats and serum potassium ($r = -0.19$), there was a similar relation with serum urate ($r = -0.18$) suggesting that the association lacked specificity. In any event, the effect of serum potassium must be very small: variation in ventricular ectopic activity attributable to serum potassium ($r^2 \times 100$), 3.4%.

In hypertensive patients treated with hydrochlorothiazide the frequency of ventricular extrasystoles was reported to correlate with serum magnesium, changes in serum magnesium and the product of change in serum magnesium and change in serum potassium [40]. This work does not appear to have been published in a refereed journal and detail is scant. Other studies in hypertension have failed to confirm a correlation between the frequency of ventricular extrasystoles and serum magnesium or changes in serum magnesium, nor do increases in serum magnesium appear to be associated with changes in ventricular ectopic activity [22].

Patients with underlying cardiac abnormalities such as ischaemic heart disease or left ventricular hypertrophy might be expected to be more susceptible to any arrhythmogenic potential of diuretic-induced hypokalaemia. During 24-hour ECG monitoring in hypertensive patients attending the Glasgow Blood Pressure Clinic [41], the frequency of ventricular arrhythmias of all grades was increased in those with left ventricular hypertrophy but was unrelated to diuretic treatment of hypokalaemia. In a series of prospective within-patient comparisons conducted by Papademetriou *et al.* [35,42], individuals with left ventricular hypertrophy had no increase in ventricular ectopy after diuretics as assessed by 24–48-hour ECG monitoring.

The role of diuretic-induced hypomagnesaemia in the genesis of cardiac arrhythmias is based largely on case reports, in many of which other causes are equally likely [43] and on the suppression of arrhythmias by magnesium salts [20]. Correction of arrhythmias by elevating serum magnesium is non-specific and does not prove that the arrhythmia was caused by hypomagnesaemia. Low plasma magnesium is not associated with significant ECG alterations and there exist no animal models which link magnesium deficiency with cardiac arrhythmias or sudden death [43].

Many of the studies linking diuretic therapy to cardiac arrhythmias have serious design flaws [22], notably the preselection of patients with low frequency of extrasystoles before treatment. Since there is marked intraindividual variability in ectopic activity [44], preselection of patients without ectopy makes it probable that regression to the mean is responsible for much of the supposed thiazide-induced ectopic activity. Often the studies lacked adequate controls, they were analyzed inappropriately and presentation was incomplete. Finally, the same material appears to have been published repeatedly without acknowledgement or peer review.

DRUG INTERACTIONS

Diuretic-induced hypokalaemia increases the QT prolongation caused by several drugs [45]. A prolonged QT interval is associated with a tendency to develop the polymorphic ventricular tachycardia, torsade de pointes, and this propensity is exaggerated by hypokalaemia caused by diuretics. Diuretic-induced hypokalaemia is potentially dangerous in patients treated with many antiarrhythmic drugs and with the β-blocker sotalol. When diuretics are used with these drugs, effective prophylaxis against hypokalaemia must be ensured by prescribing an adequate dose of a potassium-sparing drug. It should be noted that potassium supplements, and the doses of potassium-sparing agents contained in most combination products, may *not* be sufficient in these circumstances. Adequate prophylaxis against hypokalaemia is also essential in patients treated with digoxin, again to prevent serious arrhythmias.

DIURETICS AND ARRHYTHMIAS AFTER MYOCARDIAL INFARCTION

There is much speculation that diuretic-treated patients are at increased risk of serious cardiac arrhythmias after myocardial infarction, as a result of disturbances in potassium metabolism [46–53]. Representative studies are summarized in Table 2.

Hypokalaemic patients have a higher incidence of serious ventricular ectopic beats, ventricular tachycardia and ventricular fibrillation but, crucially, the frequency of arrhythmias, and in particular ventricular fibrillation, is not related to prior diuretic use. The study reported by Ramsay *et al.* [51] deserves particular comment. In 277 patients with acute myocardial infarction, low serum potassium was associated with a high risk of ventricular fibrillation but a significant relation was present in those who had never taken diuretics. Previous diuretic treatment was associated with a two-fold increased incidence of ventricular fibrillation, but this was independent of serum potassium and was due entirely to an excess in diuretic users of secondary ventricular fibrillation complicating the failing heart.

Hypokalaemia after myocardial infarction (and other serious illnesses) is probably caused by high circulating levels of catecholamines [54]. Ventricular fibrillation could be triggered by hypokalaemia, by high

Table 2 Diuretics and arrhythmias after myocardial infarction

	Association with	
Reference	Hypokalaemia	Diuretics
[46]	Yes	Yes
[47]	Yes	No
[48]	Yes	Yes
[49]	Yes	No
[50]	Yes	No
[51]	Yes	No
	No*	Yes*
[52]	Yes	No
[53]	Yes	No

* Excess of secondary ventricular fibrillation in failing heart.

adrenaline levels, or by extensive myocardial infarction accompanied by hypokalaemia as an epiphenomenon. However, normalization of serum potassium after myocardial infarction does not affect ventricular ectopic activity [55], and catecholamines promote arrhythmias independent of any hypokalaemic effect [56]. Thus, the consistent relation between hypokalaemia and arrhythmias in acute myocardial infarction does not necessarily indicate a causal role for hypokalaemia. It seems clear that diuretics are innocent bystanders, as the relation is independent of diuretic use and there is no consistent relation between diuretic use and arrhythmias.

In the Glasgow Blood Pressure Clinic [57,58] 750 deaths occurred in 3783 hypertensive patients over 6.5 years of observation. There was no association between death and hypokalaemia. In fact, the reverse was seen. Age-adjusted mortality and death related to ischaemic heart disease did not correlate with serum potassium. Serum potassium was not lower in those who died of ischaemic heart disease than in those who survived; 3.71 mmol/l and 3.72 mmol/l, respectively. Hypokalaemia failed to predict outcome in univariate or multivariate analyses which included cigarette smoking, renal function and ECG findings. Low serum potassium had no adverse effect on prognosis in those with left ventricular hypertrophy. Observations from this clinic indicate that hypokalaemia is not a risk factor in treated hypertensive patients.

Hypomagnesaemia was associated with ventricular arrhythmias in one survey of 343 patients after myocardial infarction [59] but diuretic-treated patients had higher, not lower, serum magnesium concentrations. In another cross-sectional study [52], arrhythmias were unrelated to serum magnesium which was again not lower in patients taking diuretics.

OUTCOME TRIALS

The controversy concerning the cardiotoxicity of diuretics can be resolved only by examining the results of long-term controlled clinical trials which have directly compared clinical outcome in patients treated with thiazides and those treated with placebo or another drug. If the hypothesis that diuretics are cardiotoxic were true, the cumulative evidence should show an increased incidence of fatal myocardial infarction or sudden death. Critical scrutiny of all the available data indicates that diuretic treatment of mild to moderate hypertension reduces fatal and not-fatal myocardial infarction and appears to be equally effective as treatment with a β-blocker [22,60]. However, despite these convincing results, doubts about the safety of diuretics continue to be expressed on the basis of findings from isolated trials.

Multiple Risk Factor Intervention Trial (MRFIT)

The data cited most frequently in support of cardiotoxic effect of diuretics emerged from MRFIT [61]. In that trial, intensive intervention including diuretic therapy (SI) did not reduce coronary heart disease risk when compared to usual care (UC). This negative outcome prompted several retrospective analyses of subgroups in one of which [62] men in the SI group with an abnormal ECG at rest (but not in exercise) had higher coronary mortality manifest mainly as sudden death: 36 deaths among 1299 in SI versus 21 among 1185 in UC.

The relationship between intensive diuretic treatment and increased cardiovascular mortality has been ascribed to diuretic-induced hypokalaemia but there is no direct supporting evidence and there are many imponderables. The difference in thiazide use between SI and UC was relative rather than absolute (75% versus 55%). In SI, higher doses were used and hypokalaemia was more common but neither hypokalaemia nor diuretic dose predicted death from coronary heart disease. Coronary deaths were more frequent after hydrochlorothiazide than following chlorthalidone, despite more pronounced hypokalaemia with chlorthalidone. Mortality was *lowest* in patients with the greatest degree of hypokalaemia on high dose diuretics, whether or not they had abnormal ECG. These findings provide no support for the suggestion that arrhythmias related to hypokalaemia were responsible for the excess coronary heart disease deaths in the group managed intensively.

In another MRFIT subgroup with abnormal exercise ECG at entry [63], patients had a better outcome if treated intensively (SI). This casts serious doubt on the suggestion that MRFIT demonstrated a cardiotoxic effect of diuretic in patients with myocardial ischaemia prior to therapy. Furthermore, patients with abnormal ECG in the UC group had a lower mortality rate than those with a normal ECG, an observation at variance with all other hypertension studies and very difficult to explain. The MRFIT controversy illustrates the hazards of subgroup analysis.

The MRFIT speculations gained no support from the Hypertension Detection and Follow-Up Programme [64], The International Prospective Primary Prevention Study in Hypertension [65] or Systolic Hypertension in the Elderly Programme (SHEP) [66]. In SHEP, subjects with abnormal resting ECG experienced a 31% reduction in fatal and non-fatal coronary heart disease events when treated with a diuretic compared with placebo.

Metoprolol Atherosclerosis Prevention in Hypertension (MAPHY) trial

Only in the MAPHY study [67] were fatal myocardial infarctions and sudden deaths significantly more frequent in men randomized to a diuretic compared with those receiving a β-blocker (metoprolol). In fact, the MAPHY study population was a subset of the much larger Heart Attack Primary Prevention in Hypertension (HAPPHY) trial [68], followed up for an extended period. The HAPPHY trial reported no difference between thiazides and metoprolol or atenolol in the incidence of coronary events. Thiazides were at least as good as the β-blockers in each quartile of risk at entry and, despite hypokalaemia in 12%, sudden cardiac death and fatal myocardial infarction did not occur more frequently in diuretic-treated patients. The advantage of metoprolol over thiazides reported in MAPHY did not emerge only in the extended follow-up but was already present during HAPPHY which found no difference between diuretics and both β-blockers. Therefore, patients treated with atenolol in HAPPHY must have fared worse than those treated with thiazide and much worse than those treated with metoprolol. There was no prior hypothesis nor is there a plausible explanation for this difference between the β-blockers. The apparent advantage of metoprolol in MAPHY was probably a chance finding produced by *post hoc* subgroup analysis. It is certainly unsafe to incriminate diuretics on the basis of these findings.

A meta-analysis [69] of the 14 unconfounded trials of antihypertensive drugs (chiefly diuretics and β-blockers) up to 1990 in which about 37 000 individuals were studied for a mean duration of 5 years indicated that coronary events fell significantly by 14% (95% CI 4, 21%), representing just over half the benefit (20–25%) anticipated from prospective epidemiological studies. For subjects who died, however, mean treatment duration was only 2–3 years suggesting that the observed advantage occurred rapidly and might be an underestimate of the long-term value of treatment. An overview including results from trials reported in 1991–92 [70] indicated a 16% reduction in fatal coronary events with treatment. The shortfall in expected prevention of coronary heart disease might easily be due to chance.

DIURETIC DOSE AND METABOLIC EFFECTS

Most of the information on the metabolic effects of diuretics comes from studies employing high doses. Soon after their introduction it was recognized that biochemical changes are less at low doses and that the dose-response for blood pressure reduction is shallow [71]. The most recent and best evidence for a dissociation of the metabolic and antihypertensive effects of thiazides indicated similar blood pressure reduction after doses of bendrofluazide 1.25–10 mg daily but a clear dose-response for biochemical variables [72]. After bendrofluazide 2.5 mg daily, only changes in potassium, triglycerides and urate were significant compared to placebo. Similar dissociation has been reported with other diuretics. In The

Treatment of Mild Hypertension Study [73], after one year of chlorthalidone 15 mg daily, antihypertensive efficacy was equivalent to that of other drugs but the only significant metabolic changes were a modest reduction in serum potassium and increase in total cholesterol. There is little justification for using thiazides at doses greater than the equivalent of bendrofluazide 2.5 mg daily. The optimal dose may be even less.

CONCLUSIONS

The biochemical changes which accompany therapy with diuretics have been widely publicized. Reduction in plasma potassium is common but sound studies are consistent in showing that diuretics do not deplete body potassium or cause potassium deficiency. Most reviews of the effects of diuretics on magnesium metabolism are uncritical and extrapolate unacceptably from the little sound evidence that is available. Long-term thiazide treatment causes a small fall in plasma magnesium within the normal range; competent investigations do not support a reduction in intracellular magnesium due to diuretics. Diuretic-induced disturbances of magnesium metabolism do not cause depletion of intracellular potassium. The influence of thiazides on serum lipids is largely transient and in the long-term total cholesterol is raised only slightly. There is strong evidence that thiazides interfere with glucose metabolism and that diuretics can cause hyperuricaemia. All metabolic effects are greatly reduced at low doses.

The risks of diuretic-induced metabolic changes have been greatly exaggerated with much unwarranted speculation and extrapolation. The evidence linking thiazide-induced hypokalaemia with arrhythmias and sudden death is indirect and tenuous at best. Even in patients with left ventricular hypertrophy and concomitant coronary heart disease, the association is unconvincing. Diuretics are not responsible for the relation between hypokalaemia and ventricular fibrillation in acute myocardial infarction. No single clinical study has shown clearly a relation between thiazides, hypokalaemia, malignant arrhythmias and sudden death. However, even mild diuretic-induced hypokalaemia is dangerous in patients taking digoxin or drugs known to markedly prolong the QT interval, because of the real risk of serious arrhythmias and sudden death. Such combinations should be used with caution, and in patients at risk for hypokalaemia must be prevented by concomitant use of adequate dosage of a potassium-sparing agent. The clinical significance of the small diuretic-induced alterations in magnesium status, if any, is obscure. There is no satisfactory evidence that diuretic-induced magnesium disturbances cause or predispose to cardiac arrhythmias in general or after myocardial infarction. The argument that modest long-term effects of diuretics on lipid levels may blunt the beneficial influence on blood pressure is difficult to sustain. Such changes are likely to account for at most only a tiny fraction of any shortfall in coronary prevention. In any case, it is not known whether diuretic-induced cholesterol changes carry the same prognostic significance as naturally occurring hypercholesterolaemia. Elevation of cholesterol is avoided entirely by prescribing thiazides at the low doses now in standard use. The clinical trials do not indicate a major risk of developing diabetes mellitus even with high dose diuretics and prospective studies have not demonstrated that glucose intolerance short of diabetes, or elevated insulin levels, are independent risk factors for coronary heart disease. Hyperuricaemia secondary to diuretics carries the risk of gout but is not an independent risk factor for coronary heart disease.

In contrast, controlled clinical trials have demonstrated decisively the benefits of diuretics. Regardless of dose or metabolic disturbances there is no valid evidence that diuretics contribute to myocardial infarction, sudden death, or to a failure of antihypertensive treatment or other risk factor interventions to prevent coronary deaths. An association between diuretics and sudden death has been suggested only in selected subset analyses which allow no valid conclusions. Even in subjects with ECG abnormalities before therapy, there is no sound or consistent evidence to support the suggestion that diuretics predispose to sudden death. Unconfounded comparisons have demonstrated equivalence of thiazides and β-blockers with regard to sudden coronary deaths (Table 3). If thiazides

Table 3 Coronary heart disease events in comparative treatment trials in mild to moderate hypertension

		β-Blocker based		Thiazide based	
Trials (Reference)		*n*	Events	*n*	Events
Fatal					
MRC	[74]	4403	47	4297	59
IPPPSH	[65]	3185	40	3172	46
HAPPHY	[68]	3297	54	3272	50
MAPHY	[67]	1609	36	1625	43
MRC-2	[75]	1102	52	1081	33
Total		13596	229	13447	231
Non-fatal					
MRC	[74]	4403	56	4297	60
IPPPSH	[65]	3185	56	3172	60
HAPPHY	[68]	3297	84	3272	75
MAPHY	[69]	–	NR	–	NR
MRC-2	[75]	1102	28	1081	15
Total		11987	224	11822	210
All events*		11987	417	11822	399

* Excluding MAPHY.

have an adverse effect on coronary heart disease this adverse effect must be common to β-blockers – a group of drugs which has been shown repeatedly to substantially *reduce* coronary events and sudden death when used for secondary prevention after myocardial infarction. The case for a malign cardiotoxic influence of diuretics has been overstated repeatedly. It simply does not withstand critical scrutiny.

The various charges brought against diuretics have little substance. No other class of drugs has undergone more intensive and prolonged surveillance. More than 30 years of wide clinical use has established the safety of diuretics beyond all reasonable doubt. Careful inspection of the available data allows only one conclusion. Diuretic-induced cardiotoxicity is a myth.

REFERENCES

1 Kaplan NM. Problems with the use of diuretics in the treatment of hypertension. *Am J Nephrology* 1986;6:1–5.

2 Robertson JIS. Hypertension and coronary risk: possible adverse effects of antihypertensive drugs. *Am Heart J* 1987;114:S1051–S1054.

3 Weinberger MH. Diuretics and their side-effects. Dilemma in the treatment of hypertension. *Hypertension* 1988;11(Suppl II):16–20.

4 Morgan DB, Davidson C. Hypokalaemia and diuretics: an analysis of publications. *Br Med J* 1980;280:905–908.

5 Dyckner T, Wester PO. Potassium/magnesium depletion in patients with cardiovascular disease. *Am J Med* 1987;82 (Suppl 3A):11–17.

6 Wester PO, Dyckner T. Problems with potassium and magnesium in diuretic-treated patients. *Acta Pharmacol Toxicol* 1984;54(Suppl 1):59–65.

7 Flear CTG, Quirton A, Carpenter RED, *et al.* Exchangeable body potassium and sodium in patients with congestive heart failure. *Clin Chim Acta* 1986;13:1–12.

8 White RJ, Chamberlin DA, Hamer J, *et al.* Potassium depletion in severe heart disease. *Br Med J* 1969;ii:606–610.

9 Kassirer JP, Harrington JT. Diuretics and potassium metabolism: A reassessment of the need, effectiveness and safety of potassium therapy. *Kidney Int* 1977;11:505–515.

10 Smith WO. The influence of various diuretic agents on the urinary excretion of magnesium in non-oedematous subjects. *Clin Res* 1959;7:162.

11 Laerum E. Metabolic effect of thiazide versus placebo in patients under treatment for recurrent urolithiasis. *Scand J Urol Nephrol* 1984;18:143–149.

12 McVeigh G, Galloway D, Johnston D. The case for low dose diuretics in hypertension: comparison of low and conventional doses of cyclopenthiazide. *Br Med J* 1988;297: 95–98.

13 Murdoch DL, Forrest G, Davies DL, McInnes GT. A comparison of the potassium and magnesium-sparing properties of amiloride and spironolactone in diuretic-treated normal subjects. *Br J Clin Pharmacol* 1993;35:373–378.

14 Papademetriou A, Notargiacomo A, Heine D, *et al.* Effect of diuretic therapy and exercise-related arrhythmias in systemic hypertension. *Am J Cardiol* 1989;64:1152–1156.

15 Hollifield JW. Magnesium depletion, diuretics and arrhythmias. *Am J Med* 1987; 82(Suppl 3A):30–37.

16 Martin BJ, Milligan K. Diuretic-associated hypomagnesaemia in the elderly. *Arch Intern Med* 1987;147:1768–1771.

17 Lim P, Jacob E. Magnesium deficiency in patients on long-term diuretic therapy for heart failure. *Br Med J* 1972;ii:620–622.

18 Bergstrom J, Hultman E, Solheim SB. The effect of frusemide on plasma and muscle

electrolytes and blood pressure in normal subjects and in patients with essential hypertension. *Acta Med Scand* 1973;194:427–432.
19 Whang R, Welt LG. Observations in experimental magnesium depletion. *J Clin Invest* 1963;42:305–313.
20 Dyckner T, Wester PO. Ventricular extrasystoles and intracellular electrolytes before and after potassium and magnesium infusions in patients on diuretic therapy. *Am Heart J* 1979;97:12–18.
21 Ames RP. The effects of antihypertensive drugs on serum lipids and lipoproteins. 1. Diuretics. *Drugs* 1986;32:260–278.
22 McInnes GT, Yeo WW, Ramsay LE, Moser M. Cardiotoxicity and diuretics: much speculation–little substance. *J Hypertens* 1992;10:317–335.
23 Lasser NL, Grandits G, Caggiula AW, *et al.* Effects of antihypertensive therapy on plasma lipids and lipoproteins in the Multiple Risk Factor Intervention Trial. *Am J Med* 1984;74(Suppl 2A):52–66.
24 Thompson WG. Review: An assault on old friends: thiazide diuretics under siege. *Am J Med Sci* 1990;300:152–158.
25 Moser M. Update on some hypertension treatment controversies. *Cardiovasc Risk Factors* 1991;1:413–426.
26 Murphy MB, Lewis PJ, Kohner E, *et al.* Glucose intolerance in hypertensive patients treated with diuretics: A fourteen year follow-up. *Lancet* 1982;ii:1293–1295.
27 Grunfeld C, Chappell DA. Hypokalaemia and diabetes mellitus. *Am J Med* 1983;75: 553–554.
28 Shapiro AP, Benedeck TG, Small JL. Effect of thiazides on carbohydrate metabolism in patients with hypertension. *N Engl J Med* 1961;265:1028–1033.
29 Pollare T, Lithell H, Berne C. A comparison of the effects of hydrochlorothiazide and captopril on glucose and lipid metabolism in patients with hypertension. *N Engl J Med* 1989;321:868–873.
30 Eschewege E, Richard JL, Thibult N, *et al.* Coronary heart disease mortality in relation with diabetes, blood glucose and plasma insulin levels: The Paris Prospective Study, ten years later. *Horm Metab Res* 1985;15(Suppl 15):41–46.
31 Pyorala K, Savolainen E, Kaukola S, Haapokoski J. Plasma insulin as coronary heart disease risk factor: relationship to other risk factors and predictive value during 9½-year follow-up of the Helsinki Policemen Study population. *Acta Med Scand* 1985; (Suppl 701):38–52.
32 The Hypertension Detection and Follow-Up Program Co-operative Research Group: Mortality findings for stepped-care and referred-care participants in the Hypertension Detection and Follow-Up Program stratified for other risk factors. *Prevent Med* 1985; 14:312–335.
33 Langford HG, Blaufox D, Borhani NO, *et al.* Is thiazide-produced uric acid elevation harmful? Analysis of data from the Hypertension Detection and Follow-Up Program. *Arch Intern Med* 1987;147:645–649.
34 Holland OB, Nixon JV, Kuhnert L. Diuretic-induced ventricular ectopic activity. *Am J Med* 1981;70:762–768.
35 Papademetriou V, Price M, Gottdiener J, *et al.* Effect of diuretic therapy on ventricular arrhythmias in patients with or without left ventricular hypertrophy. *Am Heart J* 1985;110:595–599.
36 Lief PD, Belizon I, Matos J, *et al.* Diuretic-induced hypokalaemia does not cause ventricular ectopy in uncomplicated essential hypertension. *Proc Am Soc Nephrol* 1983; 16:A66.
37 Madias JE, Madias NE, Gavras HP. Nonarrhythmogenicity of diuretic-induced hypokalaemia. Its evidence in patients with uncomplicated hypertension. *Arch Intern Med* 1984;144:2171–2176.
38 Medical Research Council Working Party on Mild to Moderate Hypertension: Ventricular extrasystoles during thiazide treatment: Sub-study of MRC mild hypertension trial. *Br Med J* 1983;287:1249–1253.
39 Narayan P, Colleran J, Kokkinos P, *et al.* Hydrochlorothiazide therapy and ventricular arrhythmias in hypertensive patients with advanced left ventricular hypertrophy. *J Am Coll Cardiac* 1992;19(Suppl A):196A.

40 Hollifield JW. Potassium and magnesium abnormalities: diuretics and arrhythmias in hypertension. *Am J Med* 1984;77(Suppl 5A):28–32.
41 McLenachan JM, Henderson E, Morris KI, Dargie HJ. Ventricular arrhythmias in patients with hypertensive left ventricular hypertrophy. *N Engl J Med* 1987;308: 787–792.
42 Papademetriou V, Burris ZF, Notargiaecomo A, *et al.* Thiazide therapy is not the cause of arrhythmias in patients with systemic hypertension. *Arch Intern Med* 1988;148: 1272–1276.
43 Surawicz B. Is hypomagnesaemia or magnesium deficiency arrhythmogenic? *J Am Coll Cardiol* 1989;14:1093–1096.
44 Michelson EL, Morganroth J. Spontaneous variability of complex ventricular arrhythmias detected by long-term electrocardiographic recording. *Circulation* 1980;61:690–695.
45 McInnes GT, Brodie MJ. Drug interactions that matter. A critical reappraisal. *Drugs* 1988;36:83–110.
46 Dyckner T, Helmers C, Lundman T, Wester PO. Initial serum potassium level in relation to early complications and prognosis in patients with acute myocardial infarction. *Acta Med Scand* 1975;197:207–210.
47 Dyckner T, Helmers C, Wester PO. Cardiac dysrhythmias in patients with acute myocardial infarction – relation of serum potassium level and prior diuretic therapy. *Acta Med Scand* 1984;216:127–132.
48 Nordrehaug JE, Van der Lippe G. Hypokalaemia and ventricular fibrillation in acute myocardial infarction. *Br Heart J* 1983;50:525–529.
49 Nordrehaug JE, Johnssen K, Van der Lippe G. Serum potassium concentration as a risk factor of ventricular arrhythmias early in acute myocardial infarction. *Circulation* 1985;71:645–649.
50 Thomas RD. Ventricular fibrillation and initial plasma potassium in acute myocardial infarction. *Postgrad Med J* 1983;59:354–356.
51 Ramsay LE, Toner JM, Camerson HA. Diuretic use, serum potassium and ventricular fibrillation in patients with myocardial infarction. *Br J Clin Pharmacol* 1984;17:605P.
52 Boyd JC, Bruns DE, Di Marco JP, *et al.* Relationship of potassium and magnesium concentrations in serum to cardiac arrhythmias. *Clin Chem* 1984;30:754–757.
53 Cooper WD, Kuan P, Reuben SR, Vandenburg MJ. Cardiac arrhythmias following acute myocardial infarction: association with the serum potassium level and prior diuretic therapy. *Eur Heart J* 1984;5:464–469.
54 Brown MJ, Brown DC, Murphy MB. Hypokalaemia from beta 2-receptor stimulation by circulating epinephrine. *N Engl J Med* 1983;309:1414–1419.
55 Fletcher GF, Hurst JW, Schlant RC. Polarizing solutions in patients with acute myocardial infarction. *Am Heart J* 1968;75:319–324.
56 Nordrehaug JE. Hypokalaemia, arrhythmias and early prognosis in acute myocardial infarction. *Acta Med Scand* 1985;217:299–306.
57 Isles CG, Walker LM, Beevers DG, *et al.* Mortality in patients of the Glasgow Blood Pressure Clinic. *J Hypertens* 1986;4:141–156.
58 Robertson JWK, Isles CG, Brown I, *et al.* Mild hypokalaemia is not a risk factor in treated hypertensives. *J Hypertens* 1986;4:603–608.
59 Dyckner T. Serum magnesium in acute myocardial infarction. Relation to arrhythmias. *Acta Med Scand* 1980;207:59–66.
60 McInnes GT. Results of trials of antihypertensive therapy: a plan for action. In: Lorimer AR, Shepherd J, eds. *Preventive Cardiology*. Oxford: Blackwell Scientific Publications, 1991:107–135.
61 Multiple Risk Factor Intervention Trial Research Group. Multiple Risk Factor Intervention Trial: risk factor changes and mortality rate. *JAMA* 1982;245:1465–1477.
62 Cohen JD, Neaton JD, Prineas RJ, Daniels KA. Diuretic-induced ventricular tachycardia: diuretics, serum potassium and ventricular arrhythmias in the Multiple Risk Factor Intervention Trial. *Am J Cardiol* 1987;60:548–554.
63 Mutiple Risk Factor Intervention Trial Research Group. Exercise electrocardiogram and coronary heart disease mortality in the Multiple Risk Factor Intervention Trial. *Am J Cardiol* 1985;55:16–24.

64 Hypertension Detection and Follow-Up Program Co-operative Group. Five year findings of the Hypertension Detection and Follow-Up Program. 1. Reduction in mortality of persons with high blood pressure, including mild hypertension. *JAMA* 1979;252: 2562–2571.

65 The IPPPSH Collaborative Group. Cardiovascular risk and risk factors in a randomized trial of treatment based on the beta-blocker oxprenolol: The International Prospective Primary Prevention Study in Hypertension (IPPPSH). *J Hypertens* 1985;3:379–392.

66 SHEP Co-operative Research Group. Prevention of stroke by antihypertensive drug treatment in older persons with isolated systolic hypertension: Final results of the Systolic Hypertension in the Elderly Program (SHEP). *JAMA* 1991;265:3255–3264.

67 Wikstrand J, Warnold I, Olsson G, *et al.* Primary prevention with metoprolol in patients with hypertension. Mortality results from the MAPHY study. *JAMA* 1988; 259:1976–1982.

68 Wilhelmsen L, Berglund G, Elmfeldt D, *et al.* Beta-blockers versus diuretics in hypertensive men: main results from the HAPPHY Trial. *J Hypertens* 1987;5:561–572.

69 Collins R, Peto R, MacMahon S, *et al.* Blood pressure, stroke and coronary heart disease. Part 2, short-term reductions in blood pressure: overview of randomised drug trials in their epidemiological context. *Lancet* 1990;335:827–838.

70 McInnes GT. Hypertension: effects of therapy on reducing mortality. *Int Pharm J* 1992;6:120–121.

71 Cranston WI, Juel-Jensen BE, Semmence AM, *et al.* Effects of oral diuretics on raised arterial pressure. *Lancet* 1963;ii:966–970.

72 Carlsen JE, Kober L, Torp-Pedersen C, Johansen P. Relation between dose of bendrofluazide, antihypertensive effect and adverse biochemical effects. *Br Med J* 1990;300: 975–978.

73 The Treatment of Mild Hypertension Research Group. The Treatment of Mild Hypertension Study. A randomised, placebo-controlled trial of a nutritional-hygienic regimen along with various drug monotherapies. *Arch Intern Med* 1991;151:1413–1423.

74 Medical Research Council Working Party. MRC trial of treatment of mild hypertension: principal results. *Br Med J* 1985;291:97–104.

75 MRC Working Party. Medical Research Council trial of treatment of hypertension in older adults: principal results. *Br Med J* 1992;304:405–412.

Pharmacogenetics: can the therapeutic key objective be accomplished?

M. C. S. HALL, W. L. GREGORY & J. R. IDLE

Diseases desperate grown,
By desperate appliance are relieved,
Or not at all.

Shakespeare: Hamlet

PHARMACOGENETICS

Pharmacogenetics is a word unfamiliar to many, if not most, physicians. Relegated over the years to a paragraph or table in undergraduate textbooks, the subject is still broadly regarded as one of academic interest only. Resistance to the concept that the genetic constitution of a patient may contribute in an essential way to both the pattern and extent of response to drug therapy is rooted in a social conditioning that all are born of equal potential. However, from a therapeutic standpoint, nothing could be further from the truth. The lack of response of some patients to standard treatments and the occurrence of unwanted side-effects in others are both testimonies to the bald fact that ideal drug therapy can be difficult to accomplish, frustrating to manage and wasteful of resources, when interpatient variability is at play. Although laboratory monitoring of drug plasma levels has improved the use of drugs such as gentamicin, digoxin and the anticonvulsants, it is worth noting that therapy is always initiated without the knowledge of how the drug will behave in a given patient. Cyclosporin and warfarin are both eminent examples of how regular monitoring of either plasma concentration or therapeutic response is an essential component of the therapeutic plan. This is itself not without economic consequences, as any large transplant centre knows.

What if, prior to inception of new drug therapy, a test could broadly predict whether or not the patient is likely to respond appropriately, adversely or not at all? Another common therapeutic manoeuvre, blood transfusion, depends both upon serology and, amongst other things, HIV testing, to protect the interests of the patient. Not to carry out such testing may be catastrophic. So should not drug therapy aspire to the same standards, those based upon discerning at the outset which patients are suitable and which unsuitable for a particular therapy? The therapeutic key objective of pharmacogenetics should be to proscribe therapy in patients identified as likely to be non-responders or adverse responders. To accomplish this, readily-performed non-invasive tests are needed. Here we shall seek to demonstrate that this is both desirable and now achievable for a growing number of drugs, using DNA-based assays to determine phenotypes which can radically alter the extent of metabolism, and thus the plasma pharmacokinetics, of a number of widely used drugs. The rate of progress in this field has of late been so considerable that the list of drugs where this technology will be of assistance is expected to enlarge.

POLYMORPHISMS OF DRUG METABOLISM

Although the myriad of receptors, membrane channels and enzymes which provide the ultimate molecular targets for drug action are likely to harbour examples of genetic variability between patients, there has sadly been all too little research in this potentially fertile field. The vast majority of investigators have restricted themselves to the genetics of drug disposition, where differences between subjects in drug metabolism can be identified in the laboratory using techniques merely dependent upon the chemistry of small molecules. Table 1 summarizes the drug metabolizing enzymes for which genetic polymorphism has been found. Since metabolism is the principal process by which the pharmacological action of a drug is terminated *in vivo*, it is easy to envisage how extremes of drug metabolism may lead to unfavourable therapeutic outcomes. When genetic variability underlies these extremes of metabolism, this has a number of important and obvious consequences for an individual patient, as follows:

1 the metabolic phenotype of the patient (compare with blood group) will be predictable and stable over time;

2 knowledge of the metabolic phenotype may predict the metabolism of a number of drugs in that patient;

3 knowledge of the metabolic phenotype may predict susceptibility to adverse drug reactions or therapeutic failure;

4 DNA-based tests should predict phenotype and thus therapeutic outcomes.

The importance of the above four points in relation to the therapeutic key objective of pharmacogenetics will be returned to after a brief description of the CYP2D6 genetic polymorphism, which gives rise to the highly variable metabolism of a wide range of clinically important drugs.

CYP2D6: THE ARCHETYPAL GENETIC POLYMORPHISM

The first example of genetic polymorphism in the most ubiquitous pathway of drug biotransformation, namely hydroxylation, was that of the cytochrome P450 isozyme now referred to as CYP2D6 [1]. Early observations with nortriptyline in Sweden [2] and sparteine in Germany [3], both in MD theses, showed all the hallmarks of what we would recognize today as genetic polymorphism. But it was not until the observations with debrisoquine 4-hydroxylation [4] that a genetic polymorphism of metabolic hydroxylation was established. Eichelbaum and Gross [5] have reviewed 37 population studies where either debrisoquine, sparteine or dextromethorphan (all CYP2D6 substrates) have been administered to a total of 7274 healthy volunteers in 14 ethnic groups, of which 415 persons could be identified as being deficient in the metabolism of the

Table 1 Genetic polymorphisms of drug metabolizing enzymes of relevance to clinical practice

Enzyme	Drug substrate	Adverse outcomes in susceptible patients
Pseudocholinesterase	Succinylcholine (suxamethonium)	Prolonged apnoea
Aldehyde dehydrogenases	Cyclophosphamide	?
	Ifosfamide	?
CYP1A2	Theophylline	?
CYP2A6	Coumarin	?
$CYP2C_{MP}$	Omeprazole	Grossly elevated plasma levels
CYP2C9	Warfarin	?
CYP2D6	β-Blockers	Multiple (see text)
	Tricyclic antidepressants	
	Neuroleptics	
	Antidysrhythmics	
	Monoamine oxygenase inhibitors	
	Antihypertensives	
	Opiates	
CYP3A4	Nifedipine	Exaggerated responses in some CF patients
UDP-glucuronosyl transferases (UDPGTs)	Paracetamol	?
N-Acetyltransferase 2 (NAT 2)	Isoniazid	Neuropathy
	Hydralazine	SLE
	Sulphonamides	Stevens–Johnson syndrome
	Dapsone	
Thiopurine methyl transferase (TPMT)	6-Mercaptopurine	Therapeutic failure
	Azathioprine	Myelosuppression

CYP, Cytochrome P450; CF, cystic fibrosis; SLE, systemic lupus erythematosus.

administered drug. Such persons are called poor metabolizers (PMs) and comprise up to almost 20% of certain populations. In the UK, one might expect 1 in every 10 or 12 patients to be phenotypically PM. The deficient PM phenotype is recessive [6] and thus not apparent from family histories. A significant number of drugs, used particularly in cardiovascular medicine and in psychiatry, show genetically variable metabolism due to the CYP2D6 polymorphism. Because the CYP2D6 complementary DNA (cDNA) has been cloned and characterized [7] and the structure of the gene elucidated [8], it has been possible to develop DNA-based tests which determine, with high certainty, the individual's genotype, and thus predict phenotype [9–11]. This now obviates the administration of probe drugs to patients, as will be seen below.

STABILITY OF THE METABOLIC PHENOTYPE

One very important characteristic of monogenic traits is their chronic stability. From the point of view of drug doses and pharmacokinetics, it is an advantage when the metabolism of a drug is largely determined by a single allelomorphic gene, such as the examples given in Table 1. Once the dose a particular patient requires has been determined, this will remain stable over time. Whereas, when the metabolism of another drug is capricious, because physiological, environmental and lifestyle factors are the principal determinants of the rate of metabolism, it is easy to see how the intrasubject variance in dose requirement may be significant. An example of this is theophylline which is metabolized by three inducible cytochromes P450, namely CYP1A2, CYP2E1 and CYP3A4 [12]. Alteration of tobacco usage or alcohol drinking will thus significantly alter the metabolic clearance of theophylline [13,14]. This would not be so for a polymorphically metabolized drug such as debrisoquine [15,16] and, by implication (see below) many others.

PREDICTION OF METABOLISM OF OTHER DRUGS FROM METABOLIC PHENOTYPE

Populations of healthy volunteers who have been phenotyped with debrisoquine have often been used to establish whether or not another drug displays polymorphic metabolism. Very strong correlations are sometimes found where knowledge of the extent of debrisoquine 4-hydroxylation in the individual (measured by the parameter 'metabolic ratio', per cent of dose in urine excreted as debrisoquine/per cent of dose excreted as 4-hydroxy-debrisoquine) can quite accurately forecast the degree of metabolism of a second drug, or indeed some other pharmacokinetic parameter. Examples of drugs with such strong correlations with debrisoquine metabolic ratio include timolol [17], codeine [18,19]

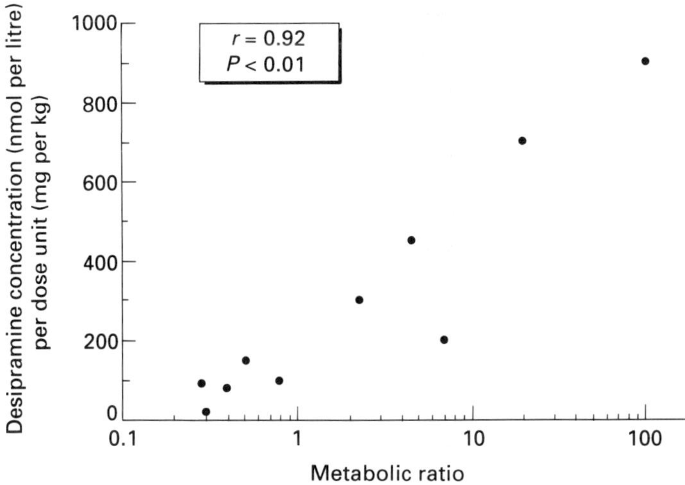

Fig. 1 Strong correlation between polymorphic debrisoquine metabolism (represented by the logarithmic expression of the metabolic ratio) and the plasma concentrations of desipramine. (Data redrawn from Dahl and Bertilsson [26], with permission of Chapman & Hall.)

desipramine [20] (Fig. 1), zuclopenthixol [21], nortriptyline [22], sparteine [23] and phenformin [24]. The list of CYP2D6 substrates, drugs whose metabolism will be impaired in approximately 10% of the population, is around 30 in number [5,25] However, some of these have fallen into disuse (e.g. sparteine and debrisoquine), whilst others never made it through clinical trials (e.g. encainide and bufuralol) and another group have been actively restricted by regulatory authorities due to unacceptable incidences of life-threatening side-effects (e.g. phenformin and perhexiline). These are the innate characteristics of drugs which harbour large interpatient variability in pharmacokinetics, rendering their use difficult. However, a 'hard core' of polymorphically metabolized CYP2D6 substrates enjoys widespread clinical usage. These drugs, numbering at present some 15–20, but whose ranks will gradually swell, share both structural and physicochemical properties and thus fall into a restricted number of therapeutic groups as shown in Table 2. Whilst it is possible to avoid a CYP2D6 substrate when prescribing an antidysrhythmic drug or β-blocker, it is not so simple to avoid prescribing a neuroleptic drug or tricyclic antidepressant which will not have impaired metabolism, and thus grossly elevated plasma concentrations, in some 10% of patients to whom it is given. As has been discussed elsewhere [5], in the pharmacokinetic and metabolism studies which make up an important part of a drug's preregistration clinical development, only a limited number of volunteers or patients are in general recruited, insufficient to account for pharmacogenetic variability. Were such a small panel to include a PM

Table 2 CYP2D6 substrates in clinical practice. (Data from references [25,26])

Cardiovascular drugs	
Antidysrhythmics	β-Blockers
Flecainide	Timolol
Mexiletine	Metoprolol
Propafenone	Propranolol
Psychoactive drugs	
Neuroleptics	Tricyclic antidepressants
Clozapine	Amitriptyline
Fluphenazine	Clomipramine
Haloperidol	Desipramine
Perphenazine	Imipramine
Remoxipride	Nortriptyline
Thioridazine	
Trifluperidol	
Zuclopenthixol	

subject, his/her aberrant metabolic behaviour might be dismissed and, as has already occurred [27], in an early study of the antihypertensive guanoxan, the subject's data excluded from the statistical evaluation of that drug's disposition. Accordingly, there are many polymorphically metabolized drugs in clinical practice for which the recommended dose range underrepresents the polymorphic population variance. An excellent example, quoted before [5], is that of the tricyclic antidepressant nortriptyline: it was shown a quarter of a century ago [28] that patients given the same dose of nortriptyline display a 30-fold range of steady-state plasma concentrations. Nortriptyline was shown to be a CYP2D6 substrate in 1980 [29]. The daily maintenance dose recommended in the *British National Formulary* is 30–75 mg. One must assume that the impact of pharmacogenetics upon the drug treatment of depressive illness in this country has been nil! Despite the availability over 15 years of non-invasive tests which employed an innocuous probe drug to derive data which could be used to forecast the behaviour of other drugs in that same patient, the technology was not applied in clinical practice. A significant number of patients have obviously been both under- and over-dosed with the drugs in Table 2. It appears that the therapeutic key objective of pharmacogenetics is not being met, at least not with metabolic phenotyping.

PREDICTION OF ADVERSE DRUG REACTIONS OR THERAPEUTIC FAILURE FROM METABOLIC PHENOTYPE

Most studies examining the relationship between CYP2D6 phenotype and clinical response have either examined the pharmacodynamic response in a small panel of extensive metabolizers (EMs) and PMs (the earliest studies with hypotensive responses to debrisoquine [30] or blood lactate changes after phenformin [31] were performed in this way, and similar protocols are still used today) or studied debrisoquine metabolism in patients exhibiting adverse drug reactions compared with control patients. The earliest and perhaps most compelling example is that of perhexiline, a first generation calcium entry blocker used predominantly to treat angina. As perhexiline usage increased from the mid-1970s an alarming pattern of adverse reactions began to emerge, including peripheral neuropathy and hepatic cirrhosis. Serious side-effects were associated with higher plasma levels and longer elimination half-lives of perhexiline [32]. An explanation was soon to emerge from the study of 20 neuropathic patients and 14 well-controlled non-neuropathic patients [33]. The neuropathy was associated with impaired metabolism of the probe drug debrisoquine and, by implication, impaired metabolism of perhexiline [33]. As the perhexiline story unfolded pharmacogenetics took a giant step, acquiring a predictive and preventative basis. In view of the findings above, the St Mary's group began to recruit patients newly treated with perhexiline. It is worthwhile to quote from the report of one such patient, a 60-year-old man with angina [34].

> The patient began receiving perhexiline, 100 mg twice daily, and in view of encouraging therapeutic response and normal liver function tests 4 weeks later, the dose was increased to 100 mg three times a day. At regular follow-up visits, he reported considerable reduction in anginal episodes and had no neurological complaints . . . Following a total of 33 weeks of perhexiline therapy, the patient's phenotype was determined with 10 mg oral debrisoquine for his hydroxylation status . . . He was found to have a metabolic ratio of 18.1, confirming that he was of poor metabolizer phenotype. In view of this finding, an electromyogram (EMG) was obtained 3 days later, and it revealed definitive evidence of subclinical demyelinating, predominantly sensory, neuropathy. Perhexiline was therefore discontinued . . . The plasma elimination half-life of perhexiline in this patient was estimated to be 9.5 days.

As can be seen from this account, a serious adverse drug reaction was averted because routine debrisoquine phenotyping had been introduced at St Mary's. The Product Licence for perhexiline maleate (Pexid) was not renewed in 1985.

DNA-BASED TESTS TO PREDICT CYP2D6 PHENOTYPE

In the 15 years following the introduction of debrisoquine hydroxylation phenotyping [4], a number of limitations of the metabolic test had surfaced. Whilst the administration of a single oral 10 mg dose of de-

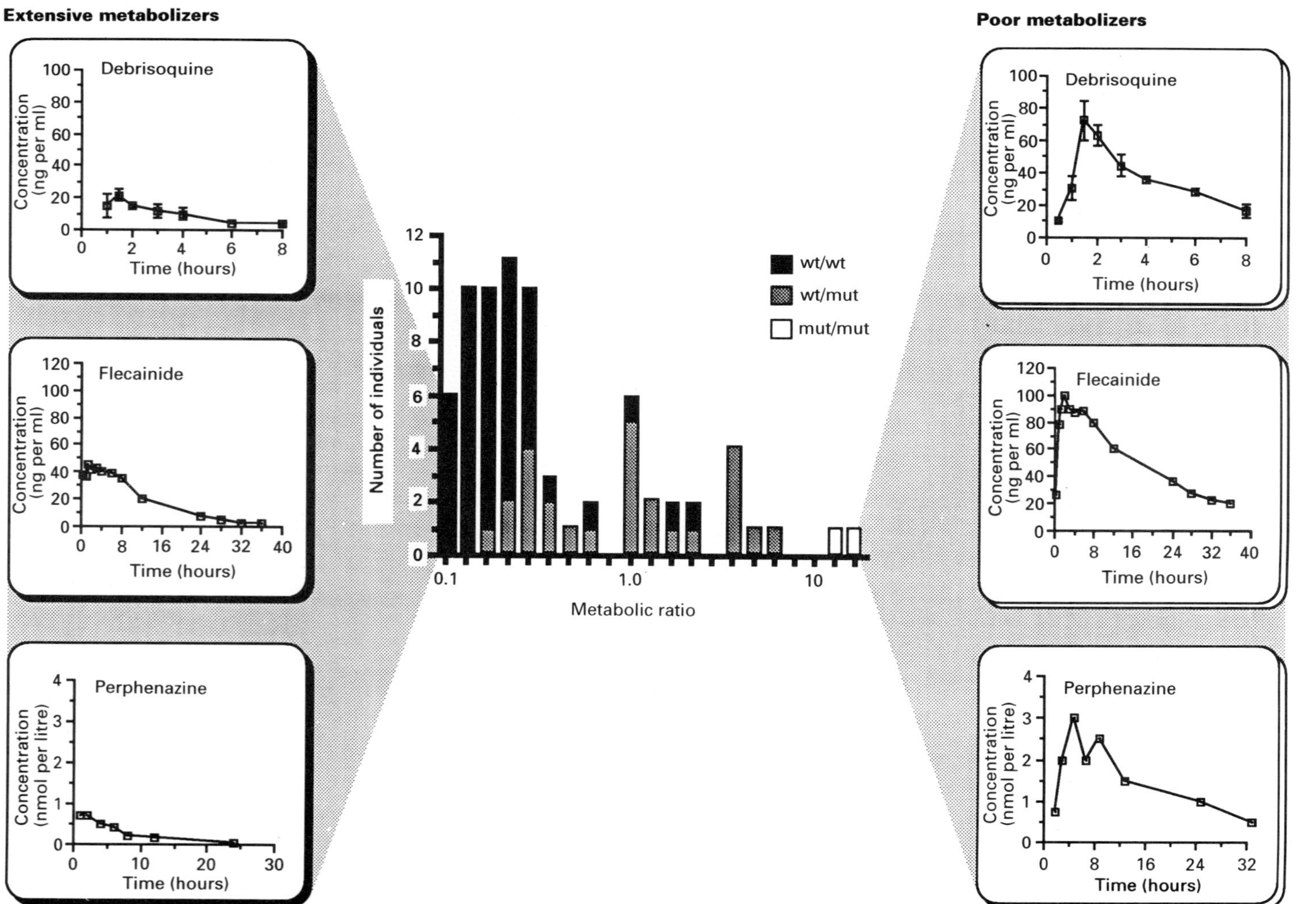
Extensive metabolizers
Debrisoquine
Flecainide
Perphenazine
Concentration (ng per ml)
Concentration (nmol per litre)
Time (hours)
Number of individuals
Metabolic ratio
0.1
1.0
10
wt/wt
wt/mut
mut/mut
Poor metabolizers
Debrisoquine
Flecainide
Perphenazine
Concentration (ng per ml)
Concentration (nmol per litre)
Time (hours)

brisoquine was undoubtedly a safe procedure, for patients or for healthy volunteers, the test nevertheless demanded a bulked urine collection over a period up to 8 hours. This in general presented few problems for in-patients, but it was impracticable to incarcerate out-patients or volunteers for 8-hour periods. More serious was the commonly encountered problem of metabolic drug interactions, whereby the drug of interest currently being taken by the patient, would inhibit the metabolism of the test dose of debrisoquine, making the outcome meaningless. For years the only way around this problem was to withhold drug therapy both before and during the debrisoquine test. As can readily be envisaged, this rendered many interesting clinical situations impossible to investigate. It was clear to many investigators that the future would lie in a 'blood test', a DNA-based assay which would predict the phenotype of the patient. Such tests are now with us [9–11], having taken surprisingly little time to emerge after the original report of the cloning of the *CYP2D6* cDNA [7], despite the need to develop a somewhat complex assay for the multiple mutated alleles which cause the PM phenotype [35]. The central part of Fig. 2 shows the power of such tests. Individuals can be genotyped with great certainty (98–99%) as having no, one or two *CYP2D6* mutations. Those with two mutations ('mut/mut') comprise the PM phenotype and, most importantly, the EM phenotype can be subdivided into homozygotes (no mutations, wild-type or 'wt/wt') and heterozygotes (one mutation or 'wt/mut'). The central graph clearly shows that there is a gene dose effect, meaning that being a heterozygote causes partially impaired metabolism of debrisoquine, manifested as an intermediate metabolic ratio. The very few individuals who have been genotyped as wt/wt, but who have metabolic ratios in the heterozygote range (particularly the two subjects with values of 3 and 4), are likely to harbour as yet undiscovered mutations in heterozygous copy. As such, they provide a useful resource for the characterization of new mutations and indeed new mutations have been described when there was a discrepancy between apparent genotype and debrisoquine metabolism [36].

Hardly surprisingly, because the DNA-based tests predict phenotype, they also predict the pharmacokinetics of debrisoquine (Fig. 2). The PM subjects have peak plasma concentrations of debrisoquine four-

Fig. 2 (*Opposite*) (*Centre*) Relationship between *CYP2D6* genotype, determined by polymerase chain reaction and Southern blotting [11], and debrisoquine metabolism in a population of healthy volunteers. The open bars (metabolic ratio, MR, less than 10) are poor metabolizers with two mutations (mut/mut), the stippled bars are heterozygous extensive metabolizers (wt/mut) and the black bars are homozygous extensive metabolizers (wt/wt). (*Edges*) Prediction of plasma levels of debrisoquine, flecainide and perphenazine using DNA-based genotyping assays. Homozygous wild-type extensive metabolizers (wt/wt) are the commonest genotype; homozygous poor metabolizers with two *CYP2D6* mutations (mut/mut) have plasma levels four to five times higher.

fold higher than EM subjects. The total body burden of drug, expressed as area under the plasma concentration–time curve (AUC), is also four-fold higher in PMs. In theory then, the DNA-based genotyping assay should be able to predict those patients who might develop postural hypotension when treated with debrisoquine, a phenomenon associated with the PM phenotype [30]. However, this is of little practical interest today, since so few patients are treated with debrisoquine. What is of intense interest is to be able to preselect patients who will have higher than expected plasma levels of drugs such as antidysrhythmics or neuroleptics and in so doing identify the patients at greatest risk of adverse drug reactions. This is one of the critical objectives of pharmacogenetics. Figure 2 shows how the antidysrhythmic drug flecainide has approximately a four-fold higher AUC in PMs than in EMs, how the neuroleptic drug perphenazine displays an even greater interphenotype difference in its pharmacokinetics. These major deviations in pharmacokinetics, seen in PM patients, can be predicted using genotyping.

Another critical objective of pharmacogenetics is to identify therapeutic failures. Much work is going on in the important area of cancer chemotherapy [37]. In the case of the CYP2D6 polymorphism, where the molecular genetics has been worked out, therapeutic failures can also be predicted on the basis of forecasting excessively fast metabolism of a given drug. There has recently been described a *CYP2D6* allele which confers 'ultrarapid' metabolism. The allele, known as *CYP2D6L* [38], causes therapeutic failure when its carriers are treated for disturbances of their mental health with drugs such as nortriptyline (30–75 mg per day normal) and clomipramine (30–50 mg per day normal). One patient with the *CYP2D6L* allele required 500 mg per day of nortriptyline to attain therapeutic plasma levels and treat her depression, whilst a second genotypically *CYP2D6L* patient needed 300 mg of clomipramine for stable treatment of agoraphobia [38]. We suspect strongly that many psychiatric patients who are difficult to manage with neuroleptic drugs and antidepressants would benefit from screening with DNA-based tests of *CYP2D6* genotype and consequent rationalization of their therapy. The same arguments apply to the other drugs, particularly the antidysrhythmics, listed in Table 2.

MOLECULAR PHARMACOGENETIC TESTING IN A HEALTH SERVICE CONTEXT

The drugs most widely used and most affected by the CYP2D6 polymorphism are largely prescribed by general practitioners. However, therapy is usually initiated by specialist clinics. Chronically sick patients, whether requiring psychiatric or cardiological treatments, may over the course of many years be tried on several different drugs from the same therapeutic category. This is especially true for problem patients, those difficult to manage because, unbeknown to the treating physician, they have either excessively slow or excessively fast metabolism of the given drugs. In order to reduce the incidence of side-effects, predominantly in the use of neuroleptic agents and tricyclic antidepressant drugs in psychiatry and antidysrhythmic drugs in cardiology, we propose the following courses of action:

1 establishment of pilot schemes, initially at regional level to provide a *pharmacogenotyping service* to specialist clinics;

2 funding of regionally based research projects to determine the health economic benefits of *pharmacogenotyping*;

3 inclusion of the interpretation of *pharmacogenotyping* data in relation to management in training programmes for clinical pharmacologists, psychiatrists and cardiologists.

CONCLUDING REMARKS

The past 5 years has witnessed a quantum leap in our understanding of the discrete enzymic processes responsible for the disposition of drugs in humans, and why these should vary from patient to patient. This has been made possible by the fusion of pharmacogenetics with molecular biology. In particular, our understanding of the molecular genetics of the human cytochromes P450 [39], which are responsible for such a significant proportion of drug metabolism [25], has improved dramatically. The most completely understood system, in terms of the sources of interpatient variability, is CYP2D6 (debrisoquine hydroxylase). DNA-based tests are now available which can predict with high certainty the metabolic phenotypes of extensive (EM) and poor (PM) metabolism. This now permits forecasting of the likely pharmacokinetic behaviour of widely-used groups of drugs on an individual patient basis. More than anything else, the importance of the availability of such tests is that the physician can now hope to reduce both therapeutic failures and adverse drug reactions, by *getting the dose right*. What is urgently required is both the broader availability of, what we have called here, *pharmacogenotyping*, and its evaluation in health economic terms. CYP2D6 is the first system in which the new technologies can impact upon therapeutic practice. As the science unfolds, other systems will follow on its heels. By accomplishing the therapeutic key objective of pharmacogenetics, we should improve significantly the lot of patients, initially in cardiological and psychiatric settings, and reduce the uncertainties in the minds of the treating physician.

ACKNOWLEDGEMENTS

The development of pharmacogenotyping technologies in this Unit has been accomplished by our colleagues, Dr Ann Daly and Martin Armstrong, with the support of a grant from British American Tobacco Limited. The support to these laboratories over a sustained period by Bayer plc is gratefully acknowledged. WLG is in receipt of an MRC Training Fellowship. MH is in receipt of an MRC Studentship.

REFERENCES

1 Nebert DW, Nelson DR, Adesnik M, *et al.* The P-450 superfamily: update on listing of all genes and recommended nomenclature of the chromosomal loci. *DNA* 1989;8:1–13.

2 Alexanderson B. *On Interindividual Variability in Plasma Levels of Nortriptyline and Desmethylimipramine in Man: a Pharmacokinetic and Genetic Study.* [Medical Dissertation No. 6]. Linköping, Sweden: Linköping University, 1972.

3 Eichelbaum M. *Ein Neuendeckter Defekt im Artzneimittel-Stoffwechsel des Menschen: Die Fehlende N-Oxidation des Spartein. Habilitationsschrift.* Bonn, Germany: Medizinische Fakultät Rheinischen Friedrich-Wilhelms-Universität, 1975.

4 Mahgoub A, Idle JR, Dring LG, *et al.* Polymorphic hydroxylation of debrisoquine in man. *Lancet* 1977;ii:584–586.

5 Eichelbaum M, Gross AS. The genetic polymorphism of debrisoquine/sparteine metabolism – clinical aspects. In: Kalow W, ed. *Pharmacogenetics of Drug Metabolism.* New York: Pergamon Press, 1992:625–648.

6 Evans DAP, Mahgoub A, Sloan TP, *et al.* A family and population study of the genetic polymorphism of debrisoquine oxidation in a white British population. *J Med Genet* 1980;17:102–105.

7 Gonzalez FJ, Skoda RC, Kimura S, *et al.* Characterization of the common genetic defect in humans deficient in debrisoquine metabolism. *Nature* 1988;331:442–446.

8 Kimura S, Umeno M, Skoda RC, *et al.* The human debrisoquine 4-hydroxylase (CYP2D) locus sequence and identification of the polymorphic CYP2D6 gene, a related gene and a pseudogene. *Am J Hum Genet* 1989;45:889–904.

9 Heim M, Meyer UA. Genotyping of poor metabolisers of debrisoquine by allele-specific PCR amplification. *Lancet* 1990;336:529–532.

10 Wolf CR, Moss JE, Miles JS, *et al.* Detection of debrisoquine hydroxylation phenotypes. *Lancet* 1990;336:1452–1453.

11 Daly AK, Armstrong M, Monkman SC, *et al.* Genetic and metabolic criteria for the assignment of debrisoquine 4-hydroxylation (cytochrome P4502D6) phenotypes. *Pharmacogenetics* 1991;1:33–41.

12 Gu L, Gonzalez FJ, Kalow W, Tang BK. Biotransformation of caffeine, paraxanthine, theobromine and theophylline by cDNA-expressed human CYP1A2 and CYP2E1. *Pharmacogenetics* 1992;2:73–77.

13 Hunt SN, Jusko WJ, Yurchak AM. Effects of smoking on theophylline disposition. *Clin Pharmacol Ther* 1976;19:546–551.

14 Iber FL. Drug metabolism in heavy consumers of ethyl alcohol. *Clin Pharmacol Ther* 1977;22:735–742.

15 Crothers M, Cartmel B, Idle J. Chemical and biological stability of the debrisoquine metabolic ratio. *Acta Pharmacol Toxicol* 1986;(Suppl V):313 (Abstract).

16 Oates NS, Ayesh R, Cartmel B, Idle JR, Influence of smoking on the distribution of the debrisoquine metabolic ratio. *Proc Xth Int Congr Pharmacol (Sydney)* 1987:91 (Abstract).

17 Lennard MS, Lewis RV, Brown LA, *et al.* Timolol metabolism and debrisoquine oxidation polymorphism: a population study. *Br J Clin Pharmacol* 1989;27:429–434.

18 Yue QY, Svensson JO, Alm C, *et al.* Codeine *O*-demethylation co-segregates with polymorphic debrisoquine hydroxylation. *Br J Clin Pharmacol* 1989;28:639–645.

19 Johansson I, Yue QY, Dahl ML, *et al.* Genetic analysis of the interethnic difference between Chinese and Caucasians in the polymorphic metabolism of debrisoquine and codeine. *Eur J Clin Pharmacol* 1991;40:553–556.
20 Bertilsson L, Åberg-Wistedt A. The debrisoquine hydroxylation test predicts steady-state plasma levels of desipramine. *Br J Clin Pharmacol* 1983;15:388–390.
21 Dahl M-L, Ekqvist B, Widen J, Bertilsson L. Disposition of the neuroleptic zuclopenthixol cosegregates with the polymorphic hydroxylation of debrisoquine in humans. *Acta Psychiatr Scand* 1991;84:99–102.
22 Woolhouse N, Adjepon-Yamoah KK, Mellström B. Nortriptyline and debrisoquine hydroxylations in Ghanaian and Swedish subjects. *Clin Pharmacol Ther* 1984;36: 374–378.
23 Evans DAP, Harmer D, Downham DY, *et al.* The genetic control of sparteine and debrisoquine metabolism in man with new methods of analysing bimodal distributions. *J Med Genet* 1983;20:321–329.
24 Woolhouse NM, Eichelbaum M, Oates NS, *et al.* Dissociation of co-regulatory control of debrisoquin/phenformin and sparteine oxidations in Ghanaians. *Clin Pharmacol Ther* 1985;37:512–521.
25 Cholerton S, Daly AK, Idle JR. The role of individual human cytochromes P450 in drug metabolism and clinical response. *Trends Pharmacol Sci* 1992;13:434–439.
26 Dahl ML, Bertilsson L. Genetically variable metabolism of antidepressants and neuroleptic drugs in man. *Pharmacogenetics* 1993;3:61–70.
27 Jack DB, Stenlake JB, Templeton R. The metabolism and excretion of guanoxan in man. *Xenobiotica* 1972;2:35–43.
28 Hammer W, Sjöqvist F. Plasma levels of monomethylated tricyclic antidepressants during treatment with imipramine-like compounds. *Life Sci* 1967;6:1895–1903.
29 Bertilsson L, Eichelbaum M, Mellström B, *et al.* Nortriptyline and antipyrine clearance in relation to debrisoquine hydroxylation in man. *Life Sci* 1980;27:1673–1677.
30 Idle JR, Mahgoub A, Lancaster R, Smith RL. Hypotensive response to debrisoquine and hydroxylation phenotype. *Life Sci* 1978;22:979–984.
31 Oates NS, Shah RR, Idle JR, Smith RL. Influence of oxidation polymorphism on phenformin kinetics and dynamics. *Clin Pharmacol Ther* 1983;34:827–834.
32 Singlas E, Govjet MA, Simon P. Pharmacokinetics of perhexiline maleate in anginal patients with and without peripheral neuropathy. *Eur J Clin Pharmacol* 1978;14: 195–201.
33 Shah RR, Oates NS, Idle JR. *et al.* Impaired oxidation of debrisoquine in patients with perhexiline neuropathy. *Br Med J* 1982;284:295–299.
34 Shah RR, Oates NS, Idle JR. Prediction of subclinical perhexiline neuropathy in a patient with inborn error of debrisoquine hydroxylation. *Am Heart J* 1983;105: 159–161.
35 Idle J. Enigmatic variations. *Nature* 1988;331:391–392.
36 Armstrong MA, Idle JR, Daly AK. A polymorphic *Cfo*I site in exon 6 of the human *CYP2D6* gene detected by the polymerase chain reaction. *Hum Genet* 1993;91:616–617.
37 Boddy AV, Idle JR. The role of pharmacogenetics in chemotherapy: modulation of tumour response and host toxicity. *Cancer Surveys* 1993;17:79–103.
38 Bertilsson L, Dahl M-L, Sjöqvist F, *et al.* Molecular basis for rational megaprescribing in ultrarapid hydroxylators of debrisoquine. *Lancet* 1993;341:63 (Letter).
39 Gonzalez FJ. Human cytochromes P450: problems and prospects. *Trends Pharmacol Sci* 1992;13:346–352.

Cardiovascular and skeletal effects of hormone replacement therapy

J. C. STEVENSON, D. CROOK & I. F. GODSLAND

The acute effects of oestrogen deficiency due to loss of ovarian function at the menopause include vasomotor, psychological and genitourinary symptoms. However, the major importance of the long-term effects of the menopause, particularly on the cardiovascular system and the skeleton, is now being recognized. Thus, the use of hormone replacement therapy (HRT) is no longer confined to the relief of classical menopausal symptoms, and it is important to consider its effects on cardiovascular disease and osteoporosis.

MENOPAUSE AND CARDIOVASCULAR DISEASE RISK

Cardiovascular disease, particularly coronary heart disease (CHD), is well known to be the major cause of death in men. Yet it is often not appreciated that overall cardiovascular mortality is slightly greater in women than in men [1], or that anginal-type chest pain is more common in middle-aged and elderly women than in men of the same age [2]. CHD is thus a major cause of death as well as of morbidity in women.

Whilst the incidence of cardiovascular disease rises with age in both sexes, the menopause has a substantial and additional effect in women [3]. Indeed, it has long been recognized that premature menopause results in premature CHD [4]. Although it is not possible to reverse the ageing process, it is possible to reverse the menopause with HRT. Thus, there is considerable scope for reducing a significant proportion of the increased incidence of cardiovascular disease seen in postmenopausal women. Evidence from a number of epidemiological studies confirms that a substantial reduction in cardiovascular disease can be achieved with postmenopausal oestrogen usage [5].

It is clearly important to try to establish the mechanisms whereby the menopause affects cardiovascular disease risk. Oestrogen deficiency leads to potentially adverse changes in certain metabolic parameters such as lipids and lipoproteins, insulin secretion and metabolism, body fat distribution and arterial blood flow.

In a study of over 540 healthy non-obese British women, we found a marked effect of the menopause on lipids and lipoproteins which was independent of ageing, body mass, and other confounding factors such as smoking and exercise [6]. In comparison with premenopausal women, postmenopausal women have significantly higher total cholesterol, triglycerides, low-density lipoprotein (LDL) cholesterol, and high-density lipoprotein subfraction 3 (HDL_3) cholesterol, whilst they have significantly lower total high-density lipoprotein (HDL) and high-density lipoprotein subfraction 2 (HDL_2) cholesterol. Although lipoprotein changes are clearly of importance in the pathogenesis of CHD in women, they only account for perhaps a quarter of the incidence. Other factors must therefore be of importance.

It has been proposed that reduced tissue sensitivity to the action of insulin – insulin resistance – with accompanying hyperinsulinaemia is a pivotal metabolic disturbance in the pathogenesis of CHD [7]. Insulin resistance may be associated with disturbances in lipoproteins, coagulation and fibrinolysis, hypertension and obesity. An increase in insulin secretion is related to time since menopause [8], and there is evidence for reduced insulin elimination [9].

Obesity is a well recognized risk factor, but it is the android (male pattern) or upper body segment distribution which is associated with disease, whilst the gynoid (female pattern) or lower body segment fat appears to carry no appreciable risk [10]. In preliminary studies, we have found that android fat distribution correlates with an adverse lipid and lipoprotein profile [11]. Thus, android fat may be an important metabolic mechanism in the development of CHD. In studies of body composition in healthy non-obese women, we have found that the menopause results not only in an increase in total body fat mass but also that there is a redistribution of fat from the gynoid to the android region. Body fat mass increases following the menopause, and the proportion of fat in the android distribution significantly increases whilst that in the gynoid distribution significantly decreases [12]. This is in keeping with the adverse changes in lipoproteins seen after the menopause.

Finally, as well as atheroma and thrombosis, vessel spasm and changes in arterial tone may also be important in the pathogenesis of both angina and myocardial infarction. Evidence that arterial blood flow decreases postmenopausally is suggested by the relationship between arterial wave form velocity (an index of arterial resistance to flow) and time since menopause [13]. Indeed, it seems likely that the arterial tree is a target for direct oestrogen action.

All these factors, many of which are interrelated, would be expected to produce adverse changes and increase the cardiovascular disease risk.

CARDIOVASCULAR BENEFITS OF HRT

Many epidemiological studies have looked at the effect of postmenopausal oestrogen usage and cardiovascular disease incidence [5]. Case-control studies have shown fairly uniformly that the relative risk for cardiovascular disease decreases with postmenopausal oestrogen replacement. This effect is seen even more clearly in cohort studies, where the majority of studies show a reduction in risk of up to 50%. However, most of these studies were conducted in women using unopposed oestrogen therapy, predominantly with conjugated equine oestrogens, and it has been suggested that the addition of a progestin will negate all the benefit of oestrogen therapy on cardiovascular risk. This concept is largely based on the results of a multivariate analysis of oestrogen effects on a limited selection of metabolic risk markers. From this analysis, an increase in HDL cholesterol appeared to be the single protective factor against cardiovascular disease [14], and certain androgenic progestins negate any oestrogen-induced rise in HDL cholesterol. But it is biologically rather implausible that HDL cholesterol alone is independent of changes in other risk factors such as LDL cholesterol and triglycerides, since these various lipoproteins are intimately related. Furthermore, these lipoproteins are also related to other metabolic risk factors for cardiovascular disease. A recent epidemiological study [15] of opposed oestrogen replacement showed that progestin addition did not negate the benefit of oestrogen replacement on cardiovascular disease risk in postmenopausal women. Furthermore, animal studies have shown that combined oestrogen–progestin treatment still prevents the development of atheroma [16].

HRT is beneficial in reducing cardiovascular disease risk not only in healthy postmenopausal women but also in women with established coronary heart disease. Sullivan *et al.* [17] showed an impressive effect of oestrogen usage on increased 10-year survival in women with angiographically-defined severe coronary artery disease. Such findings should encourage the use of HRT as mainline therapy for the prevention and treatment of coronary heart disease in postmenopausal women.

Effects of HRT on lipids and lipoproteins

Postmenopausal oestrogen administration results in a fall in total and LDL cholesterol in the order of 10–15%, whilst there may be a variable increase in HDL cholesterol of up to 5%, irrespective of the route of administration. The addition of the more androgenic progestins may prevent the oestrogen-induced rise in HDL although it does not negate the lowering of LDL [18]. Since most postmenopausal women have higher levels of HDL compared with men, the fact that there is no further increase when oestrogen is given with such progestins may not

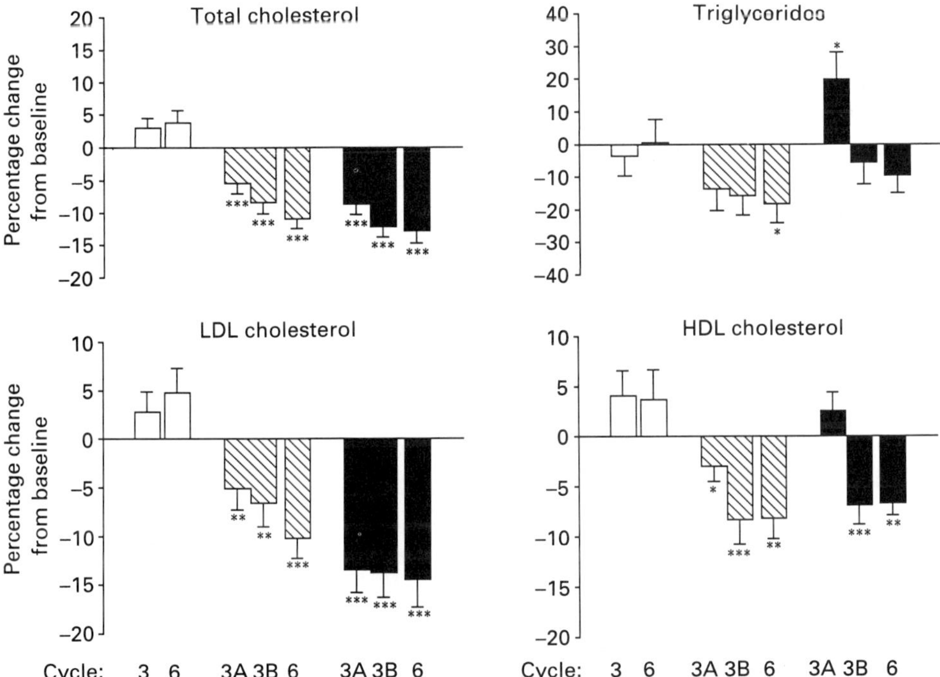

Fig. 1 Lipid and lipoprotein changes (mean ± SE) in postmenopausal women. Open bars represent untreated controls, hatched bars are those on transdermal HRT, whilst solid bars are those on oral HRT. Measurements were performed during the combined phase of treatment (cycles 3B and 6) and in the oestrogen-alone (cycle 3A) at 3 and 6 months. (By permission from Crook *et al.* [19].) $^{*}P < 0.05$, $^{**}P < 0.01$, $^{***}P < 0.001$ compared with untreated controls.

be of any real clinical significance. Furthermore, the use of progestins of the pregnane group does not prevent any increase in HDL.

Orally administered conjugated equine oestrogens increase triglyceride levels by around 15%, whilst the more androgenic progestins lower triglycerides [19]. The lowering of triglycerides may be beneficial since triglycerides themselves may be an independent risk factor for CHD in women [20].

It had been thought that only orally administered gonadal hormones would produce changes in lipids and lipoproteins through the hepatic first-pass effect. However, we have shown that this is not the case in a comparative study of the metabolic effects of transdermal HRT and oral HRT in postmenopausal women [19] (Fig. 1). We used transdermal oestradiol 17-β 0.05 mg daily continuously with the cyclical addition of transdermal norethisterone acetate 0.25 mg daily for 14 out of every 28 days. Oral therapy was given as continuous conjugated equine oestrogens 0.625 mg daily with the cyclical addition of *dl*-norgestrel 0.15 mg for 12 out of every 28 days. Transdermal therapy lowered total and LDL cholesterol in much the same way as oral therapy, and these findings were confirmed by the appropriate changes in apolipoprotein B levels. However, in contrast to oral oestrogens, transdermal oestrogen administration resulted in a fall in triglycerides. This different effect on triglycerides between oral and transdermal administration may be of relevance in terms of CHD risk benefit. HDL cholesterol levels and those of apolipoprotein AI fell with the transdermal HRT, but the decrease was in the HDL_3 subfraction, and no overall change was seen in HDL_2, the subfraction considered to be of greater clinical importance. Thus, the net changes seen with combined HRT were a fall in LDL and triglycerides, with no change in HDL_2, and this would seem to be a beneficial profile for CHD risk.

It must be remembered that other lipoproteins may be of greater importance in terms of cardiovascular risk. For example, lipoprotein (a) (Lp(a)) levels appear to independent risk markers for the development of CHD, with high levels being associated with increased risk [21]. Apolipoprotein (a) has a similar structure to plasminogen and may therefore interact with the plasminogen receptor. Androgenic steroids, such as danazol [22], norethisterone acetate [23], and tibolone [24] result in a lowering of Lp(a), and this may be another potentially beneficial effect of progestins, although it is currently not known whether altering Lp(a) levels has any influence on CHD development. Other lipoproteins, such as the LDL subtypes A and B, may also be more relevant to CHD risk than the traditional lipoprotein markers [25], and further studies of HRT effects on these markers are clearly needed.

Effects of HRT on body fat distribution

We have found that HRT results in a reversal of the changes seen in fat distribution following the menopause. Whilst little change in total body fat is seen with HRT, a redistribution of regional fat occurs with a relative reduction in android fat and a relative increase in gynoid fat.

Insulin resistance

We have observed differences in the glucose and insulin responses to our transdermal and oral HRT regimens [26]. No overall effect was seen with the transdermal therapy, but there was a small adverse change in glucose response to a glucose load seen in women taking oral HRT (Fig. 2). This appeared to be due to an inadequate initial pancreatic response of insulin secretion which resulted in an increase in insulin secretion in later stages of the test. The progestin addition in the oral HRT caused a significant increase in insulin resistance.

Insulin resistance may be associated with hypertension, and is also related to certain coagulation and fibrinolytic parameters. The usual

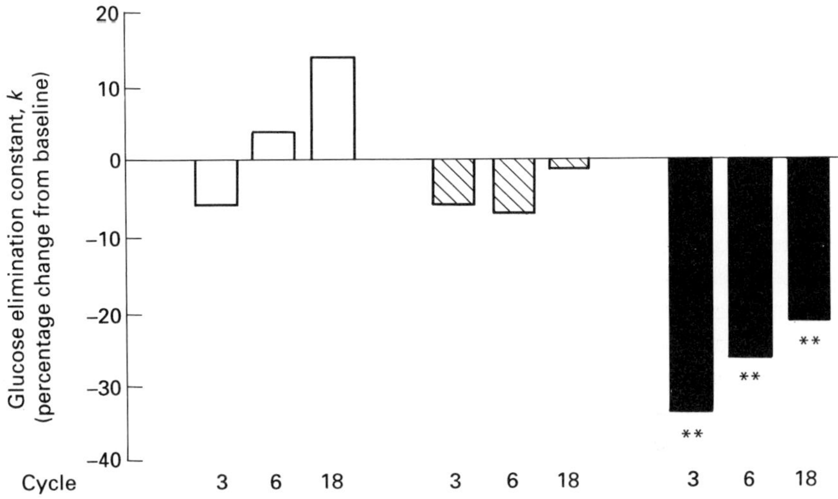

Fig. 2 Changes in mean glucose elimination constants (k) in postmenopausal women. Open bars represent untreated controls, hatched bars are those on transdermal HRT, whilst solid bars are those on oral HRT. Measurements were performed during the combined phase of treatment at 3, 6 and 18 months. (By permission from Godsland *et al.* [26].) $^{**}P < 0.01$ compared with untreated controls.

effect of HRT on blood pressure is to cause a small fall, and HRT does not usually cause any overall adverse perturbation of haemostasis, particularly when given by the transdermal route [27]. However, further detailed studies of specific effects of different HRT formulations and routes of administration on coagulation and fibrinolysis are needed.

Whilst all these various cardiovascular risk factors may be influenced by HRT, there is also evidence for direct arterial effects of oestradiol.

Arterial tone

Oestradiol receptors can be found in the arterial wall throughout the vascular tree in humans, suggesting direct effects of oestradiol on blood vessels. Recent studies have demonstrated effects of oestrogen deficiency and replacement on arterial wave form velocity, suggesting changes in arterial resistance and perhaps blood flow. The increase in arterial wall impedance with time after the menopause is reversed when transdermal oestradiol is given [13]. The subsequent addition of progestin only reduces this effect to a small extent. The mechanism whereby oestradiol brings about such changes is not yet fully established, but could be through changes in local cytokines and neurotransmitters such as calcitonin gene-related peptide (CGRP) [28]. Oestradiol also appears to act as a calcium antagonist thereby causing arterial dilatation [29].

MENOPAUSE AND OSTEOPOROSIS RISK

Loss of ovarian function at the menopause leads to increased bone turnover, with resorption exceeding formation. The net result is loss of bone which eventually leads to structural failure – osteoporotic fracture. At least 50% of women achieving full life expectancy will have evidence of osteoporosis by the time they die [30]. The classical osteoporosis fractures occur in the distal forearm, vertebral bodies and proximal femur, sites of relatively higher trabecular bone content. Hip fracture is an important cause of both morbidity and mortality, with 20% of women who sustain such a fracture dying as a result [31]. Indeed, the lifetime risk of hip fracture for a woman is greater than the combined lifetime risk of developing carcinoma of the breast, cervix, ovary or uterus. Two basic factors determine a woman's risk of developing postmenopausal osteoporosis, peak adult bone mass and subsequent bone loss. The former is largely genetically determined, but the latter primarily occurs in relationship to the loss of ovarian function at the menopause.

Skeletal benefits of HRT

HRT with oestrogen, and progestin when indicated, is effective in preventing bone loss and subsequent osteoporosis with its attendant fractures, even in the long term. Early prospective studies of oophorectomized women established that oestrogen could prevent bone loss and the development of osteoporosis in the long term [32,33]. Similar long-term studies [34] in women following natural menopause also confirmed the benefit suggested by retrospective population studies [35–37]. Orally administered oestrogens include conjugated equine oestrogens, oestradiol 17-β, and oestrone sulphate. The bone-conserving doses of these oestrogens have been established: conjugated oestrogens 0.625 mg daily [38,39], oestradiol 17-β 2 mg daily [40], and oestrone sulphate 1.5 mg daily [41]. Oestrogens can also be administered by non-oral routes, which have the advantage of avoiding the hepatic 'first-pass' effect. Oestradiol 17-β can be administered transdermally through adhesive skin patches; the bone-conserving dose is 50 μg daily [39] (Figs 3 and 4). Oestradiol 17-β can also be given as a subcutaneous implant which lasts for around 6 months. The bone-conserving dose is 50 mg [42]. HRT is equally effective in elderly women and in those who already have established osteoporosis [43]. Not only is there bone conservation, but also small increases in bone density can be achieved. Withdrawal of HRT leads to loss of bone, but only at the same rate as normal postmenopausal loss [44,45]. Thus, any period of treatment with HRT buys time for the skeleton. Indeed, it has been estimated, for example, that just 5 years' therapy would reduce the overall incidence of hip fracture by 50% [46].

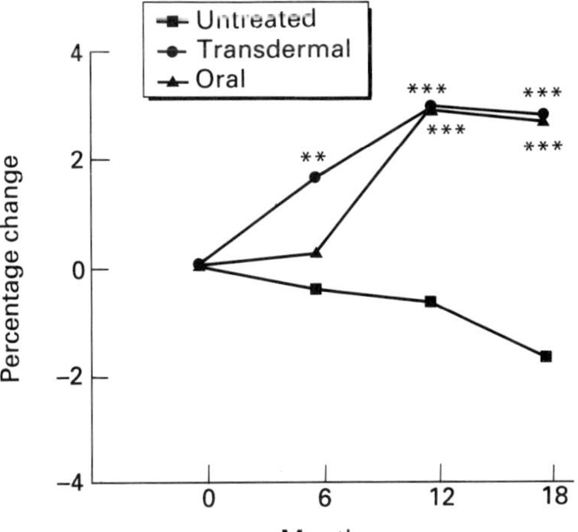

Fig. 3 Changes in mean bone density in the lumbar spine over 18 months in postmenopausal women. (By permission from Stevenson *et al.* [39].) $^{**}P < 0.01$, $^{***}P < 0.001$ compared with untreated controls.

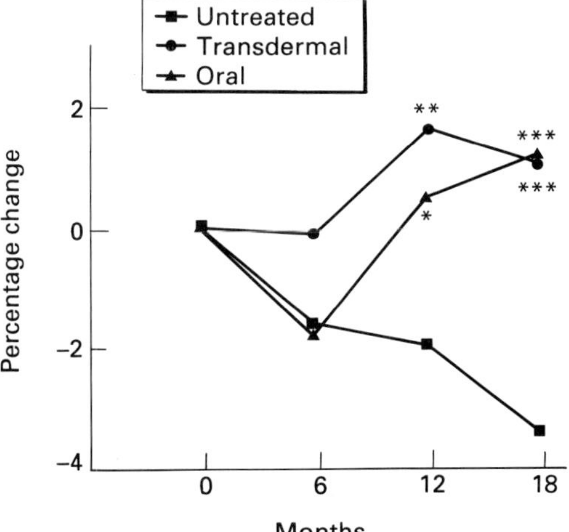

Fig. 4 Changes in mean bone density in the femoral neck over 18 months in postmenopausal women. (By permission from Stevenson *et al.* [39].) $^{*}P < 0.05$, $^{**}P < 0.01$, $^{***}P < 0.001$ compared with untreated controls.

Since HRT has many other benefits, including relief of menopausal symptoms and reduction of cardiovascular disease risk, it is the therapy of choice for both prevention and treatment of osteoporosis. However, there may be some women who are unable or unwilling to take HRT. In these patients effective alternatives are necessary and other antiresorptive agents may prove useful [47].

CONCLUSIONS

Although in the past, the main indication for use of HRT has been for relief of menopausal symptoms, it is now being used increasingly for the prevention and treatment of postmenopausal osteoporosis. In the future, it seems likely that another major indication for HRT will be the prevention of CHD by reduction of cardiovascular disease risk factors.

REFERENCES

1 Stevenson JC. Osteoporosis and cardiovascular disease in women: converging paths? *Lancet* 1990;336:1121–1122.

2 LaCroix AZ, Haynes SG, Savage DD, Havlink RJ. Rose questionnaire angina among United states black, white and Mexican-American women and men. *Am J Epidemiol* 1989;129:669–686.

3 Gordon T, Kannel WB, Hjortland MC, McNamara PM. Menopause and coronary heart disease. The Framingham Study. *Ann Intern Med* 1978;89:157–161.

4 Snazdjerman M, Oliver MF. Spontaneous premature menopause, ischaemic heart disease, and serum lipids. *Lancet* 1963;i:962–964.

5 Knopp RH. The effects of postmenopausal estrogen therapy on the incidence of arteriosclerotic vascular disease. *Obstet Gynecol* 1988;72:23S–30S.

6 Stevenson JC, Crook D, Godsland IF. Effects of age and menopause on lipid metabolism. In: Christiansen C, Overgaard K, eds. *Osteoporosis 1990*. Copenhagen: Osteopress ApS, 1990:1826–1828.

7 Reaven GM. Role of insulin resistance in human disease. *Diabetes* 1988;37:1595–1607.

8 Proudler AJ, Felton C, Stevenson JC. Aging and the plasma insulin, glucose and C-peptide response to intravenous glucose in postmenopausal women. *Clin Sci* 1992; 83:489–494.

9 Walton C, Godsland IF, Proudler AJ, *et al.* The effects of the menopause on carbohydrate metabolism in non-obese, healthy women. *Eur J Clin Invest* 1993;23:466–473.

10 Vague J. The degree of masculine differentiation of obesities: a factor determining predisposition to diabetes, atherosclerosis, gout and uric calculus disease. *Am J Clin Nutr* 1956;4:20–34.

11 Stevenson JC, Lees B, Bruce R, *et al.* Influence of body composition on lipid metabolism in postmenopausal women. In: Christiansen C, Overgaard K, eds. *Osteoporosis 1990*. Copenhagen: Osteopress ApS, 1990:1837–1838.

12 Ley CJ, Lees B, Stevenson JC. Sex- and menopause-associated changes in body-fat distribution. *Am J Clin Nutr* 1992;55:950–954.

13 Gangar KF, Vyas S, Whitehead M, *et al.* Pulsatility index in internal carotid artery in relation to transdermal oestradiol and time since menopause. *Lancet* 1991;338:839–842.

14 Bush TL, Barrett-Connor E, Cowan LD, *et al.* Cardiovascular mortality and noncontraceptive use of estrogen in women: results from the Lipid Research Clinics Program Follow-up Study. *Circulation* 1987;75:1102–1109.

15 Falkeborn M, Persson I, Adami H, *et al.* The risk of acute myocardial infarction after oestrogen–progesterone replacement. *Br J Obstet Gynaecol* 1992;99:821–828.

16 Adams MR, Kaplan JR, Manuck SB, *et al.* Inhibition of coronary artery atherosclerosis by 17-beta estradiol in ovariectomized monkeys. *Arteriosclerosis* 1990;10:1051–1057.

17 Sullivan JM, Zwang RV, Hughes JP, *et al.* Oestrogen replacement and coronary artery disease. *Arch Intern Med* 1990;150:2557–2562.

18 Crook D, Stevenson JC. Progestagens, lipid metabolism and hormone replacement therapy. *Br J Obstet Gynaecol* 1991;98:749–750.

19 Crook D, Cust MP, Gangar KF, *et al.* Comparison of transdermal and oral estrogen/progestin hormone replacement therapy: effects of serum lipids and lipoproteins. *Am J Obstet Gynecol* 1992;166:950–955.

20 Bengtsson C, Björklund C, Lapidus L, Lissner L. Associations of serum lipid concentrations and obesity with mortality in women: 20 year follow up of participants in prospective population study in Gothenburg, Sweden. *Br Med J* 1993;307:1385–1388.

21 Utermann G. The mysteries of lipoprotein (a). *Science* 1989;264:904–910.

22 Crook D, Sidhu M, Seed M, *et al.* Lipoprotein Lp(a) levels are reduced by danazol, an anabolic steroid. *Atherosclerosis* 1992;92:41–47.

23 Farrish E, Rolton HA, Barnes JF, Hart DM. Lipoprotein (a) concentrations in post-menopausal women taking norethisterone. *Br Med J* 1991;303:694.
24 Rymer J, Crook D, Sidhu M, *et al.* Effects of tibolone on serum concentrations of lipoprotein (a) in postmenopausal women. *Acta Endocrinol* 1993;128:259–262.
25 Krauss RM. The tangled web of coronary risk factors. *Am J Med* 1991;90:36S–41S.
26 Godsland IF, Gangar KF, Walton C, *et al.* Insulin resistance, secretion and elimination in postmenopausal women receiving oral or transdermal hormone replacement therapy. *Metabolism* 1993;42:846–853.
27 Fox J, George AJ, Newton JR, *et al.* Effect of transdermal oestradiol on the hemostatic balance of menopausal women. *Maturitas* 1993;18:55–64.
28 Stevenson JC, Macdonald DWR, Warren RC, *et al.* Increased concentration of circulating calcitonin gene related peptide during normal human pregnancy. *Br Med J* 1986;293:1329–1330.
29 Collins P, Rosano GMC, Jiang C, *et al.* Cardiovascular protection by oestrogen – a calcium antagonist effect? *Lancet* 1993;341:1264–1265.
30 Jensen GF, Christiansen C, Boesen J, *et al.* Epidemiology of postmenopausal spinal and long bone fractures: a unifying approach to postmenopausal osteoporosis. *Clin Orthop Rel Res* 1982;166:75–81.
31 Stevenson JC, Whitehead MI. Postmenopausal osteoporosis. *Br Med J* 1982;285: 585–588.
32 Lindsay R, Hart DM, Aitken JM, *et al.* Long-term prevention of postmenopausal osteoporosis by oestrogen. *Lancet* 1976;i:1038–1041.
33 Lindsay R, Hart DM, Forrest C, Baird C. Prevention of spinal osteoporosis in oophorectomised women. *Lancet* 1980;ii:1151–1154.
34 Nachtigall LE, Nachtigall RH, Nachtigall RD, Beckman EM. Estrogen replacement therapy. A 10-year prospective study in relationship to osteoporosis. *Obstet Gynecol* 1979;53:277–281.
35 Hutchinson TA, Polansky SM, Feinstein A. Postmenopausal oestrogens protect against fractures of hip and distal radius. *Lancet* 1979;ii:706–709.
36 Weiss NS, Ure CL, Ballard JH, *et al.* Decreased risk of fractures of the hip and lower forearm with postmenopausal use of estrogen. *N Engl J Med* 1980;303:1195–1198.
37 Paganini-Hill A, Ross RK, Gerkins VR, *et al.* A case-control study of menopausal estrogen therapy and hip fractures. *Ann Intern Med* 1981;95:28–31.
38 Lindsay R, Hart DM, Clark DM. The minimum effective dose of estrogen for prevention of postmenopausal bone loss. *Obstet Gynecol* 1984;63:759–763.
39 Stevenson JC, Cust MP, Gangar KF, *et al.* Effects of transdermal versus oral hormone replacement therapy on bone density in spine and proximal femur in postmenopausal women. *Lancet* 1990;335:265–269.
40 Christiansen C, Christensen MS, Larsen N-E, Transbøl I. Pathophysiological mechanisms of estrogen effect on bone metabolism. Dose-response relationships in early postmenopausal women. *J Clin Endocrinol Metab* 1982;55:1124–1130.
41 Harris ST, Genant HK, Baylink DJ, *et al.* The effects of estrone (Ogen) on spinal bone density of postmenopausal women. *Arch Intern Med* 191;151:1980–1984.
42 Studd J, Savvas M, Watson N, *et al.* The relationship between plasma oestradiol and the increase in bone density in post-menopausal women after treatment with subcutaneous hormone implants. *Am J Obstet Gynecol* 1990;163:1474–1479.
43 Lindsay R, Tohme JF. Oestrogen treatment of patients with established postmenopausal osteoporosis. *Obstet Gynecol* 1990;76:290–295.
44 Christiansen C, Christensen MS, Transbøl I. Bone mass in postmenopausal women after withdrawal of oestrogen/gestagen replacement therapy. *Lancet* 1981;i:459–461.
45 Stevenson JC, Kanis JA, Christiansen C. Bone-density measurement. *Lancet* 1992; 339:370–371.
46 Stevenson JC. Post-menopausal bone loss and osteoporosis. In: Zichella L, Whitehead MI, van Keep PA, eds. *The Climacteric and Beyond*. Carnforth: Parthenon Publishing Group, 1988:125–135.

Drug misuse: from molecule to society

D. G. GRAHAME-SMITH

INTRODUCTION

My aim here is to show how a drug molecule interacts with a receptor in the brain of humans to create a psychological state and behavioural pattern which affect profoundly the society in which we live.

Definitions in this subject are difficult and I like the saying, 'Everybody knows what time is, until they come to define it.' So we see in the field of drug misuse a collection of terms – substance misuse, abuse, addiction, tolerance, dependence, craving, withdrawal and substance-related problems. This burgeoning vocabulary is beginning to be counter-productive, causing some impatience and confusion in society. The fact is, if the taking of a drug or the use of a substance is causing, or is likely to cause, harm to the user or those around him, then there is a problem.

Craving is an important term and describes a strong psychological need for a drug that pervades the consciousness. Dependence, as Edwards [1] has pointed out in a very level-headed general discussion of drug addiction, is not an all or none phenomenon but can be of any degree from mild to severe. There is a mild dependence operating when an individual thinks how nice that drink before dinner will be after a hard day but the dependence exemplified by the heroin addict who thieves to finance his habit is severe, and would be classed as addiction. That is enough of the semantics.

Most of the drugs we shall consider affect directly the brain mechanisms of the mind. An exception is anabolic steroids and other anabolic drugs such as clenbuterol, used by sportsmen and sportswomen, and body-builders. Because of their androgenic activity, their potential hepatic toxicity, their unwanted effects upon metabolic processes, the potential to cause hypertension, and in some individuals, their possible tendency to fuel aggression – these drugs are physically dangerous to an individual. Their use in the Olympics and by sportsmen and sportswomen, whom the young admire, is a pernicious, subversive activity. It sullies a wholesome activity and promotes cheating and if that is not a bad thing for society I do not know what is.

Table 1 Common drugs of misuse

Drug	Mechanism
Opiates	Opiate receptor agonists
Cocaine	Dopamine reuptake blocked
Amphetamines	Dopamine release
Ecstasy (MDMA)	5HT and dopamine release
Cannabis	Cannabis receptors? Role
LSD	$5HT_2$ receptor agonist
Alcohol	Enhances GABA function
Nicotine	Puzzle (some dopamine release)
Benzodiazepines	Enhance GABA function
Solvents	Unknown (intoxication)

The mind-altering drugs of common misuse are listed in Table 1. Their neuropsychobiology is fascinating and tells us much about the brain–mind–behaviour interrelationship. Those who think that this discussion will solve all the problems of this interrelationship are in for a disappointment. There is an intellectual void, a complete absence of any convincing theory, which links, in a satisfying way, activities of the brain to the complexities of consciousness and feeling, even though we know they must exist [2].

It is the vulnerability of the neuropsychobiology of the brain to the effects of the hedonistic properties of the drugs in Table 1 that presents the threat to the individual and thence to society.

MECHANISMS OF ACTION OF DRUGS OF MISUSE

All the drugs in Table 1 (except perhaps for the solvents) interact with neuronal receptors to alter central neurotransmitter function. Conceptually this leads to the cascade shown in Fig. 1 which while worked out in the rat, most probably applies also to humans. Although undoubtedly too simplistic it seems that the function of dopamine in the nucleus accumbens is crucial to this cascade. In the ventral tegmental area of the brain stem are the cell bodies of dopaminergic neurones, which project to the nucleus accumbens and at the terminal of which dopamine is a major neurotransmitter. Efferents emerge from the nucleus accumbens which project to many areas of the brain but particularly to the ventral pallidum and thalamus which are thought to be important in a behavioural sense in leading to a desire to repeat the drug experience (positive reinforcement) [3,4]. It is presumed that this circuitry underlies the pleasurable feelings. Behaviourally the matter of reinforcement is important in the analysis of drug-seeking behaviour [5]. A drug is known as a reinforcer when its administration increases the probability that

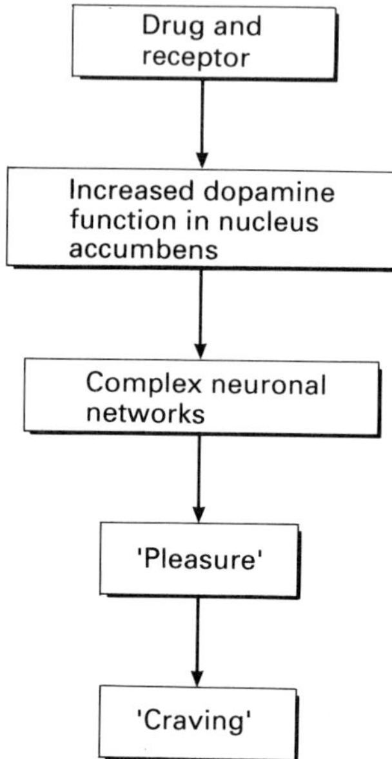

Fig. 1 Drugs of misuse: mechanism of action.

when a behaviour associated with drug administration has been learned then that behaviour will recur in order to repeat the experience. In other words if a rat is trained to press two levers and lever A administers water and lever B administers heroin, the rat will show a preference for pressing the heroin lever. Indeed, the rat will go through hell-fire and high water to press the heroin lever. This is known as positive reinforcement. It obviously applies to humans as well.

The behavioural psychologists also consider negative reinforcement [5]. Negative reinforcers act by reducing or eliminating unpleasant states. When a drug alleviates withdrawal distress, pain, anxiety, anger or depression then it becomes a negative reinforcer and its administration is sought.

The action of dopamine in the nucleus accumbens is at least one factor underlying the process of reinforcement [3,6,7].

In this context, opiates are thought to act on μ-opioid receptors, probably situated on γ-aminobutyric acid (GABA)-ergic interneurone cell bodies. Here these μ-receptors are linked to a G-protein and on stimulation of the receptor, potassium channels open, potassium ions pass out of the cell body, the neuronal membrane is hyperpolarized and the function of the GABA neurone is diminished. This GABA neurone projects to dopaminergic cell bodies in the ventral tegmental area and usually they act as tonic inhibitors of dopaminergic neuronal function. When by the action of the opiates GABA release is inhibited, dopaminergic neuronal function in the ventral tegmental area (VTA) is

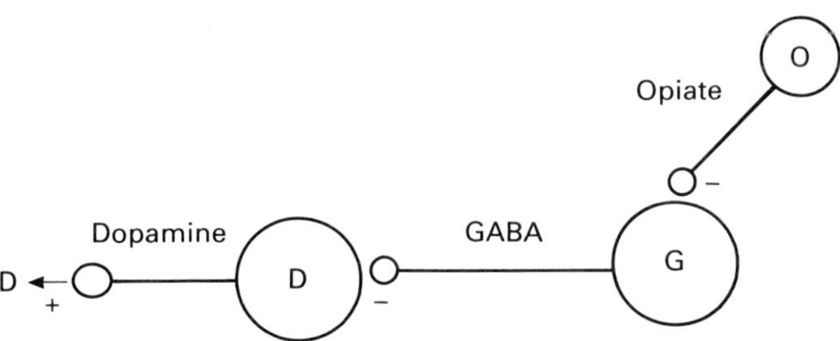

Fig. 2 In the normal brain an opiate peptide pathway projects to GABA interneurones which normally inhibit dopaminergic neurones in the ventral tegmental area, the terminals of which release dopamine in the nucleus accumbens. Opiate peptides acting as μ-receptors on GABA neurones cause hyperpolarization and inhibition of GABA function. There is therefore a diminution of inhibitory tone on the dopaminergic neurones, they fire and dopamine is released in the nucleus accumbens. O, Opiate; G, GABA (γ-aminobutyric acid); D, dopamine.

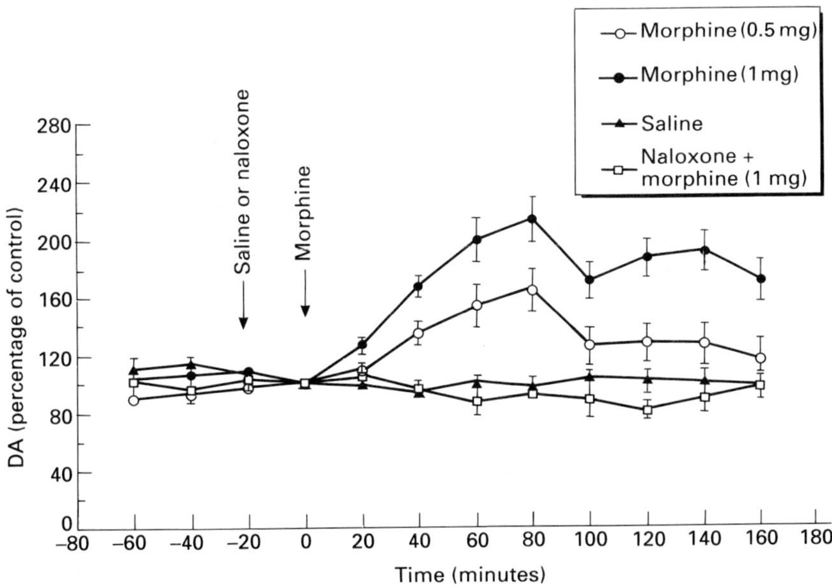

Fig. 3 Through a microdialysis probe placed in the nucleus accumbens of the rat, brain extracellular dopamine (DA) is sampled and measured by high-performance liquid chromatography with electrochemical detection. When morphine (1 mg per kg sc) is given, there is a clear rise of dopamine in the microdialysis fluid indicating dopamine release. This is inhibited by prior treatment with the opiate antagonist naloxone (1 mg per kg sc). (By permission from Pei *et al.* [9].)

increased and dopamine release at the terminals in the nucleus accumbens also increased [3,8]. This is shown in Figs 2 and 3 [9].

Neuropharmacologically this increase in dopamine function in the nucleus accumbens can be achieved in various ways [7]. The opiates act indirectly to cause increased dopamine release. Cocaine probably acts by inhibiting the reuptake of dopamine by the nerve terminals in the nucleus accumbens thus increasing synaptic concentrations of dopamine in that area. Amphetamines (and Ecstasy: MDMA) act by both releasing dopamine and inhibiting its reuptake in the nucleus accumbens. Cannabis, alcohol, barbiturates and nicotine also appear to cause some increase in dopamine function in the nucleus accumbens.

Techniques of electrical stimulation and point anatomical lesioning affect the behavioural responses to drugs of misuse in animals, which back up the neuropharmacological hypothesis that increased dopamine function in the nucleus accumbens is an important (but perhaps not the sole) action underlying the 'pleasurable feeling' resulting from the administration of such drugs. Evidence is emerging that cannabis may also act partly through this system [10].

Ecstasy (3,4-methylene dioxy methamphetamine) also releases 5-hydroxytryptamine (5HT) in various areas of the brain [11]. Although in the drugs field, it is always difficult to separate the environmental factors in a drug culture from strict neurobiology (i.e. it is generally nicer to have a drink in company than alone), nevertheless the 5HT release produced by Ecstasy is thought to be involved with the induction of the warm feeling (Love Drug) felt towards people in the 'Rave scene'. LSD (lysergic acid diethylamide) is an oddity. Its psychotomimetic effects are probably mediated through brain 5HT receptors (sub-type $5HT_2$) [12].

In addition to dopamine release in the nucleus accumbens alcohol also enhances GABA function [7] and this might be responsible for its sedative and tranquillizing actions. Benzodiazepines also enhance the functions of GABA [7] and there is a hypothesis that the mechanisms of dependence for alcohol and benzodiazepines and the withdrawal phenomena for both depend upon alterations in GABA function [13].

In recent years the phenomenon of craving and its underlying neuropsychobiology has been a focus of interest. Wise [6] analyzes the neurobiology of craving, recognizes the role of positive reinforcement and accepts much of what has been written above about the role of dopamine. Indeed he extends the role of dopamine to the reinforcing effectiveness of food and water in hungry and thirsty animals. He links craving (and here comes a conceptual jump) to the memory of past positive reinforcement and then blames addiction and relapse from prolonged detoxification on that. Unfortunately, we have no clue to the neurobiological basis of that memory.

There is a biological basis for dependence and for drug craving that does not have its roots in withdrawal distress. There appear to be different mechanisms for the craving requiring the *positive* reinforcement of the drug as compared with the craving that involves the *negative* reinforcement properties of the drug, i.e. getting rid of the withdrawal distress. In brain electrical stimulation experiments craving for stimulation in so-called 'pleasure areas' in rat brains can be demonstrated long after any post-stimulation withdrawal effects from such techniques. So strong can this craving be that under certain conflict conditions animals would rather starve to death than give up the opportunity to work for more stimulation [6].

If indeed there is a difference between the neurobiological bases of craving and withdrawal then there are implications for the treatment of addictive states.

MECHANISMS OF TOLERANCE AND WITHDRAWAL

How are withdrawal states and symptoms mediated? After the initial exposure to a reinforcing drug and with repeated administration neuroadaptive responses occur. A clear manifestation of this is tolerance, i.e. the necessity to increase doses in order to achieve required effects and related to withdrawal.

During recent years there have been some interesting pharmacological insights into opiate, benzodiazepine and alcohol withdrawal.

In rats, opiate withdrawal induced by the opiate agonist, naloxone, is an acute phenomenon accompanied by signs of the withdrawal syndrome. This is accompanied by an acute and marked release of noradrenaline in the hippocampus, and locus coeruleus. The molecular basis of the neuronal mechanism whereby noradrenergic neuronal networks are activated on withdrawal to produce the aversive experiences is not yet fully understood. In general, it is presumed that neuroadaptive responses occur in drug addictive states such that neuronal networks mediating aversive experiences such as anxiety, heightened autonomic nervous system function, dysphoria and low mood are progressively suppressed by repeated drug administration. This then leads to atrophy of the normal mechanisms of suppressive control. In other words the drug substitutes for normal endogenous suppressive control. An endocrine analogy for this is the occurrence of adrenocortical atrophy and the decrease of pituitary adrenocorticotrophic hormone (ACTH) secretion in patients being treated with exogenous glucocorticoids and the months it takes to re-establish normal hypothalamic–pituitary–adrenocortical relationships on steroid withdrawal.

Because of neuroadaptation leading to tolerance and opiate substitution for endogenous suppressive mechanisms of central noradrenergic activity in people addicted to opiates, opiate withdrawal results in excessive brain noradrenergic function.

Figure 4 shows the release of noradrenaline in rat brain hippocampus in morphine addicted animals, in response to withdrawal precipitated by naloxone.

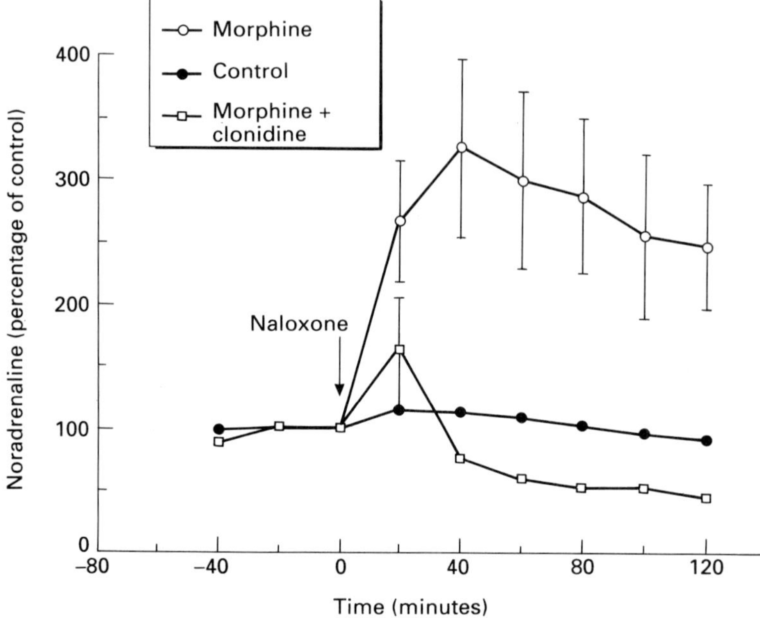

Fig. 4 Effect of opiate withdrawal on noradrenaline release in rat hippocampus. Rats pretreated with morphine 100 mg per kg sc per day for 8 days were given naloxone 1 mg per kg sc at '0' time. Extracellular noradrenaline was sampled and measured by a microdialysis technique utilizing a probe placed stereotactically in the nucleus accumbens. Naloxone produces a clear increase in hippocampal noradrenaline release, which is inhibited by prior treatment with clonidine (0.1 mg per kg sc). (By permission from Done *et al.* [14].)

Clonidine is an α_2-agonist which acts at central presynaptic noradrenergic nerve terminals to inhibit the release of noradrenaline [14] and its administration has been used in the prevention and treatment of opiate withdrawal syndromes, particularly in the USA, and in some centres it is part of the detoxification package.

Cowen and Nutt [13] proposed a neuropharmacological mechanism for benzodiazapine and alcohol withdrawal syndromes. Delirium tremens is the well known withdrawal syndrome of alcohol dependence. It is of many grades, from mild anxiety and dysphoria through to severe anxiety, disturbance of the autonomic nervous system, particularly the sympathetic nervous system, confusional organic psychosis and epilepsy.

Although benzodiazepine withdrawal is generally less severe, nevertheless the syndromes are not dissimilar, sharing anxiety, dysphoria, tremor, insomnia, shakiness, impaired concentration, depersonalization and epilepsy. The frank hallucinatory delirious state does not generally occur with benzodiazepine withdrawal. Cowen and Nutt [13] hypothesized that the acute effects of both these drugs are mediated through an increase in the function of GABAergic mechanisms, though probably at different sites on the benzodiazepine–GABA–chloride channel complex. Benzodiazepines and alcohol both exogenously produce a state akin to an increase in GABA function. This would lead to a decrease in endogenous GABA function because GABA neurones no longer have 'to work'. This neuroadaptive effect is chronic, and on withdrawal of alcohol or benzodiazepines the exogenous source of GABA function is removed, endogenous GABA function is low and takes some time to resume its normal activity. In the meantime there is a relative lack of inhibitory GABA function in various brain areas which leads to the manifestations of the two withdrawal syndromes. As GABA function returns, the acute withdrawal syndromes subside. It is of interest to note that chlormethiazole and benzodiazepines are used in the prevention and treatment of delirium tremens and that both these drugs act by enhancing GABA function and therefore 'substituting' for the alcohol.

Substitution therapy is traditionally the therapeutic approach to dependence and withdrawal. Oral long-acting opiates such as methadone, which is used in opiate misuse treatment programmes [15], act on the biological mechanisms upon which the opiates themselves act. In the well-motivated individual, methadone will cut down craving and diminish withdrawal symptoms. Patients can be maintained on methadone or it can be used in a detoxification/withdrawal treatment programme in which doses are gradually diminished allowing a gradual re-emergence of endogenous control mechanisms from the inhibitory neuroadaptive response previously incurred. This general approach is also useful for the treatment of benzodiazepine withdrawal in which gradually decreasing doses of a long-acting benzodiazepine are advocated [16].

The substitute drug should have a fairly long half-time so that the receptors are occupied for long duration, to avoid the 'ups and downs' of agonist action. The substitute drug should also be formulated usually in liquid form, to allow a very gradual reduction in dosage, e.g. diazepam, methadone.

There is, however, much more to successful drug withdrawal programmes and therapy than drug manipulation, substitution and maintenance [17].

The cocaine withdrawal syndrome consists of a chronic dysphoria and anhedonia. It is particularly notable with cocaine that even after abstinence and the disappearance of the withdrawal syndrome, craving may persist and can be triggered by environmental cues, mood change, exhaustion and boredom. There is some evidence that desipramine, which partially blocks dopamine uptake and certainly noradrenaline and 5HT uptake, may be helpful in cocaine withdrawal. Bromocriptine, a dopamine agonist, has also been used.

THE LINK BETWEEN THE NEUROBIOLOGY OF DRUGS OF MISUSE, THEIR EFFECTS IN THE INDIVIDUAL AND SOCIETY

Figure 5 shows the links between neurobiological effects of drugs of misuse and crime. It is clear that the drug seeker who is in the grip of addiction will go to great lengths to procure a supply of illicit drugs and since these are expensive he/she resorts to crime to provide the finance. Prostitution is also a source of money to finance the habit, and if the prostitute is an intravenous drug user then the spread of HIV becomes a further problem.

There are also the primary drug offences where the user is charged with possession of an illicit drug or traffickers are charged with supplying. The secondary drug offences committed to provide finance for purchase are much more numerous.

The extent of these problems should be determined by the prevalence of drug misuse. Unfortunately prevalence is extremely difficult to measure accurately because gathering data on an activity which is illegal is not easy. Drug misusers do not want to reveal their habit. Many of those

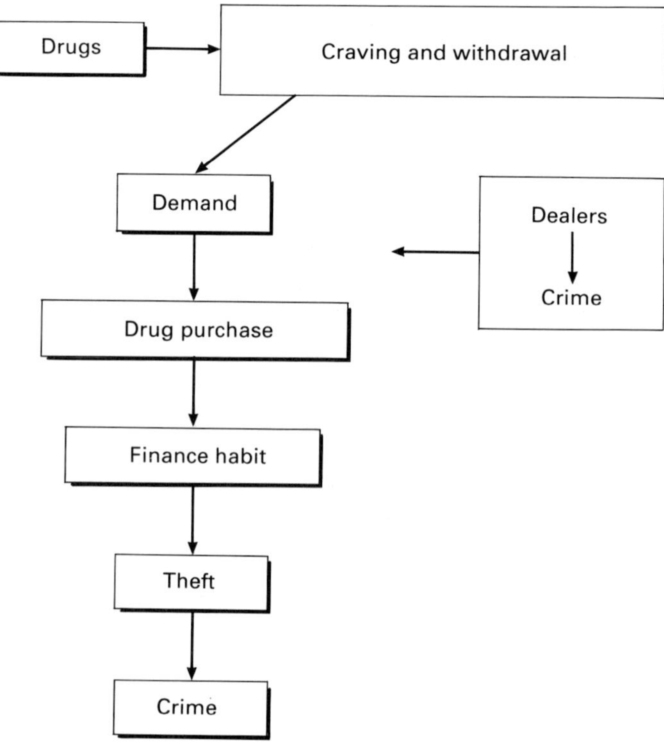

Fig. 5 Links between neurobiological effects of drugs of misuse and crime.

involved in drug misuse do not reach collective consciousness until they perceive they have a problem and decide to seek help. The helping agency is then in a position to notify the misuser in some way, preserving confidentiality. The epidemiology of drug misuse is bedevilled by inadequate data. Therefore, field work, focused surveys, and the culling of data from a multitude of sources is necessary, to construct an overall view of what is going on.

In the UK a source of such statistics is the Addicts Index, to which doctors are statutorily required to notify misusers of a number of drugs (see *British National Formulary*) amongst which are cocaine and most of the opiates including diamophine, morphine, methadone, pethidine and a number of synthetic opiates. This reporting is required by the Misuse of Drugs Act 1971 (with amendments 1985) which controls the manufacture, supply and possession of certain classes of drugs.

There is probably serious under-reporting of drug misuse to the Addicts Index, because of course, if a drug misuser does not present to a doctor he or she will not be notified. There is now the NHS Regional Drug Misuse Database which, on a regional basis, accepts notifications from a range of health staff involved in drug misuse services and which is expected to pick up and record the misusers of a larger range of drugs than that currently covered by the Addicts Index. Even so there will always be an unknown number of misusers who do not present. Various informed guesses of opiate misuse estimate that there are perhaps five times the number of opiate misusers than are notified. No sensible informed guesses can be made in regard to cocaine, amphetamines or temazepam. We know the number of offenders in regard to cannabis but have little idea of the prevalence of cannabis use.

However measurements are made, it is clear there is a huge problem of substance misuse causing great damage in society. What are the implications in society as opposed to the problems for the individual?

Table 2 Crime associated with heroin misuse

1989:
30% committed household burglaries
24% committed theft from person
41% stole from shops
If heroin users notified are 50% of true total:
3600 committed household burglary
2900 committed theft from person
5000 stole from shops
Accounts for:
6–24% burglaries
6–22% thefts from person
0.06–8% shoplifting

These can be conveniently considered under the headings: (i) crime and its influence; (ii) health and its wider effects; (iii) effects upon the family; (iv) group behaviour in society, including violence; (v) effects upon productivity.

Crime and its influence

Table 2 shows the estimates of crimes associated with heroin misuse. The extent of the involvement of drugs in crime is staggering and its background in providing the finance for the habit clear [18,19].

Health and its wider effects

Intravenous injection of opiates and some other drugs with shared needles and syringes is still widespread with the potential for the spread of HIV infection, hepatitis and other infections. HIV infection amongst drug misusers is a potential persisting nidus for the virus in society. Despite campaigns aimed at educating injectors on the dangers of HIV infection in certain areas of the country the practice is still common. Even in prisons there is a problem [20,21]. Much has been done to try and eliminate behaviour of shared 'works' but it is ingrained in the drug culture. Syringe and needle exchange schemes in communities have been created and to some extent these have been effective in cutting down sharing of syringes and needles. Prostitutes who misuse intravenous drugs may pick up HIV infection by their drug misuse and spread it by sex.

The health problems associated with alcohol and nicotine are well known and very serious. They do, however, fall into the same neurobiological context of craving, withdrawal and drug culture. Accidents due to drinking and driving are of particular concern.

Effects upon the family

Family life can be severely disrupted by drug misuse and one should not underestimate the fear and concern of parents in regard to the potential for drug misuse in their children. Once there is a drug misuser in the household, whether it be father and alcohol, a child sniffing solvents, a teenager smoking cannabis or getting Ecstasy at a rave, there is trouble, distrust and a breakdown in relationships. Opiates can destroy a family.

Group behaviour in society

In recent years, particularly in the USA, the drug culture has been seen to take over whole areas of cities. Cocaine particularly seems to have engendered a vicious, aggressive, tribalistic organizational structure for supply which can control designated regions of cities with violence amongst dealers, murder of dealers, users and the innocent, threatening behaviour on the streets, open dealing, riots (often with a background of ethnicity) and virtual 'no-go' areas.

In The Netherlands, where there is a more liberal attitude toward drug misuse, a backlash is now emerging with, for instance, the citizens of Amsterdam becoming intolerant of the unpleasantness of open drug dealing, the irresponsibility of many drug misusers in the city, and the influx of drug misusers from other European countries to gain access to much more freely available drugs.

Alcohol and violence disturb society. Soccer violence, gratuitous violence by intoxicated groups of young men in the streets of cities, is terrifying to the peaceful citizen, invoking serious policing which is disruptive of society. Drugs and alcohol are frequent factors in public disorder in the city.

Effects upon productivity

The deleterious influence of alcohol in the workplace and its effect upon productivity is well known.

There is also the fiscal aspect. The cost of health care in respect of the ravages of drug misuse including alcohol and nicotine is huge. The cost of all forms of policing add up, including Customs and Excise, the costs of prevention programmes, and the hidden costs to society of the social benefits required for drug misusers, their support, their unemployment, and the loss of productivity.

SOCIETY'S RESPONSE

What can be done about it? There is no simple, easy, single, snappy answer. The human brain is what it is and people are what they are. It is not within our power (yet) to change the wiring of the human brain but we should not despair. It is within our power to change the function of the brain in respect of the attitude of mind which predisposes the individual to the vulnerability of drug misusing.

Briefly, there are three aims: (i) reduce demand; (ii) reduce supply; (iii) minimize harm [22].

Demand reduction

There is now in place in the UK an educational programme designed to prevent drug misuse, bringing the matter into the general context of education in health, starting in schools at an early age and gradually progressing. This is a sensitive matter, difficult to pursue and not without controversy. There are from time to time national programmes to persuade the public against various aspects of drug misuse, e.g. solvent misuse or the dangers of intravenous drug injection as an agent in spreading HIV infection. Action at a national level is insufficient and local initiatives at the community level are required to create an antidrug culture. The training and placement of personnel to enact this programme is vital and community support and finance essential.

Reduction of supply

There are the activities of Customs and Excise, which will become more difficult with the abolition of border barriers and the toning down of custom procedures in the European Community. There are the activities of the Coastguard in regard to smuggling. There is a huge international intelligence operation which is active. Then, as the supply chain filters down through to the small-time street dealers, there is police activity permeating down to the street level.

An important influence on the nature of policing at street level is the criminal justice system. Policies on how to deal with drug misusers, criteria for arrest, severity of sentence, role of the probation system, rehabilitation whilst in prison, follow-up by the probation service after cautioning and introducing the offender to drug services are crucial to coping with the drug problem. At an international level, the sequestration of drug money, the problem of picking up the laundering of drug money, the design of operations to arrest the big operators – these are matters of complex international cross-border policies and international treaties.

Harm minimization

We cannot close our eyes to the fact that despite attempts to reduce demand and supply, drug dealing and drug taking is going to continue in some form. We must have in place procedures and avenues that reduce the harm that it does. Sensitive services must be available to the drug misuser who gets into trouble. They must be easily accessible and staffed by understanding people well trained in the subject. If people insist on using the intravenous route, clean needles and syringes must be made available to them to prevent the spread of HIV and other viral infections. Prostitutes who are intravenous drug misusers should be persuaded to undergo HIV screening: at least one can try.

Parents need to be educated to spot drug misuse such as solvent sniffing and cannabis smoking in their children and have ready access to non-threatening services to help out in that situation.

There is continuous activity at government level on all of these issues, trying to cope with the threat of drug misuse to society. The Advisory Council on the Misuse of Drugs advises the government on many of these issues and has published several documents dealing with various aspects of the problem such as prevention, training (of all those who may be involved in the problems of drugs misuse), AIDS and drug misuse, and involvement of the criminal justice system with the problems posed by drug misuse. These documents have had a positive influence in society.

I hope that this consideration of drug misuse from its molecular neurobiology right through to society gives a useful and perhaps different perspective on the problem, emphasizes that it will not go away, shows that strategies are available for its partial control, and at the same time, emphasizes the seriousness of the threat.

I have not considered decriminalization or legalization of the drugs of addiction. These are very complex issues which others have discussed and which will continue to be the subject of debate [23]. My serious apprehension in these issues is the very great vulnerability of the human brain to the addictive process, and its implications for the individual and at the population level, society. This vulnerability should not be dismissed lightly.

REFERENCES

1 Edwards G. Taking substance misuse seriously. *Health Hygiene* 1992;13:147–157.

2 Edelman GM. *Bright Air, Brilliant Fire: On the Matter of the Mind.* London: Allen Lane, Penguin, 1992.

3 Koob GF, Bloom FE. Cellular and molecular mechanisms of drug dependence. *Science* 1988;242:715–723.

4 Jaffe JH. Addictions: what does biology have to tell? In: Bebbington PE, Appleby L, eds. *Review of Psychiatry*, Vol. 1, No. 1/2. London: Institute of Psychiatry, Carfax Publishing Company, 1989:51–56.

5 Stolerman I. Drugs of abuse: behavioural principles, methods and terms. *Trends Pharmacol Sci* 1992;13(5):170–176.

6 Wise RA. The neurobiology of craving: implications for the understanding and treatment of addiction. *J Abnormal Psychol* 1988;97(2):118–132.

7 Koob GF. Drugs of abuse: anatomy, pharmacology and function of reward pathways. *Trends Pharmacol Sci* 1992;13(5):177–184.

8 Di Chiara G, North RA. Neurobiology of opiate abuse. *Trends Pharmacol Sci* 1992; 13:185–193.

9 Pei Q, Zetterstrom T, Leslie RA, Grahame-Smith DG. $5HT_3$ receptor antagonists inhibit morphine-induced stimulation of mesolimbic dopamine release and function in the rat. *Eur J Pharmacol* 1993;230:63–68.

10 Ng Cheong Ton JM, Gerhardt GA, Friedmemann M, *et al.* The effects of ^{9}-tetrahydrocannabinol on potassium-evoked release of dopamine in the rat caudate nucleus: an in vivo electrochemical and in vivo microdialysis study. *Brain Res* 1988; 451:59–68.

11 Schmidt CJ, Wu L, Lovenberg W. Methylenedioxymethamphetamine: a potentially neurotoxic analogue. *Eur J Pharmacol* 1986;124:175–178.

12 Glennon RA, Titeler M, MacKenney JD. Evidence of $5HT_2$ involvement in the mechanisms of action of hallucinogenic drugs. *Life Sci* 1985;35:2505–2511.
13 Cowen PH, Nutt DJ. Abstinence symptoms after withdrawal from tranquillising drugs; is there a common neurochemical pathway? *Lancet* 1982;ii:360–362.
14 Done C, Silverstone P, Sharp T. Effect of naloxone-precipitated morphine withdrawal on noradrenaline release in rat hippocampus *in vivo*. *Eur J Pharmacol* 1992;215: 333–336.
15 Department of Health, Scottish Office Home and Health Department, Welsh Office. *Drug Misuse and Dependence: Guidelines on Clinical Management. Report of a Medical Working Group*. London: HMSO, 1991.
16 Lader M. The psychopharmacology of addiction – benzodiazepine tolerance and dependence. In: Lader M, ed. *The Psychopharmacology of Addiction*. Oxford Medical Publications: Oxford, 1988:1–14.
17 Kleber HD. Treatment of drug dependence: what works. *Int Rev Psychiatry* 1989;1: 81–100.
18 Home Office. *Drug Misusers and the Criminal Justice System. Part I: Community Resources and the Probation Service. Report by the Advisory Council on the Misuse of Drugs*. London: HMSO, 1991.
19 Mott J. *7: Reducing Heroin Related Crime. Home Office Research and Planning Unit. Research Bulletin No. 26*. 1989.
20 Dye S, Isaacs C. Intravenous drug misuse among prison inmates: implications for spread of HIV. *Br Med J* 1992;302:1506.
21 Farrell M, Strang J. Drugs, HIV, and prisons: Time to rethink current policy. *Br Med J* 1991;302:1477–1478.
22 Home Office. *Tackling Drug Misuse: a Summary of the Government's Strategy*. 3rd edn. London, 1988.
23 Editorial. Your heroin, sir. *Lancet* 1991;337:402.

PART 3
NEUROLOGY

The pathogenesis of demyelinating disease

D. A. S. COMPSTON

Multiple sclerosis has a lifetime frequency of at least 1:800 for inhabitants of the UK and neighbouring parts of northern Europe and, as the commonest potentially disabling neurological disease of young adults, it represents an important challenge for contemporary clinical neuroscience. Inflammation in the nervous system depends upon migration of activated lymphocytes across the blood–brain barrier, bringing to the abluminal surface of cerebral blood vessels a variety of cellular and soluble immune mediators. The pivotal role of T-lymphocyte traffic into the nervous system as the basis for demyelination is consistent with the effects of treatments which reduce the availability of circulating lymphocytes or limit their entry into the brain, both in human and experimental disease, but the knowledge that inflammatory processes in the brain culminate in contact between microglia and the oligodendrocyte–myelin unit provides additional complexities and opens up further opportunities for treatment. Disability results both from the inflammatory process and the failure of its repair so that, in time, a combination of manoeuvres involving limitation of the inflammatory process and increased availability of glial progenitors with re-establishment of their developmental growth factor environment may be needed to treat demyelinated lesions.

GENETIC SUSCEPTIBILITY AND DEMYELINATION

The aetiology of multiple sclerosis involves an interplay between genetic and environmental factors. It is a disease of northern Europeans and occurs less frequently in other racial groups. Within the UK, the disease is more prevalent in north-east Scotland than in other parts [1]. Regional differences in the frequency throughout North America match patterns of migration from northern Europe, and correlate inversely with the distribution of American blacks. In South Africa, multiple sclerosis occurs more commonly in English speaking whites than in Afrikaaners or Coloureds and is not seen in native Africans; in Australia and New Zealand it is rarely diagnosed in Aborigines or Maoris [2]. The lifetime risk of multiple sclerosis in northern Europeans increases from approximately 1:800 to 1:50, 1:20 and 1:3 for the offspring, siblings and monozygotic twin partners of affected individuals, respectively. These occurrence risks are based on clinical expression of the disease but the figures rise somewhat if imaging abnormalities are taken as evidence for subclinical disease [3].

Pedigree analysis strongly suggests that susceptibility to multiple sclerosis is under polygenic control. Candidate genes include class II alleles of the major histocompatibility complex and there are population associations with the alleles DRw15 and DQw6; their genotypic correlates are the specificities DRB1.1501/DRB5.0101/DQA1.0102/DQB2.0602 [4]. Preliminary evidence, based on linkage analysis in large cohorts of sibling-affected pairs, indicates that germline variations in the variable regions of the T-cell receptor β-chain and the immunoglobulin heavy chain also increase the risk of multiple sclerosis, especially in individuals who possess HLA-DRw15 [5,6]. However, these findings have not consistently been reported [6–8], and population associations with polymorphisms of the immunoglobulin heavy chain genes have also yet to be confirmed [9]. The relationship between susceptibility to multiple sclerosis and DRw15/DQw6 suggests that this molecule itself has biological significance in initiating the sequence of events leading to tissue damage, but the lack of linkage in family studies and the incomplete population association show that this genetic factor is neither necessary nor sufficient for the development of multiple sclerosis. Linkage to the loci which encode components of the T-cell receptor and the immunoglobulin heavy chain demonstrates that these regions of the genome encode independent susceptibility genes. The interaction of class II molecules and the T-cell receptor in antigen processing may explain why these susceptibility genes additively confer disease susceptibility, and the role of activated T cells in providing help for B-cell responses provides a rationale for immunoglobulin genes acting as a third determinant of susceptibility. Heritability in multiple sclerosis may result entirely from genes which restrict the immune response but there is evidence that, in some populations, inherited differences in the structure of myelin also contribute to susceptibility [10].

The distribution of multiple sclerosis cannot be explained only on the basis of population genetics. In white South Africans and in Australia, prevalence rates are 50% those documented for many parts of northern Europe and there is a gradient in frequency, both in Australia and in New Zealand, which does not follow genetic clines. Multiple sclerosis occurs at a low frequency in Caribbeans but the risk increases substantially in first generation descendants of these immigrants raised in the UK. Conversely, the risk is higher for English-speaking whites migrating into South Africa as adults than in childhood [2,11].

Prospective studies have demonstrated that new episodes of demyelination are more likely to occur following viral exposure but no one triggering agent has been identified. The risk of developing multiple sclerosis is increased for individuals who are exposed to measles, mumps, rubella and Epstein–Barr virus infection relatively late in childhood or adolescence [12,13]. These studies do not implicate any one infectious agent as the exclusive cause of multiple sclerosis but suggest that a narrow and age-linked window of susceptibility to viral exposure exists in those who are constitutionally at risk of developing the disease.

NEUROPATHOLOGY: EVOLUTION OF THE PLAQUE

Inflammatory demyelinating lesions provide the pathological substrate for the symptoms, signs and disabilities which occur in patients with multiple sclerosis; four stages are recognized in the evolution of focal inflammation within the central nervous system [14]. The first is characterized by the accumulation of inflammatory cells, lymphocytes and monocytes, around venules within the central nervous system; the functional unit formed by the oligodendrocyte and its myelin sheath remains intact although inflammation indirectly causes a functional block in conduction through structurally intact myelinated axons, through mechanisms which remain to be elucidated [15]. Next, there is active destruction of the oligodendrocyte and its myelin sheath and this involves contact between macrophages or microglia and the oligodendrocyte–myelin unit. This leads to an acellular phase characterized by depletion of oligodendrocytes and the development of naked axons within lesions. Finally, the areas of inflammation heal by scar formation dependent upon astrocytic reactivity, from which multiple sclerosis gets its name. A limited degree of remyelination is seen in post-acute lesions [16], known as shadow plaques, and this coincides with the reappearance of oligodendrocytes but the remyelination rarely persists, presumably due to recurrent injury, and the contribution that it makes to functional recovery is unknown [17].

Since different inflammatory cells and their mediators are involved in separate stages of the inflammatory cascade, a range of therapeutic approaches must be taken in attempting to manage demyelination. Disability develops in multiple sclerosis not only as a result of the inflammatory insult but also through subsequent lack of remyelination. The issues involved in solving the problem of multiple sclerosis are therefore both to limit and repair the damage.

INFLAMMATION AND THE BRAIN

Cellular penetration of the blood–brain barrier is central to the pathogenesis of multiple sclerosis and provides an obvious opportunity for interfering with the cascade of events which culminates in demyelination. Alterations in vascular permeability can be visualized in life by the technique of gadolinium-enhanced magnetic resonance imaging which confirms that increased leak through the blood–brain barrier is the initial step in lesion formation [18]; this occurs more frequently than the white matter changes which subsequently are demonstrated by T_2-weighted imaging [19]. Blood–brain barrier damage begins with the passage of activated inflammatory cells across endothelial barriers in the microvasculature of the central nervous system [20,21]. Following activation, there is adhesion between lymphocytes and cerebral endothelial cells, consequent upon a change in the expression of cell surface molecules and electrostatic forces which allows their passage to the abluminal surface of blood vessels [22,23].

Cells entering the brain which fail to encounter antigen are believed to be removed by the process of apoptosis. Activated lymphocytes which recognize antigen within the nervous system establish local inflammatory responses, one consequence of which is further damage to the blood–brain barrier, amplifying the movement of potentially pathogenic inflammatory substances into the brain.

PREVENTING BLOOD–BRAIN BARRIER PERMEABILITY

Some manifestations of multiple sclerosis can be attributed to mediators entering the nervous system and not structural damage to myelinated axons; others depend upon demyelination and axonal degeneration. Events occurring at the blood–brain barrier provide sufficient rationale for attempting to treat the disease by limiting the entry of activated inflammatory cells into the central nervous system. Many treatments currently in use probably operate at this level, e.g. sequential changes in an individual gadolinium-enhancing lesion following treatment with high-dose intravenous methylprednisolone show rapid reduction in enhancement, indicating that the blood–brain barrier is impermeable, but within a few days there is further enhancement indicating that the blood vessels are once again leaky [24].

Recently, this aspect of tissue injury in inflammatory brain disease has been managed by the use of monoclonal antibodies, which target specific components of the immune system, in the hope that these will prove effective and less toxic than non-specific immunological treatments. Experimental allergic encephalomyelitis can be prevented by the use of an antibody directed against the α-4-β-1 integrin adhesion molecule which interferes with lymphocyte–endothelial cell adhesion [25]. Antibodies used in humans include those which deplete the circulation of lymphocytes by targeting the CD4 or CDw52 antigen [26]; these can be engineered to produce chimaeric or humanized antibodies, which carry the theoretical advantage of limiting antiidiotypic responses [27]. It would be premature to draw any conclusions from these studies but preliminary observations show a reduction in the accumulation of new gadolinium-enhancing magnetic resonance imaging abnormalities, implying a significant alteration in blood–brain barrier permeability; subjectively, these imaging changes are associated with clinical stability and even improvement in the few patients treated to date (D.A.S. Compston, *et al.*, unpublished observations). In the acute phase, each patient has experienced a severe but temporary increase in symptoms, analogous to Uthoff's phenomenon and probably due to release of cytokines, coinciding with extensive lysis of cells having a high surface density of the CDw52 antigen.

This cytokine release syndrome of monoclonal antibody therapy has previously been described [28] and the most likely candidate is tumour necrosis factor α, which is released in large quantities as lymphocytes are lysed and can be detected systemically in increased concentrations during the few hours of increased symptomatology that follows treatment with anti-CDw52 (CAMPATH-1H) antibody. These observations may prove informative with respect to mechanisms of symptom production in inflammatory brain disease and relate to the basis for interactions between macrophages and microglia which lead to digestion of the oligodendrocyte and its myelin sheath [29,30].

OLIGODENDROCYTES AND MICROGLIA

During development, glial progenitors proliferate and migrate so as to be widely distributed throughout the central nervous system before terminally differentiating and adopting their specialist roles [31]. *In vitro* studies in rodents implicate one cell type, the oligodendrocyte-type 2A astrocyte (O-2A) progenitor and glial growth factors in myelination; in tissue culture, O-2A progenitors undergo a limited number of divisions and, in the absence of platelet-derived and basic fibroblast growth factors, differentiate constitutively into oligodendrocytes [32]. As O-2A cells contact the axons which they will myelinate, a further proliferative signal is provided by platelet-derived growth factor β-chain, so that most precursor cells aligned along axons are in a mitotic phase [33,34]. Terminal differentiation occurs with formation of compact myelin lamellae along a short segment of several neighbouring axons. Alteration in the growth factor conditions under which O-2A progenitors differentiate stimulates the development of type 2 astrocytes which in cocultures also contact axons between the territory of each oligodendrocyte [35]. The O-2A progenitor is therefore capable, at least *in vitro*, of generating both cell types which form the cellular architecture of the node of Ranvier, and this structure provides the basis for saltatory conduction in the central nervous system.

Bone marrow-derived macrophages migrating into the brain during development function as immunocompetent cells [36] and these brain macrophages or microglia play a crucial role in development by removing cells which have undergone programmed cell death; microglia are also involved in tissue removal during inflammatory processes.

Two principles emerge from tissue culture studies aimed at understanding the late stages of brain inflammation. Oligodendrocytes are especially vulnerable amongst glia to inflammatory mediators and they have an inherent capacity for repair at the cellular level [37]. One model system for studying inflammatory events within the central nervous system involves interactions between oligodendrocytes and complement [38,39]. Rodent oligodendrocytes express a cell surface molecule during development which fixes C1q and activates the classical complement pathway but in the absence of antibody [40]; the neonatal rat oligodendrocyte also lacks the complement regulatory protein CD59 which normally prevents assembly of the membrane attack complex of complement following the conversion of C3 [41]. Exposure to normal serum as a source of complement leads to formation of membrane pores on the surface of neonatal rat oligodendrocytes, and these act initially as calcium ionophores [42].

Dynamic studies of oligodendrocytes exposed to pore-forming molecules show a calcium transient which peaks at about 7 minutes and then returns to normal, restoring calcium homeostasis in the target cell. Single cell studies show that this calcium transient depends upon a series of complex oscillations resulting from entry and buffering of extracellular calcium together with some release from intracellular stores [43]. Calcium oscillations are critical for repair of the permeabilized oligodendrocyte membrane. This involves the accumulation of membrane pores into vesicles which are shed from the cell surface restoring its integrity [37] and leaving the cell capable of functioning as a myelinating cell.

Survival from the direct effects of inflammatory injury may expose repaired oligodendrocyte to cell damage mediated by microglia or macrophages. Macrophages and microglia possess receptors for C1q, C3b (CR1) and iC3b (CR3), amongst other ligands, which bind target cells [44,45]. Some of these receptors are constitutively expressed, whereas others require activation by liposaccharide, present as part of the carbohydrate moiety of bacteria, or cytokines, including interferon γ. Cell activation with interferon γ increases either the number, mobility or affinity of these receptors. Adherence occurs occasionally between resting oligodendrocytes and microglia, *in vitro*, but cytotoxicity is rare. With microglial activation following exposure to interferon γ, and opsonization of oligodendrocyte targets with corresponding complement ligands, there is adherence, cytotoxicity and phagocytosis. The lethal signal for cytotoxicity is local release of tumour necrosis factor α [29]; although suprapharmacological

macological doses of soluble tumour necrosis factor α lyse oligodendrocytes *in vitro* [46], short range killing of opsonized oligodendrocytes by activated microglia requires the high concentration of cytokine available at the cell surface [29].

Although the complement receptor–ligand combination has proved informative with respect to microglial–oligodendrocyte interaction *in vitro* using neonatal rat oligodendrocytes, preliminary evidence suggests that autologous complement activation is not a property of human oligodendrocytes [47]. Oligodendrocytes recovered from samples obtained at craniotomy are not susceptible to contact with normal human serum and these cells stain positively for the complement regulatory protein CD59, which is missing from the surface of neonatal rat cells. Other interactions may therefore be more important in mediating damage to human oligodendrocytes by microglia. Of particular relevance to multiple sclerosis is the demonstration that antibody in low concentration, coating the surface of the oligodendrocyte or its myelin sheath, opsonizes the target cell for lytic damage by microglia using Fc receptors [30].

Although the analysis of molecules involved in microglial injury of human oligodendrocytes awaits detailed characterization, these tissue culture studies have identified several stages in the process of demyelination at which inflammatory damage could be limited. Apart from preventing the entry of T lymphocytes into the central nervous system, local release of interferon γ, which activates microglial receptors, antibody synthesis against antigen present on the oligodendrocyte cell surface or its myelin sheath, and release of tumour necrosis factor near opsonized oligodendrocyte targets all merit consideration as therapeutic targets for limiting tissue damage in inflammatory brain disease.

RESTORING GLIAL–NEURONAL ARRANGEMENTS IN THE BRAIN

Restricting the consequences of inflammatory damage in the central nervous system will not improve structure and function in patients with persistent disabilities. Here, there is need to restore, in the postinflammatory lesion, the complex glial–neuronal interactions established during development.

Regeneration has traditionally not been considered a property of the central nervous system, due to lack of precursors in the adult brain, loss of growth factor signals which orchestrate cell movement during development, and the stabilization imposed by inhibitory or repellent molecules on the mature central nervous system [48–51]. Now, it appears that the adult nervous system does contain glial progenitors which can proliferate and migrate [52–54]; there is morphological evidence that repopulation of oligodendrogliopaenic regions occurs following demyelination [17] and sustained repair might be possible if these adult progenitors could be recruited in larger numbers and protected from recurrent injury. Preliminary studies of glial lineages in the human nervous system now suggest that oligodendrocyte precursors may be present in the normal adult brain [55]. One possibility is that these cells are injured by the same process which causes oligodendrocyte depletion in inflammatory brain lesions, but their failure to remyelinate postinflammatory lesions could also result from lack of appropriate growth factor signals [56] or failure to penetrate astrocyte scars. Astrocytes represent a physical barrier to the movement of many cell types but changes in local production of proteases and other degradative enzymes permit traffic across these otherwise impenetrable tissue planes [57,58]. It is also possible that cells penetrating gliopaenic areas, *in vivo*, might encounter naked axons but in the context of inappropriate growth factor signals differentiate into astrocytes and not the oligodendrocytes required for remyelination [34].

If lack of precursors or physical impediments to migration through astrocytic scars prove insuperable obstacles to endogenous remyelination of postinflammatory lesions, an alternative strategy for repair is cellular implantation. Transplantation of gliotoxic lesions in the spinal cord with mixed glial cell grafts can achieve extensive oligodendrocyte remyelination. Apart from the immunological considerations of transplantation, three conditions have to be met for successful grafting: (i) astrocytes are required to establish the microarchitecture of the damaged region, providing the scaffold for cell migration and preventing inward migration of Schwann cells which compete successfully for naked axons in the spinal cord but fail to achieve widespread remyelination; (ii) grafts need to contain sufficient numbers of O-2A lineage cells capable of oligodendrocyte differentiation and remyelination of naked axons; and, (iii) grafts must act as a source of growth factors which ensure that cellular implants differentiate appropriately and perform their specialist roles [59–62].

Complex strategies for repairing the central nervous system make little sense unless combined with effective regimens for limiting the consequences of inflammatory damage. This should be possible by exploiting the opportunities of modern therapeutic immunology, which avoid punishing the entire immune system for the misdemeanours of a few constituent cells. But settling for immunological strategies which merely limit the damage seems a poor ambition in the face of major disabilities and handicaps; the combination of limiting the inflammatory process and repairing demyelinated axons is needed to solve the problems of preventing and reversing disability in patients with multiple sclerosis.

REFERENCES

1 Swingler RJ, Compston DAS. The distribution of multiple sclerosis in the United Kingdom. *J Neurol Neurosurg Psychiatry* 1986;49:1115–1124.

2 Compston DAS. The dissemination of multiple sclerosis; The Langdon Brown Lecture for 1989. *J Roy Coll Phys* 1990;24:207–218.

3 Mumford CJ, Wood N, Kellar-Wood H, *et al.* The British Isles survey of multiple sclerosis in twins. *Neurology* 1994;44:11–15.

4 Olerup O, Hillert J. HLA class II associated genetic susceptibility in multiple sclerosis; a critical evaluation. *Tissue Antigens* 1991;38:1–15.

5 Seboun E, Robinson MA, Doolittle TH, *et al.* A susceptibility locus for multiple sclerosis is linked to the T cell receptor beta-chain complex. *Cell* 1989;57:1095–1100.

6 Wood N, Kellar Wood H, Holmans P, *et al.* A susceptibility gene for multiple sclerosis linked to the immunoglobulin heavy chain variable region. *Am J Hum Genet* 1994 (in press).

7 Hillert J, Leng C, Olerup O. No association with germline T cell receptor beta chain gene alleles or haplotypes in Swedish patients with multiple sclerosis. *J Neuroimmunol* 1991;31:141–147.

8 Lynch SG, Rose LW, Petterjan JH, *et al.* Discordance of T cell receptor beta chain genes in familial multiple sclerosis. *Ann Neurol* 1991;23:402–410.

9 Walter MA, Gibson WT, Ebers GC, Cox DW. Susceptibility to multiple sclerosis is associated with the proximal immunoglobulin heavy-chain variable region. *J Clin Invest* 1991;87:1266–1273.

10 Tienari PJ, Wikstrom J, Sajantila A, *et al.* Genetic susceptibility to multiple sclerosis linked to myelin basic protein gene. *Lancet* 1992;340:987–991.

11 Elian M, Nightingale S, Dean G. Multiple sclerosis among United Kingdom-born children of immigrants from the Indian subcontinent, Africa and the West Indies. *J Neurol Neurosurg Psychiatry* 1990;53:906–911.

12 Compston DAS, Vakarelis BN, Paul E, *et al.* Viral infection in patients with multiple sclerosis and HLA-DR matched controls. *Brain* 1986;109:325–344.

13 Martyn CN, Cruddas M, Compston DAS. Symptomatic Epstein–Barr virus infection and multiple sclerosis. *J Neurol Neurosurg Psychiatry* 1993;56:167–168.

14 Adams CWM. The onset and progression of the lesions of multiple sclerosis. *J Neurol Sci* 1975;25:165–182.

15 Youl BD, Turano G, Miller DH, *et al.* The pathophysiology of acute optic neuritis: an association of gadolinium leakage with clinical and electrophysiological deficits. *Brain* 1991;114:2437–2450.

16 Prineas JW, Kwon EE, Goldenberg PZ, *et al.* Multiple sclerosis. Oligodendrocyte proliferation and differentiation in fresh lesions. *Lab Invest* 1989;61:489–503.

17 Prineas JW, Barnard RO, Kwon EE, *et al.* Multiple sclerosis: remyelination of nascent lesions. *Ann Neurol* 1993;33:137–151.

18 Kermode AG, Thompson AJ, Tofts P, *et al.* Breakdown of the blood brain barrier precedes symptoms and other MRI signs of new lesions in multiple sclerosis. *Brain* 1990;113:1477–1489.

19 McDonald WI, Barnes D. Lessons from magnetic resonance imaging in multiple sclerosis. *Trends Neurosci* 1989;12:376–379.

20 Wekerle H, Engelhardt B, Risau W, Meyermann R. Interaction of T lymphocytes with cerebral endothelial cells *in vitro*. *Brain Pathol* 1991;1:107–114.

21 Male DK, Pryce G, Hughes CCW, Lantos PL. Lymphocyte migration into the brain modelled *in vitro*: control by lymphocyte activation, cytokines and antigen. *Cell Immunol* 1990;127:1–11.

22 Hickey WF. Migration of hematogenous cells through the blood brain barrier and the initiation of CNS inflammation. *Brain Pathol* 1991;1:97–105.

23 Lassmann H, Rossler K, Zimprich F, Vass K. Expression of adhesion molecules and histocompatibility antigens at the blood brain barrier. *Brain Pathol* 1991;1:115–123.

24 Miller DH, Newton MR, van der Poel JC. Magnetic resonance imaging of the optic nerve in optic neuritis. *Neurology* 1988;38:175–179.

25 Yednock TA, Cannon C, Fritz LC, *et al.* Prevention of experimental allergic encephalomyelitis by antibodies against alpha-4-beta-1-integrin. *Nature* 1992;356:63–66.

26 Hale G, Xia M-O, Tighe HP, *et al.* The CAMPATH-1 antigen (CDw52). *Tissue Antigens* 1990;35:118–125.

27 Winter G, Milstein C. Man-made antibodies. *Nature* 1991;349:293–299.

28 Chatenoud L, Ferran C, Legendre C, *et al. In vivo* cell activation following OKT3 administration; cytokine release and modulation by corticosteroids. *Transplantation* 1990;49:697–702.

29 Zajicek JP, Wing M, Scolding NJ, Compston DAS. Interactions between oligodendrocytes and microglia: a major role for complement and tumour necrosis factor in oligodendrocyte adherence and killing. *Brain* 1992;115:1611–1631.

30 Scolding NJ, Compston DAS. Oligodendrocyte macrophage interactions *in vitro* triggered by specific antibodies. *Immunology* 1991;72:127–132.

31 Miller RH, ffrench Constant C, Raff MC. The macroglial cells of the rat optic nerve. *Ann Rev Neurosci* 1989;12:517–534.

32 Noble M, Murray K, Stroobant P, *et al.* Platelet derived growth factor promotes division and motility and inhibits premature differentiation of the oligodendrocyte/type 2 astrocyte progenitor cell. *Nature* 1988;333:560–562.

33 Dutly F, Schwab ME. Neurons and astrocytes influence the development of purified O-2A progenitor cells. *Glia* 1991;4:559–571.

34 Zajicek J, Compston DAS. The influence of axons on the differentiation of oligodendrocyte progenitors. *Journal of Neurology* 1992;239(Suppl 2):97(abstract).

35 Miller RH, Fulton BP, Raff MC. A novel type of glial cell associated with nodes of Ranvier in rat optic nerve. *Eur J Neurosci* 1989;1:172–180.

36 Perry VH, Gordon S. Macrophages and microglia in the nervous system. *Trends Neurosci* 1988;11:273–277.

37 Scolding NJ, Morgan BP, Houston WAJ, *et al.* Vesicular removal by oligodendrocytes of membrane attack complexes formed by complement. *Nature* 1989;339:620–622.

38 Scolding NJ, Morgan BP, Houston WAJ, *et al.* Normal rat serum cytotoxicity against syngeneic oligodendrocytes: complement activation and attack in the absence of anti-myelin antibodies. *J Neurol Sci* 1989;89:289–300.

39 Wren DR, Noble M. Oligodendrocytes and adult specific O-2A progenitor cells are uniquely susceptible to the lytic effects of complement in the absence of antibody. *Proc Natl Acad Sci USA* 1989;86:9025–9029.

40 Zajicek JP, Wing M, Lachmann PJ, Compston DAS. Oligodendrocyte interactions with human serum – the simultaneous demonstration of antibody independent classical pathway complement activation and abnormal sensitivity to terminal complement attack. *J Neurol Sci* 1992;108:65–72.

41 Wing MG, Zajicek JP, Seilly DJ, *et al.* Oligodendrocytes lack glycolipid anchored proteins which protect them against complement lysis; restoration of resistance to lysis by incorporation of CD59. *Immunology* 1992;76:140–145.

42 Scolding NJ, Morgan BP, Campbell AK, Compston DAS. The role of calcium in rat oligodendrocyte injury and repair. *Neurosci Lett* 1992;135:95–97.

43 Wood A, Wing MG, Benham CD, Compston DAS. Specific induction of intracellular calcium oscillations by complement membrane attack on oligodendroglia. *J Neurosci* 1993;13:3319–3332.

44 Adams DO, Hamilton TA. The cell biology of macrophage activation. *Ann Rev Immunol* 1984;2:283–318.

45 Griffin FM. Activation of macrophage complement receptors for phagocytosis. In: Adams DO, Hanna MG, eds. *Contemporary Topics in Immunobiology*. New York: Plenum Press, 1984;13:57–70.

46 Selmaj K, Raine CS. Tumour necrosis factor mediates myelin and oligodendrocyte damage in vitro. *Ann Neurol* 1988;23:339–346.

47 Zajicek JP, Wing MG, Compston DAS. Normal human oligodendrocyte susceptibility to complement and the expression of complement regulatory proteins on their surface. *J Neurol* 1992;239(Suppl 2):97(abstract).

48 Fawcett JW, Rokos J, Bakst I. Oligodendrocytes repel axons and cause axonal growth cone collapse. *J Cell Sci* 1989;92:93–100.

49 Caroni P, Schwab ME. Two membrane protein fractions from rat central myelin with inhibitory properties for neurite growth and fibroblast spreading. *J Cell Biol* 1988;106: 1281–1288.

50 Caroni P, Schwab ME. Antibody against myelin associated inhibitor of neurite growth neutralises non-permissive substrate properties of CNS white matter. *Neuron* 1988;1: 85–96.

51 Schnell L, Schwab ME. Axonal regeneration in the rat spinal cord produced by an antibody against myelin associated neurite growth inhibitors. *Nature* 1990;343:269–272.

52 ffrench Constant C, Raff MC. Proliferating bipotential glial progenitor cells in adult rat optic nerve. *Nature* 1986;319:499–502.

53 Wolswijk G, Noble M. Identification of an adult specific glial progenitor cell. *Development* 1989;105:387–400.

54 Noble M. Points of controversy in the O-2A lineage: clocks and type 2 astrocytes. *Glia* 1991;4:157–164.

55 Armstrong RC, Dorn HH, Kufta CV, *et al.* Pre-oligodendrocytes from adult human CNS. *J Neurosci* 1992;12:1538–1547.

56 Bogler O, Wren D, Barnett SC, *et al.* Co-operation between two growth factors promotes extended self-renewal and inhibits differentiation of oligodendrocyte-type 2 astrocytes (O-2A) progenitor cells. *Proc Natl Acad Sci USA* 1990;87:6368–6372.

57 Fawcett JW, Housden E, Smith-Thomas L, Myer RL. The growth of axons in 3 dimensional astrocyte cultures. *Dev Biol* 1989;135:449–458.

58 Fawcett JW, Housden E. The effects of protease inhibitors on axon growth through astrocytes. *Development* 1990;109:59–66.

59 Blakemore WF, Crang AJ. Extensive oligodendrocyte remyelination following injection of cultured central nervous system cells into demyelinating lesions in the adult central nervous system. *Dev Neurosci* 1988;10:1–11.

60 Blakemore WF, Crang AJ. The relationship between type 1 astrocytes, Schwann cells and oligodendrocytes following transplantation of glial cell cultures into demyelinating lesions in the adult rat spinal cord. *J Neurocytol* 1989;18:519–528.

61 Blakemore WF, Franklin RJM. Transplantation of glial cells into the CNS. *Trends Neurosci* 1991;14:323–327.

62 Franklin RJM, Crang AJ, Blakemore WF. Transplanted type-1 astrocytes facilitate repair of demyelinating lesions by host oligodendrocytes in adult rat spinal cord. *J Neurocytol* 1991;20:420–430.

Parkinson's disease

G. STERN

INTRODUCTION

In 1817 when our College was less salubriously located in Warwick Lane, a short distance from the latest Newgate building, James Parkinson published an essay on 'The Shaking Palsy'. He was neither a licentiate, member nor fellow of the Royal College of Physicians, but a simple surgeon–apothecary, a mere member of the Royal College of Surgeons, but these apparent disadvantages did not prevent him achieving international eponymous and enduring distinction – alas posthumously. At a time when this College was concerned with pressing government requests for medical advice including the management of infectious disorders (in this case undulant fever in Gibraltar) and the problems of medical advertising (a licentiate was reprimanded for having a board publicly exhibited to advertise his prescribing hours) – *plus ça change* [1] – Dr James Parkinson drew attention to the clinical features of a degenerative disabling disease of the central nervous system now known to be common and ubiquitous. While he failed to recognize rigidity and erroneously considered that the 'senses were preserved' he succinctly described the salient features of an illness [2] the nature of which continues to challenge neuroscientists and clinical neurologists.

As far as treatment was concerned, Parkinson was limited to prevailing physical methods '. . . blood should be first taken from the upper part of the neck, unless contraindicated by any particular circumstances. After which vesicatories should be applied to the same part and a purulent discharge obtained by the appropriate use of the Sabine Liniment . . . .' He was clearly aware of these limitations. 'Until we are better informed respecting the nature of this disease, the employment of internal medicine is scarcely warrantable; unless analogy should point out some remedy the trial of which rational hope might authorise.'

This remarkable prescience was fulfilled in the 1950s when it was shown that in parkinsonian brains there was a focal depletion of certain neurotransmitters and enzymes. This was most conspicuous for dopamine [3], which led to now conventional oral levodopa replacement therapy; it was also shown that there are deficiencies of noradrenaline, glutamic acid decarboxylase, serotonin and choline acetyltransferase as well as others which have yet to be therapeutically exploited. Over the past two decades considerable experience of levodopa therapy has accumulated [4] and *pari passu* there has been an explosion of interest and research into the nature of the illness as well as symptomatic relief of its symptoms. There are reasons to believe that there is a presymptomatic phase when the crucial dopamine degenerating cells of the nigrostriatal pathway are undergoing still inexplicable deterioration followed by a symptomatic phase when symptoms and signs emerge and when levodopa treatment permits reasonable containment of these disabilities. This is unfortunately succeeded by a third phase of gradual loss of control [5] – the so-called chronic levodopa syndrome. The disease continues to deteriorate, psychiatric problems appear in about 40% of patients and a bizarre group of motor disorders including 'on–off' fluctuations and a diminishing threshold for levodopa-induced movements (dyskinesias) emerge. Little is known of the underlying mechanisms responsible for this constellation of neurological problems and unfortunately they remain largely refractory despite much speculation and a wide variety of therapeutic strategies. As Parkinson predicted, while the cause or causes of the disease, its deterioration and its pathophysiology remain obscure and until we enjoy 'rational hope', it seems unlikely that we shall have truly effective treatments to prevent, delay or control the inevitable deterioration which remains a feature of the illness.

THE CONCEPT OF NEUROPROTECTION

L-Deprenyl (selegiline), a selective monoamine oxidase type B inhibitor, was originally introduced to therapeutics as a 'psychic-energizer' and early trials indicated that it had a mild antidepressant effect. It was then used in conjunction with levodopa on the basis that it might slow down oxidative deamination of endogenous and exogenous levodopa and prove to have a mild levodopa-sparing effect and to be beneficial in ameliorating mild 'wearing-off effects' or end-of-dose akinesia. The results in several trials were modest but unequivocal. However, in 1985 Birkmayer *et al.* [6] proposed that the addition of L-deprenyl resulted in increased life expectancy for parkinsonian patients already taking conventional levodopa. This was an open uncontrolled retrospective study of 941 patients observed for up to 9 years. Their figures indicated that those treated with L-deprenyl lived an average of 15.3 months longer than those who were treated only with conventional levodopa. While this trial – like all trials – was subject to criticism (e.g. there were substantial demographic differences in the two groups of patients in age when commencing treatment, in the interval between diagnosis and treatment and indeed in the mean dose of levodopa in each group) it was suggested that L-deprenyl retarded dopaminergic neurone degeneration. This concept and its therapeutic possibilities provoked great interest but also some uncritical and unbridled enthusiasm.

A major multicentred trial was initiated in the USA by the Parkinson's Study Group to try and determine whether deprenyl and also vitamin E (an agent that may trap free radicals) might favourably influence the natural history of early Parkinson's disease [7]. The results were awaited with considerable interest. Initially it was claimed that 10 mg of L-deprenyl a day, but not vitamin E (2000 IU of α-tocopherol), delayed the onset of disability associated with early, otherwise untreated Parkinson's disease.

Unfortunately this trial was planned without sufficient consideration being given to the symptomatic benefits of neat L-dopa, an observation well established in Europe before the USA study was initiated. Clearly it is extremely difficult if not impossible to measure a protective effect when the agent under scrutiny has a symptomatic benefit. This difficulty was admirably analyzed in a penetrating and – exceptional for a learned scientific paper – amusing study by Landau [8] entitled 'Clinical neuromythology. Pyramid sale in a bucket shop: DATATOP bottoms out'. Understandably this critique promoted lively responses from enthusiasts and sceptics and those who followed the field could barely wait for the next edition of the neurological journal concerned to read the correspondence.

The problem was tackled in a scholarly manner by another group of clinical pharmacologists: 'Can we differentiate symptomatic and neuroprotective effects in parkinsonism?' and the authors' conclusion was 'No' [9]. In the past year even the most fervent advocates of the L-deprenyl-protection hypothesis appear to be losing their enthusiasm and are beginning to concede that the greater part if not all of the beneficial response must be due to symptomatic relief of parkinsonian symptoms and not due to neuronal sparing.

What then is the current view about the value of L-deprenyl in the management of Parkinson's disease? It is well tolerated, side-effects are few, and when given to patients with early Parkinson's disease about 50% will report some benefit. The remainder show no change in symptoms or signs and if so there is no convincing evidence to justify continuation of the drug at this stage of the illness. If the disease becomes more advanced and a decision is made that it is now necessary to introduce levodopa in one of its several forms, it could then be argued that the addition of L-deprenyl could be justified because of its levodopa-sparing effect. However, if the addition of L-deprenyl to a levodopa regimen failed to produce unequivocal benefit appreciated by the patient in a practical sense, the justification for giving L-deprenyl indefinitely should be seriously questioned. Not only are the issues of polypharmacy and degree of therapeutic value to be considered, but in these days of increasing economic frugality all long-term medications must be scrutinized.

PRESENT PROBLEMS

Predicted prevalence of the illness, allowing for increasing life expectation, indicates that there will be more patients presenting with Parkinson's disease with commensurate pressures – clinical, pharmaceutical and social – upon diminishing resources. For the time being our task is limited to exploiting with optimal efficiency the available medications. This is determined not only by clinical results when therapeutic principles continue to be worthwhile: improvement in disabilities with smallest amounts of the fewest drugs and the least side-effects and, increasingly careful consideration of cost. The disadvantages of polypharmacy have often been prosyletized in this College; in the management of Parkinson's disease we are considering not weeks or months of therapy, but years and decades. It is still difficult not to incur Voltaire's stricture that 'doctors prescribe medicines of which they know very little to patients of whom they know even less'.

Levodopa combined with a peripheral decarboxylase inhibitor is now available in a number of different preparations. In some, controlled-release technology has been employed to effect a slower rise and fall of plasma levodopa levels with a blunter dose–response peak curve [10], in the hope of diminishing dyskinesia and even reducing dose frequency and 'off' phases. Only a minority of patients with 'end-of-dose' akinesia report significant improvement and after a trial they usually opt for conventional preparations. In addition there is a group of dopamine agonists including bromocriptine, lisuride, cabergoline and apomorphine which are usually used as adjuvants to conventional oral levodopa therapy to try and obtain a smoother control of fluctuating symptoms. This field of therapeutic endeavour has received much attention in recent years and many differing claims for the superiority of one treatment regimen over another have been made.

Our experience in the UK [11] suggests that when overall control of disabilities and survival from time of initiating treatment are the determining criteria, there is little to choose between conventional oral levodopa with a peripheral decarboxylase inhibitor with or without a monoamine oxidase B inhibitor (L-deprenyl) and (for those who are able to tolerate it) neat bromocriptine in an effective dose. It seems that whatever treatment is prescribed *ab initio* the illness continues to progress at very much the same rate. Currently there is interest in the possible advantages of a treatment strategy in which conventional levodopa is first given and the dose is not increased as the illness progresses, but instead a small dose of an agonist is added. This combined low-dose strategy [12] is based upon the expectation that fewer early and late complications of therapy will emerge. This has yet to be proved [13] and if there is an advantage, the degree of benefit and its financial implications will have to be judiciously evaluated.

One modest advance in the control of those patients with very severe 'on–off' fluctuations has been the reintroduction of apomorphine – it was first proposed by Weil in 1884 that it might have a role in the treatment of Parkinson's disease – in subcutaneous form. When given by intermittent injections or continuous subcutaneous infusion utilizing the techniques of insulin therapy it is possible to diminish significantly – by at least 50% – the number of 'off' hours when patients are severely disabled [14]. Experience indicates that this improvement can be sustained for beyond 7 years.

THE FUTURE

Leaving aside the intricacies of day-to-day management of the illness and its complications, in recent years we have witnessed burgeoning interest into possible causes of the illness [15] and to what extent these might be congenital or environmental. Considerable publicity with the usual media hyperbole has been addressed to the potential of foetal implants of dopamine-producing cells into the damaged nigrostriatal system of patients with severe Parkinson's disease [16]. While these strategies are exciting and unquestionably replete with potential, the results reported so far indicate that transplant surgery for the treatment of Parkinson's disease remains experimental and there are still no signs that such measures in the predictable future will become part of routine medical practice. These approaches raise many exciting questions including factors determining graft viability, immunological privilege, the mechanisms of improvement, patient selection, and concern as to whether initially surviving implanted cells will later become vulnerable to the same unknown factors responsible for the deteriorating idiopathic disease.

At this stage clinical neurologists usually recall James Parkinson's needlessly modest apology for writing his essay: 'The writer will repine at no censure which the precipitate publication of mere conjectural suggestions may incur; but shall think himself fully rewarded by having excited the attention of those who may point out the most appropriate means of relieving a tedious and most distressing malady.' Despite all the achievements of the past three decades, James Parkinson's description of the nature of this illness remains true.

REFERENCES

1 Clark G. *A History of the Royal College of Physicians of London*, Vol. 2. Oxford: Clarendon Press, 1966:614–650.
2 Parkinson J. *An Essay on the Shaking Palsy*. London: Sherwood Neely & Jones, 1817.
3 Ehringer H, Hornykiewicz O. Verteilung von Noradrenalin und Dopamin (3-hydroxytyramin) im Gehirn des Menschen und ihr Verhalten bis Erkrankungen des extrapyramidalen Systems. *Klin Wschr* 1960;38:1236–1240.
4 Bernheimer H, Birkmayer W, Hornykiewicz O. Vertelung des 5-hydroxytryptamins (Serotonin) im Gehirm des Menschen und sein Verhalten bei Patienten mit Parkinson-Syndrom. *Klin Wschr* 1961;39:1056–1059.
5 Marsden CD, Parkes JD. 'On–off' effects in patients with Parkinson's disease on chronic levodopa therapy. *Lancet* 1976;i:292–296.
6 Birkmayer W, Knoll J, Riederer P, *et al.* Increased life expectancy resulting from addition of L-deprenyl to Madopar treatment in Parkinson's disease: a long-term study. *J Neural Transm* 1985;64:113–127.
7 Effect of deprenyl on the progression of disability in early Parkinson's disease. Parkinson's Study Group; *N Engl J Med* 1989;321:1364–1371.
8 Landau WM. Clinical neuromythology IX. Pyramid sale in a bucket shop: DATATOP bottoms out. *Neurology* 1990;40:1337–1339.
9 Runge I, Horowski R. Can we differentiate symptomatic and neuroprotective effects in Parkinsonism? *J Neural Transm* 1991;4:273–283.
10 Poewe WH, Lees AJ, Stern GM. Treatment of motor fluctuations in Parkinson's disease with an oral sustained-release preparation of L-dopa: clinical and pharmacological observations. *Clin Neuropharmacol* 1987;9:430–439.
11 Parkinson's Disease Research Group in the United Kingdom. Comparisons of therapeutic effects of levodopa; levodopa and selegiline; and bromocriptine treatment regimens in early, mild Parkinson's disease: three year interim report. *Br Med J* 1993;307: 469–472.
12 Rinne UK. Early combination of bromocriptine and levodopa in the treatment of Parkinson's disease: a 5 year follow-up. *Neurology* 1987;37:826–828.
13 Weiner WJ, Factor SA, Sanchez-Ramos JR, *et al.* Early combination therapy (bromocriptine and levodopa) does not prevent motor fluctuations in Parkinson's disease. *Neurology* 1993;43:21–27.
14 Stibe CMH, Kempster PA, Lees AJ, Stern GM. Subcutaneous apomorphine in parkinsonian on–off oscillations. *Lancet* 1988;i:403–406.
15 Jenner P, Schapira AHV, Marsden CD. New insights into the cause of Parkinson's disease. *Neurology* 1992;42:2241–2250.
16 Fahn S. Fetal-tissue transplants in Parkinson's disease. *N Engl J Med* 1992;327:1589–1590.

Update on muscular dystrophy

V. DUBOWITZ

INTRODUCTION

When I first became interested in muscle diseases in the late 1950s, one could probably give an update of all the neuromuscular disorders in the course of one lecture. Now one cannot really do full justice even to a single disease such as Duchenne dystrophy, following the explosive advances made by the application of molecular genetics in the past few years and the rapidly continuing further evolution. Within a space of little more than 10 years we have seen the transition from the localization, isolation and characterization of the gene through the recognition of its previously unknown protein, dystrophin, to a stage where there is already a dramatic momentum aimed at potential treatment with gene therapy or cell therapy.

THE CLINICAL PHENOTYPE

It is over 130 years since Duchenne gave his classical description of the severe childhood form of muscular dystrophy, which is well characterized and readily recognized. These children have a relentlessly progressive weakness with clinical onset usually around the time they start walking and loss of ambulation before their thirteenth birthday.

On the other hand the milder type of dystrophy, Becker dystrophy, is of relatively recent recognition although undoubtedly existing for many years before. It has a similar distribution of weakness to Duchenne dystrophy, and in fact looks like a photocopy of Duchenne, but is less severe and has a more protracted course. By definition one would expect Becker dystrophy patients to remain ambulant beyond the age of 16. This helps to segregate the two clinical phenotypes from each other, which is helpful from both a diagnostic and prognostic point of view. One can also recognize intermediate cases that bridge the gap between the two defined phenotypes and lose ambulation between 14 and 16 years.

Following the localization of the Duchenne gene to the Xp21 position on the short arm of the X chromosome, it was then shown that the gene for Becker dystrophy in fact was located at the same locus, so that these were not separate muscle disorders but due to alleles of the same gene.

THE MOLECULAR GENETICS

The gene for muscular dystrophy is a gigantic one with over two million base pairs. It encodes a very large protein, named dystrophin because of its association with muscular dystrophy, which is over 400 kDa in size and is intimately attached to the inner aspect of the sarcolemmal membrane of the muscle fibre.

One of the early questions to resolve was the remarkable variability in clinical phenotype related to this single gene with some cases of Duchenne dystrophy losing the ability to walk as early as 6 or 7 years and at the other extreme some patients with Becker dystrophy remaining ambulant into their 60s. Once complementary DNA (cDNA) probes became widely available from Kunkel's laboratory at Harvard, it soon became apparent that deletions in the gene were commonly present. It was initially anticipated that possibly the location of these deletions or their size might relate to the clinical severity but it soon became apparent that very large deletions (even up to 50% of the total gene) might occur in association with very mild disorder and similarly deletions in various regions of the gene did not necessarily relate to consistent clinical phenotype.

The important point was not the size or location of the deletion but whether the residual bases after removal of the deletion were still inframe or not, as described by Monaco [1]. Thus, if the residual nucleotides remain inframe, the triplet codons can still code for amino acids and produce a functional protein which may be smaller in size but is still functional. On the other hand if the deletion is out of frame, this results in a stop codon and a functional protein can then not be produced. With few exceptions this theory has proved to hold good for well over 90% of cases. The exceptions have mainly been out of frame deletions, particularly in one or two regions of the gene, which have still been associated with a milder phenotype and where alternative compensatory mechanisms have been operative to overcome the effect of the frame shift.

DYSTROPHIN

The expression of dystrophin in the muscle has also proved useful from a diagnostic point of view and in general also to correlate with the prognosis. As a general rule dystrophin is completely absent in cases of the Duchenne type dystrophy and present in the milder Becker forms, although either reduced in size or amount. The dystrophin can be assessed both biochemically using Western blot analysis or immunocytochemically with demonstration in tissue sections. The latter also illustrates the variability between individual fibres.

Of importance in the context of the dystrophin studies is to use antibodies to different parts of the molecule, in order to get information on both ends of the protein as well as some of the intermediate parts. This is particularly so in cases that may have a large deletion, where an antibody related to the deleted area would give a negative result whereas antibodies to other parts of the protein might be positive.

These major advances rapidly opened the way for accurate carrier detection in families with affected boys and also for prenatal diagnosis on chorionic villus biopsy early in pregnancy. There was also understandably a rapid wave of optimism, among both the scientists and the affected families, about the possibility of therapeutic advances.

ANIMAL MODELS OF X-LINKED Xp21 DYSTROPHIES

A number of animal models of the Xp21 dystrophies have been identified in recent years and provided an immediate avenue of research, from both an investigative and a therapeutic point of view.

The mdx mouse

An X-linked dystrophy in the mouse was picked up purely by chance during a mutagenesis screen of serum enzymes [2]. Following a period of necrosis of the muscle at about 2–3 weeks of age there is active regeneration and recovery and the mouse then remains essentially normal and has a normal lifespan [3]. The gene for the mouse dystrophy is homologous to the human dystrophin gene [4], and dystrophin is also absent in the mdx mouse muscle [5]. It has recently been shown that the genetic abnormality is a point mutation at nucleotide position 3185, with the replacement of the nucleotide cytosine by a thymine, resulting in a termination codon (TAA) in place of a glutamine codon (CAA) [6].

The xmd dog

An X-linked muscular dystrophy has been discovered in a Golden Retriever strain of dog which is also genetically homologous to the human disease and lacks dystrophin in the muscle [7,8]. Clinically the dog manifests a severe weakness with an early onset and steady progression, comparable to the Duchenne type. From an early stage there is also marked wasting of the muscles, but none of the prominence and apparent enlargement of the muscles one sees in the human disease. The histological picture is identical to that in Duchenne dystrophy, including the early proliferation of endomysial connective tissue. Selective involvement of some muscles at an earlier stage than others has been demonstrated in the neonatal period [9], comparable to the selective involvement from an early stage in Duchenne dystrophy.

THERAPEUTIC POSSIBILITIES

Given the large size of dystrophin and its intimate connection with the muscle membrane, it seemed highly unlikely that it was going to be possible to replace the deficient protein or to find some biochemical means of compensating for its function, which is still not fully understood. The alternative approach of gene therapy also posed major hurdles in relation to handling such a gigantic gene, with over two million base pairs, way beyond the capacity of vectors such as retroviruses. On top of all this there was still the problem of how to target the gene or its product to the widely distributed musculature.

Somatic cell therapy (myoblast transfer) seemed to offer a possible shortcut for delivering the normal gene or its product direct to the muscle. It entailed transplanting normal muscle cells directly into the diseased muscle, with a view to obtaining fusion of the donor myoblasts with host myoblasts, the so-called satellite cells, which are normally quiescent in muscle until activated to proliferate, divide and fuse. This should then produce a mixture of dystrophin-positive and dystrophin-negative fibres, comparable to the heterozygote female carrier of the Duchenne gene.

In a key experiment, Partridge *et al.* [10] were able to demonstrate that direct injection of myoblasts from dissociated normal neonatal muscle into the muscle of an mdx/nude mouse produced dystrophin-positive fibres. However, only a very small proportion of these immunodeficient mice had a significant degree of fusion of donor host myoblasts and in addition could be shown to express the dystrophin in a significant number of fibres. The authors thus expressed some caution in trying to extrapolate this to therapeutic applications in relation to the human disease.

There were obviously major problems in trying to extend this study, based on a very small muscle in an immunodeficient mouse, to the human disease, with its very large muscles, or to the dystrophic dog, which was much more comparable to the human disease both pathologically and clinically than the mouse. In a similar approach, Karpati *et al.* [11] introduced suspensions of cultured normal human myoblasts into the quadriceps muscle of mdx mice and were able to demonstrate clusters of dystrophin-positive fibres comprising about 5% of fibres.

In order to define a strategy for potential myoblast therapy the

American Muscular Dystrophy Association organized a workshop in June 1989 aimed at providing a scientific basis for clinical trials of myoblast transfer therapy [12]. Despite the words of constraint expressed by several contributors to this workshop, a number of centres, perhaps fired still by a sense of optimism in the potential of the technique and perhaps also feeling the pressures from the parents of these children, opted for experiments on the Duchenne disease itself.

In the most comprehensive study to date Karpati *et al.* [13] in Montreal recruited into a double-blind study eight young boys with Duchenne dystrophy, all of whom had a deletion in the gene and absence of dystrophin in the muscle. Ten million cultured myoblasts from the father's muscle, of proven purity by cell sorting, were injected into each of 55 sites in one biceps, whereas a comparable injection, but without myoblasts, was made into the other biceps as a control. Neither patient nor personnel were aware which side was which. Immunosuppression was provided with cyclophosphamide. The power of the muscle was assessed by sequential myometry and the dystrophin status of the muscle on repeat biopsy at 3 and 12 months by Western blot and immunocytochemistry. At the end of a 1 year follow-up, there were no significant differences between the two sides in the individual cases at either a clinical level or in the dystrophin status.

In an uncontrolled study, Tremblay *et al.* [14] in Quebec performed myoblast transfer with repeated injections into several different muscles in four advanced, non-ambulant, cases of Duchenne dystrophy. Meticulous attention was paid to histocompatibility of the donor and recipient for HLA classes I and II-DR. No immunosuppression was used. In one case the donor was a brother, in the other three sisters, including one Duchenne carrier. Three of the four patients were shown to form antibodies against the donor's myotubes. Muscle biopsies of the injected tibialis anterior showed some degree of dystrophin immunostaining in 80%, 75%, 25% and 0% respectively of the muscle fibres, and in the contralateral uninjected muscle in 16% of the first case and none in the other three.

In another phase 1 study, Law *et al.* [15] in Memphis, Tennessee, injected 8 million cultured myoblasts into eight foci in the extensor digitorum brevis muscle of the foot in three boys with Duchenne dystrophy, obtained from a 1 g biopsy from the father or brother. In the first patient, the donor was the non-biological adoptive father. A comparable volume of carrier fluid without myoblasts was sham-injected into the other side. In the second and third patients this was double-blinded. After 3 months there was an increase in twitch tension, measured in the flexor hallucis longus, in the myoblast-injected side compared with a reduction on the sham-injected side. Bilateral open biopsy showed the presence of dystrophin by immunoblot and immunocytochemistry on the myoblast-injected side only. Eight further patients were also included in this study but were not analyzed.

Fired by the success of this limited series of experiments, Law established a Cell Therapy Research Foundation and proceeded to his phase 2 therapeutic trials of myoblast transfer into several major muscles in Duchenne dystrophy. He recently reported the results of a 3-month follow-up on 18 of their 21 phase 2 cases, which included the 11 from the phase 1 study [16]. Five billion cultured, normal myoblasts were transferred via 48 intramuscular injections into 22 major muscles of both lower limbs. Immunosuppression was provided by cyclosporin. Dynamometer measurements of the isometric tension in the knee flexors, knee extensors and plantar flexors before and 3 months after myoblast transfer in 18 subjects showed a mean increase of 41% in 30 of the total 69 muscle groups measured, no change in 26, and a reduction of 23% in 13. Interpretation of these statistics is difficult, given the short period of follow-up and the uncontrolled nature of the study. When Law presented these results at the first meeting of the newly established Society of Cell Transplantation in June 1992, he came under considerable fire from his scientific colleagues about the validity of his data in such an uncontrolled study [17].

Blau and colleagues [18] in Stanford studied the tibialis anterior muscle from eight cases of Duchenne dystrophy, with a documented deletion in the dystrophin gene, 1 month after the injection of 100 million cultured myoblasts into 80–100 injection sites. In three of the eight patients they were able to show by polymerase chain reaction the expression of dystrophin messenger RNA (mRNA) derived from the donor myoblast DNA. Given the extreme sensitivity of the polymerase chain reaction technique, this result presumably reflects the persistence at 1 month of donor DNA from a few of the implanted myoblasts. Immunocyto-chemically the number of dystrophin-positive fibres was only about 10 per 1000 fibres counted, which was no greater than the frequency of spontaneously occurring dystrophin-positive 'revertant' fibres in some of the control side muscles. Although *Nature* hailed this as a 'Transplant Success' in its contents page, from a clinical point of view it is no more than a fleabite in the ocean and an unequivocal therapeutic failure.

Comparative studies of myoblast transfer in 11 dystrophic dogs have also proved negative on the basis of conversion to dystrophin-positive fibres (Dux, Sewry, Cooper and Dubowitz, unpublished observations).

ANIMAL EXPERIMENTAL STUDIES

Meanwhile there have been a number of interesting developments in relation to more fundamental studies in animals. A detailed study of the regenerative potential of the dystrophic muscle in 6-month-old dogs, following toxin-induced necrosis, has shown this to be comparable to that of normal muscle [19]. This at least suggests that Duchenne muscle should potentially be capable of regeneration.

Another recent approach to therapy has been to try and introduce the gene directly into muscle. In an interesting experiment, Wolff *et al.* [20] demonstrated that injection of plasmid DNA directly into rodent skeletal muscle expressed reporter genes such as β-galactosidase or luciferase, suggesting one might be able to circumvent the need for viral or other vectors for the DNA. In a similar study, Wolff *et al.* have recently shown that non-human, primate muscle is also able to take up and express intramuscularly injected plasmid DNA, but the level of expression of luciferase was considerably lower than in rodent muscle [21]. This does not augur well for this approach in human muscle.

Meanwhile, a number of laboratories have now succeeded in producing constructs of the 12 kb full-length human dystrophin cDNA gene, containing all the 70-odd exons necessary for protein production. This provided the possibility for attempting to introduce the dystrophin gene into the muscle cell.

Lee *et al.* [22] were able to introduce DNA constructs of mouse dystrophin into cultured COS cells (a kidney cell line) which then expressed dystrophin, thought to be membrane bound, in about 3–5% of cultured cells. Acsadi *et al.* [23] were subsequently able to show that either a 12 kb full-length human dystrophin cDNA gene or a 6.3 kb minigene, derived from a Becker patient with a large deletion of the gene, could be expressed in cultured cells or *in vivo*. When human dystrophin expression plasmids were injected intramuscularly into dystrophin-deficient mdx mice, the human dystrophin was present in about 1% of myofibres. From a purely technical point of view, this was a further important step in demonstrating that dystrophin could be expressed either *in vivo* or by transfection of cultured myoblasts *in vitro*. However, in spite of the wide exposure of this 'breakthrough' in both the scientific and lay press, this is still a far cry from producing any clinical benefit and it is rather frustrating that none of these sophisticated studies have surpassed nature's spontaneous correction of the defect in individual muscle fibres in Duchenne dystrophy or the mdx mouse – the so-called 'revertant' fibres. Furthermore, the mdx mouse, with its normal clinical phenotype, cannot tell us whether the dystrophin expressed is functional and therapeutically viable, and comparable experiments will have to be done in the dystrophic dog or the dystrophic human, once a greater yield of dystrophin-positive fibres can be achieved.

A number of basic questions in relation to the transplant experiments still remain to be answered. These concern the myogenicity of the grafted cells and their potential for further division and fusion; the migration of the grafted cells and their ability to cross the sarcolemmal membrane of host fibres; the control of immune rejection of the donor cells; the stability with time of converted muscle fibres; and the definition of a threshold for functional restoration of these corrected fibres.

So where do we stand in relation to myoblast transfer in Duchenne dystrophy? Could the essentially negative results merely reflect the birth pangs reminiscent of earlier transplantation procedures such as kidney, bone marrow and heart? Simple technical problems may explain the failure, which further studies could resolve. Alternatively, cell transfer may turn out to be a non-starter in the treatment of muscular dystrophy, and other experimental approaches, such as introducing gene constructs either directly into the muscle [20] or using viral vectors, may need to be pursued further. Meanwhile, it is imperative that the Duchenne boys are given optimal supportive care, including the provision of orthoses to maintain ambulation and also other potential therapeutic agents.

STEROIDS IN MUSCULAR DYSTROPHY

Of all the drugs that have fallen by the wayside over the years the only one that still seems to be holding its own is prednisolone [24,25]. Some 20 years ago, in an uncontrolled study of 14 Duchenne patients, Drachman *et al.* [26] concluded that steroids might have some palliative value and that further trials were indicated. It was 13 years before Brooke *et al.* took up the challenge [27]. In a multicentric study of 33 cases of Duchenne dystrophy, aged 5–15 years (12 of whom were unable to walk independently), they found a definite improvement in muscle function on prednisolone, at a dose of 1.5 mg per kg per day for 6 months, in comparison with the natural history of 170 historical controls from their earlier studies.

Brooke *et al.* [28] subsequently undertook two steroid dosage levels (0.75 and 1.5 mg per kg per day) with placebo. They found a definite increase in muscle strength in the two prednisone groups compared to the control at 1, 2 and 3 months, after which the strength levelled off. The rate of loss of muscle strength in the control group was similar to the natural history of the disease. They concluded, however, that the relatively short-lived beneficial effect on the muscle strength was outweighed by the not inconsiderable side-effects of prolonged steroid therapy, and did not at the time feel able to recommend steroids as a general long-term therapy for muscular dystrophy.

In a further multicentric study [29], a randomized controlled trial of daily prednisone was undertaken in 99 boys with Duchenne dystrophy, aged 5–15 years, in order to define the time course of improvement and the dose response to treatment. Prednisone at 0.75 mg per kg (n = 34), 0.3 mg per kg (n = 33) or placebo (n = 32) were given for 6 months. As early as 10 days after commencing treatment, there was a significantly higher average muscle strength score in the two groups on prednisone treatment, compared to the placebo. This improvement increased at 1 month and then reached a plateau that persisted for 6 months and contrasted with the placebo group that became steadily weaker. At 3 months the boys in the 0.75 mg per kg group showed a significantly better muscle strength than those at 0.3 mg per kg, indicating a dose response. At 10 days and 1 month of treatment there were no side-effects of the prednisone, despite improvement in muscle strength and function. At 6 months, there were significant side-effects in the group on 0.75 mg per kg, including weight gain, cushingoid appearance and excessive hair growth, whereas the 0.3 mg per kg group showed only weight gain.

An attempt was made to maintain 89 boys from these multicentric trials on continued therapy for a year or longer [30]. At the end of a year, 49 were taking at least 0.65 mg per kg per day and 40 a greater dose. The rate of decline in average muscle score (0.017 U per year) was significantly better in the first group than in the lower dosage (0.164 U per year) ($P = 0.002$) and both did better than natural history controls (0.4 U per year).

In a further controlled trial, Griggs *et al.* [31] randomized 99 boys with Duchenne dystrophy, aged 5–15 years, into one of three groups: (i) placebo; (ii) prednisone 0.3 mg per kg per day; (iii) prednisone 0.75 mg per kg per day. After 6 months azathioprine was added in groups i and ii and placebo in group iii. As in their earlier studies, the results showed an increase in muscle strength on prednisone within 10 days. It was significantly greater with 0.75 mg per kg per day and reached a maximum at 3 months and then plateaued. The beneficial effect was maintained over the 18 months of this prednisone therapy but there were significant side-effects, particularly weight gain and growth retardation. Azathioprine had no effect on muscle strength. The authors now conclude that prednisone is of sufficient benefit to be recommended for ambulatory patients over age 5, and continued if side-effects are not severe.

Statistics are of obvious importance these days to get papers published in scientific journals, but from a clinical point of view, it is difficult to translate into actual functional benefit for the individual patient the statistically significant rise from 5.7 to 6.0 in the average muscle strength score of the whole cohort of Griggs *et al.* [31], based on the assessment of 34 muscle groups on a 10-point Medical Research Council grading. On the other hand it is extremely impressive that the score remained static over the 18 month period of treatment, compared with a decline of about 0.4 points in the placebo group, and could presumably continue to remain stable on continued treatment.

In addition to the gain in muscle strength, parallel studies in these various trials also showed an increase in muscle mass, based on creatine excretion, and a fall in the rate of muscle breakdown, based on a decreased excretion of 3-methyl histidine. There was no increase in the expression of dystrophin in the muscle or reduction in the number of necrotic fibres, but there was a significant reduction in the total number of T cells (CD2+), and selectively of the subsets of CD8+ cytotoxic suppressor T cells [32]. This suggests that the beneficial effect of prednisone might be through suppression of the immune attack on necrotic fibres.

Although muscular dystrophy is not normally considered an immunological disorder, there is considerable evidence that both humoral and cellular immune responses contribute to the pathological process. Although it has been recognized for years that necrotic fibres in muscular dystrophy were invaded by macrophages, Arahata and Engel [33] showed with selective monoclonal antibodies that many of these mononuclear cells are in fact cytotoxic T cells. In addition, complement activation with deposition of membrane attack complex is observed on necrotic fibres [34]. Furthermore, it has been found that human leucocyte antigen class I antigens are expressed in Duchenne dystrophy fibres, as in polymyositis, but not in normal muscle [35,36]. This would render the dystrophic muscle susceptible to T-cell-mediated attack. If prednisone proves to be beneficial in arresting the disease process on a long-term basis, it might be worth trying alternative therapeutic regimens aimed at achieving the benefits but avoiding the side-effects, such as an intermittent schedule of prednisone at 0.75 mg per kg per day for say 10 days each month [37].

AUTOSOMAL RECESSIVE DUCHENNE-LIKE MUSCULAR DYSTROPHY

Of special interest is the group of children with muscular dystrophy equivalent in severity to the Duchenne type but affecting both males and females and inherited through a recessive pattern. In these cases the dystrophin in the muscle is normal, suggesting that other proteins may have a similar effect on the muscle to the dystrophin itself. This has recently been resolved in one particular group of patients with a severe autosomal recessive disorder which is particularly frequent in North Africa. In recent years Campbell and his group [38,39] have demonstrated that there are a number of glycoproteins which are intimately linked to dystrophin and are involved with its attachment to the muscle membrane. The glycoproteins span the membrane and in turn link up with laminin on the outer side of the membrane. Presumably this complex helps to maintain the stability of the muscle membrane.

A recent study of these various dystrophin-associated glycoproteins ('DAGs') has revealed that one particular one (the 50 kDa) is selectively absent in relation to this particular dystrophy [38]. It has also been shown that in Duchenne dystrophy there is a general reduction of all four of these associated glycoproteins, which is probably secondary to the absence of the dystrophin itself. Campbell [38,39] has postulated that these glycoproteins may perhaps be of more importance in the actual pathogenesis of the progressive destruction of the muscle fibre than the dystrophin itself and may be a common denominator of a number of different disorders that may be associated with the dystrophin/glycoprotein complex.

A protein with a very close analogy to dystrophin but having an autosomal genetic control has been located to chromosome 6 by Davies and colleagues [40] and named dystrophin-related protein or utrophin (derived from 'ubiquitous' dystrophin). It is not expressed in the sarcolemmal membrane of normal muscle and to date there has not yet been a single form of dystrophy or related muscle disorder that has been shown to be associated with an absence of this particular protein, in spite of a very extensive search. However, in some instances, such as Duchenne dystrophy, there seems to be an upregulation of the dystrophin-related protein in the sarcolemmal membrane, in the absence of dystrophin, so that it may possibly have some compensatory effect in relation to disorders affecting the dystrophin/glycoprotein complex itself. There is much still to be learned from future research.

REFERENCES

1 Monaco AP, Bertelson CJ, Liechti-Fallati S, *et al.* An explanation for the phenotypic differences between patients bearing partial deletions of the DMD locus. *Genomics* 1989;2:90–95.

2 Bulfield G, Siller WG, Wight PAL, Moore KJ. X chromosome-linked muscular dystrophy (mdx) in the mouse. *Proc Natl Acad Sci USA* 1984;81:1189–1192.

3 Dangain J, Vrbova G. Muscle development in mdx mutant mice. *Muscle Nerve* 1984;7:700–704.

4 Hoffman EP, Monaco AP, Feener CC, Kunkel LM. Conservation of the Duchenne muscular dystrophy gene in mice and humans. *Science* 1987;238:347–350.

5 Hoffman EP, Brown RH, Kunkel LM. Dystrophin: the protein product of the Duchenne muscular dystrophy locus. *Cell* 1987;51:919–928.

6 Sicinski P, Geng Y, Ryder-Cook AS, *et al.* The molecular basis of muscular dystrophy in the mdx mouse: a point mutation. *Science* 1989;244:1578–1580.

7 Valentine BA, Cooper BJ, Cummings JF, de Lahunta A. Progressive muscular dystrophy in a golden retriever dog: light microscope and ultrastructural features at 4 and 8 months. *Acta Neuropathol* 1986;7:301–310.

8 Cooper BJ, Winand NJ, Stedman H, *et al.* The homologue of the Duchenne locus is defective in X-linked muscular dystrophy of dogs. *Nature* 1988;334:154–156.

9 Valentine BA, Cooper BJ. Canine X-linked muscular dystrophy: selective involvement of muscles in neonatal dogs. *Neuromusc Disord* 1991;1:31–38.

10 Partridge TA, Morgan JE, Coulton GR, *et al.* Conversion of mdx myofibres from dystrophin-negative to positive by injection of normal myoblasts. *Nature* 1989;337: 176–179.

11 Karpati G, Pouliot Y, Zubrzycka-Gaarn E, *et al.* Dystrophin is expressed in mdx skeletal muscle fibres after normal myoblast implantation. *Am J Pathol* 1989;134: 27–32.

12 Griggs RC, Karpati G (eds). Myoblast Transfer Therapy. *Advances in Experimental Medicine and Biology*, Vol. 280. New York: Plenum Press, 1990.
13 Karpati G, Ajdukovic D, Arnold D, *et al.* Myoblast transfer in Duchenne muscular dystrophy. *Ann Neurol* 1993;34:8–17.
14 Huard J, Bouchard JP, Roy R, *et al.* Human myoblast transplantation: preliminary results of 4 cases. *Muscle Nerve* 1992;15:550–560.
15 Law PK, Goodwin TG, Fang Q, *et al.* Pioneering development of myoblast transfer therapy. In: Angelini C, Danieli CA, Fontanari D, eds. *Muscular Dystrophy Research: From Molecular Diagnosis Toward Therapy*. Amsterdam: Excerpta Medica, 1991.
16 Law PK, Goodwin TG, Fang Q, *et al.* Feasibility, safety, and efficacy of myoblast transfer therapy on Duchenne muscular dystrophy boys. *Cell Transplant* 1992;1: 235–244.
17 Thompson L. Cell transplant results under fire. *Science* 1992;257:472–474.
18 Gussoni E, Pavlath GK, Lanctot AM, *et al.* Normal dystrophin transcripts detected in Duchenne muscular dystrophy patients after myoblast transplantation. *Nature* 1992; 356:435–438.
19 Sewry CA, Wilson LA, Dux L, *et al.* Experimental regeneration in canine muscular dystrophy. 1. Immunocytochemical evaluation of dystrophin and β-spectrin. *Neuromusc Disord* 1992;2:331–342.
20 Wolff JA, Malone RW, Williams P, *et al.* Direct gene transfer into muscle in vivo. *Science* 1990;247:1465–1468.
21 Jiao S, Williams P, Berg RK, *et al.* Direct gene transfer into nonhuman primate myofibres in vivo. *Human Gene Therapy* 1992;3:21–33.
22 Lee CC, Pearlman JA, Chamberlain JS, Caskey CT. Expression of recombinant dystrophin and its localisation to the cell membrane. *Nature* 1991;349:334–336.
23 Acsadi G, Dickson G, Love DR, *et al.* Human dystrophin expression in mdx mice after intramuscular injection of DNA constructs. *Nature* 1991;352:815–818.
24 Dubowitz V, Heckmatt J. Management of muscular dystrophy. *Br Med Bull* 1980; 36:139–144.
25 Heckmatt J, Rodillo E, Dubowitz V. Management of children: pharmacological and physical. *Br Med Bull* 1989;45:788–801.
26 Drachman DB, Toyka KV, Myer E. Prednisone in Duchenne muscular dystrophy. *Lancet* 1974;ii:1409–1412.
27 Brooke MH, Fenichel GM, Griggs RC, *et al.* Clinical investigation of Duchenne muscular dystrophy: interesting results in a trial of prednisone. *Arch Neurol* 1987;44: 812–817.
28 Mendell JR, Moxley RT, Griggs RC, *et al.* Randomised double-blind six month trial of prednisone in Duchenne's muscular dystrophy. *N Engl J Med* 1989;320:1592–1597.
29 Griggs RC, Moxley RT, Mendell JR, *et al.* Prednisone in Duchenne dystrophy. A randomised, controlled trial defining the time course and dose response. *Arch Neurol* 1991;48:383–388.
30 Fenichel GM, Florence J, Pestronk A, *et al.* Prednisone slows strength decline in Duchenne muscular dystrophy: two year observation. *Neurology* 1991;41(Suppl 1):166 (Abstract).
31 Griggs RC, Moxley RT, Mendell JR, *et al.* Duchenne dystrophy: Randomised, controlled trial of prednisone (18 months) and azathioprine (12 months). *Neurology* 1993; 43:520–527.
32 Kissel JT, Burrow K, Rammohan KW, Mendell JR, CIDD Group. Mononuclear cell analysis of muscle biopsies in prednisone-treated and untreated Duchenne muscular dystrophy. *Neurology* 1991;41:667–672.
33 Arahata K, Engel AG. Monoclonal antibody analysis of mononuclear cells in myopathies. I: Quantitation of subsets according to diagnosis and sites of accumulation and demonstration and counts of muscle fibers invaded by T-cells. *Ann Neurol* 1984;16: 193–208.
34 Engel AG, Beisecker G. Complement activation in muscle fiber necrosis: demonstration of the membrane attack complex of complement in necrotic fibers. *Ann Neurol* 1982;12: 289–296.

35 Appleyard ST, Dunn MJ, Dubowitz V, *et al.* Increased expression of HLA-ABC Class I antigens by muscle fibres in Duchenne muscular dystrophy, inflammatory myopathy, and other neuromuscular disorders. *Lancet* 1985;i:361–363.
36 Engel AG, Arahata K, Emslie-Smith AM, *et al.* Immune effector mechanisms in inflammatory myopathies. *Res Publ Assoc Res Nerv Ment Dis* 1990;68:141–157.
37 Dubowitz V. Prednisone in Duchenne dystrophy. *Neuromusc Disord* 1991;1:161–163.
38 Matsumara K, Tome FMS, Collin H, *et al.* Deficiency of the 50K dystrophin-associated glycoprotein in severe childhood autosomal recessive muscular dystrophy. *Nature* 1992; 359:320–322.
39 Matsumura K, Campbell KP. Deficiency of dystrophin-associated proteins: A common mechanism leading to muscle cell necrosis in severe childhood muscular dystrophies. *Neuromusc Disord* 1993;3:109–118.
40 Love DR, Byth BC, Tinsley JM, *et al.* Dystrophin and dystrophin-related proteins: A review of protein and RNA studies. *Neuromusc Disord* 1993;3:5–21.

The assessment of the dizzy patient

L. M. LUXON

Dizziness is a symptom that is greeted by most doctors with a degree of despair, partly because of the non-specific nature of the complaint and partly because of the plethora of diagnoses which may give rise to this symptom. By the age of 65 years, 30% of people have experienced episodes of dizziness [1] and by the age of 80 years two-thirds of women and one-third of men have suffered episodes of disequilibrium [2]. Thus, the size of the problem is considerable and clinicians in almost all medical specialties are likely to encounter patients complaining of this symptom. It is therefore the aim of this article to outline a basic diagnostic approach to dizziness, with particular emphasis upon the neuro-otological assessment.

Humans have developed a sophisticated system for maintaining balance, which relies upon the integration and modulation of visual, vestibular and proprioceptive information within the central nervous system (Fig. 1). Pathology of any one of the three sensory inputs, or of the central vestibular pathways, may disrupt the neural processing required for perfect balance and give rise to disequilibrium. As many different pathological processes may directly or indirectly affect the eye, the ear or the central nervous system, an understanding of the physiology and pathophysiology of balance [4] is of importance to many disciplines including geriatrics, cardiology, neurology, psychiatry, haematology, ophthalmology, rheumatology and endocrinology.

The vestibular receptor organs lie in the labyrinth (Fig. 2) and are anatomically paired such that head movements, involving linear and/or angular accelerations, cause displacement of the hairs of the receptor hair cells and generate equal but opposite neural activity in each ear (Fig. 3). This asymmetry of vestibular information passes via the eighth cranial nerve to the vestibular nuclei within the brain stem, and thus to the cortex, allowing cortical awareness of head and body position in space and providing the stimulus for compensatory eye (via vestibulo-ocular reflex) and body movement (via the vestibulo-spinal reflex).

Pathology which involves the peripheral labyrinth, eighth cranial nerve or central vestibular connections may also result in an asymmetry

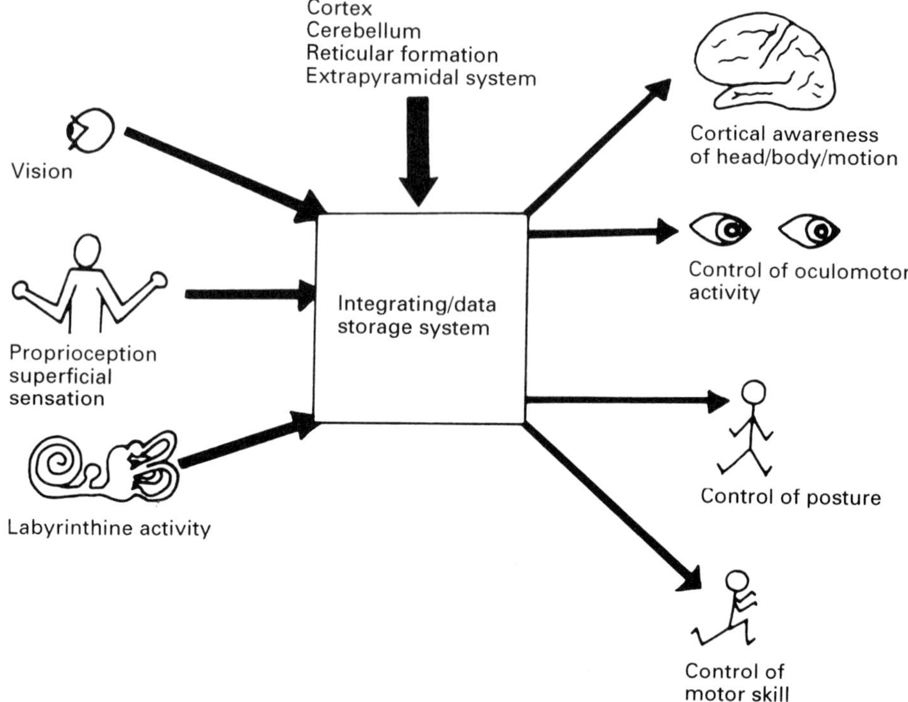

Fig. 1 Mechanism of balance in humans. (Reprinted from Luxon [3], by permission of John Wiley & Sons, Ltd.)

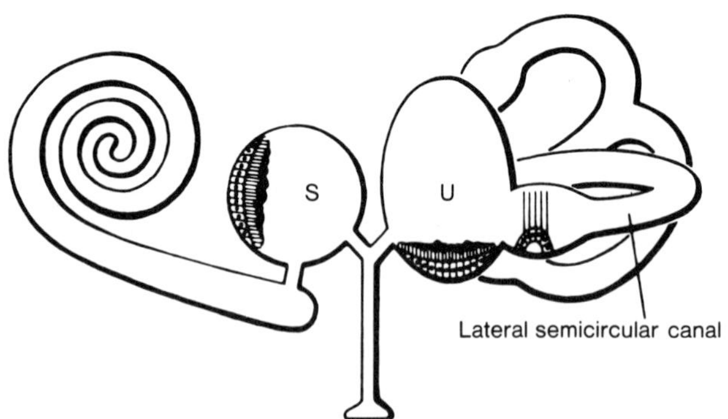

Fig. 2 Schematic diagram of vestibular receptor organs. S, Saccule; U, utricle. (By permission from Frenzel [5].)

of the resting neural activity within the vestibular system and this gives rise to vertigo, pathological spontaneous nystagmus and disordered balance. This asymmetry of vestibular activity results in a slow deviation of the eyes via the vestibulo-ocular reflex, which, for reasons that are not

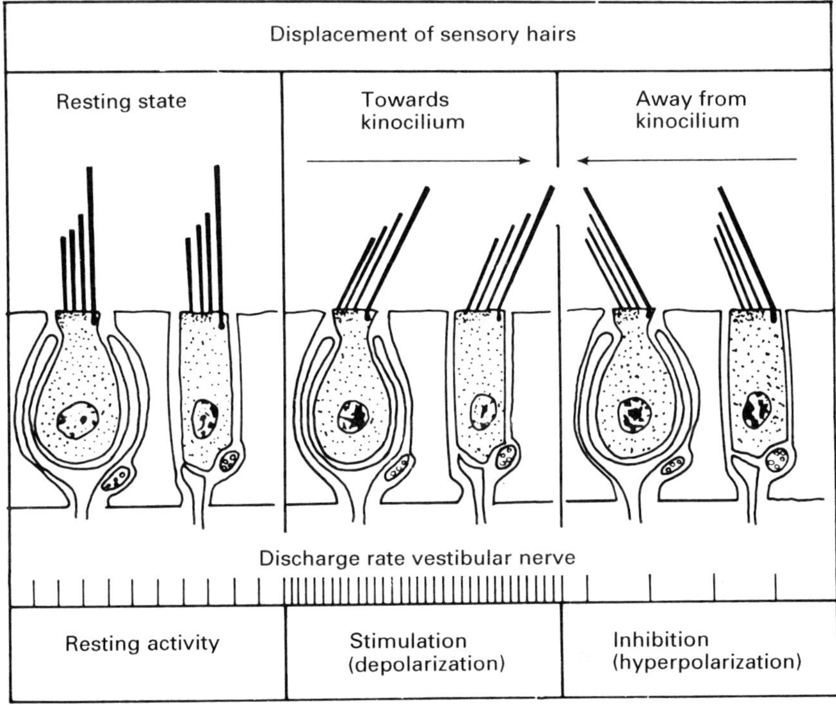

Fig. 3 Schematic illustration of the relation between hair cell orientation and the pattern of stimulation of the innervating fibres in the mammalian crista. (By permission from Wersall *et al.* [6].)

fully understood, is interrupted by a fast saccadic eye movement in the opposite direction. This is generated within the parapontine reticular formation of the brain stem. The combination of slow and fast eye movement gives rise to the characteristic saw-tooth eye movement known as spontaneous vestibular nystagmus (Fig. 4).

Physiologically the vestibular system, via the vestibulo-ocular reflex, provides one system for the control of eye movement and gaze stability. Visual stimuli provide another mechanism and, under certain circumstances, the two systems may conflict. For example, if the head is moving to watch a tennis ball flying through the air, a head movement to the right would tend to generate a vestibulo-ocular response to the left. However, the eye 'wants' to fixate the visual target, i.e. the tennis ball, and hence the visual input overrides the vestibular stimulus by modulation of neural activity at the level of the vestibulo-nuclei, and the vestibulo-ocular response is suppressed. Clinical examination of this function allows an assessment of central vestibular integrating ability (Fig. 5).

From this brief outline of vestibular dysfunction, it may be readily

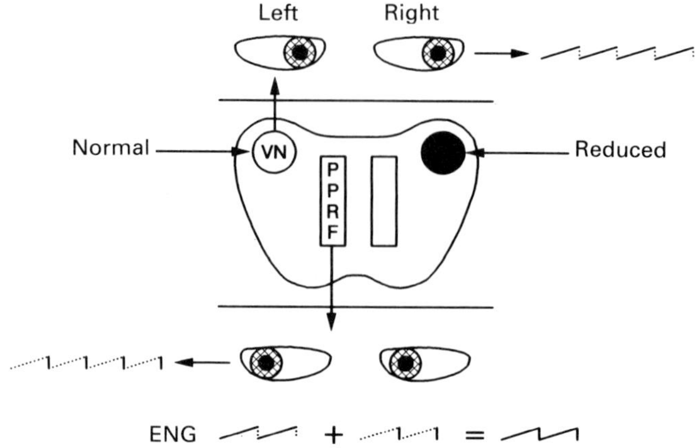

Fig. 4 Diagram of the generation of spontaneous nystagmus. VN, Vestibular nucleus; PPRF, parapontine reticular formation. (By permission from Rudge [7].)

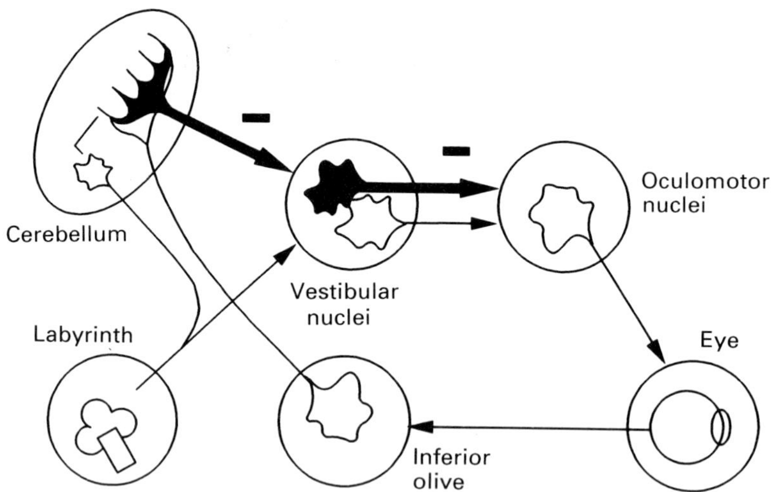

Fig. 5 Diagram to illustrate anatomical and physiological basis of visual suppression of vestibular activity. (Black neurones (–) = inhibitory neurones.)

appreciated that in response to any pathological insult, the resultant derangement in vestibular activity produces a sense of vertigo, the characteristics of which may be extremely similar from one condition to another. Hence, ischaemia to the peripheral labyrinth, a viral labyrinthitis or trauma may all give rise to the clinical syndrome of benign positional vertigo, while endolymphatic hydrops may be the end result of syphilis, vascular disease or cranial trauma. This overlap of clinical syndrome and

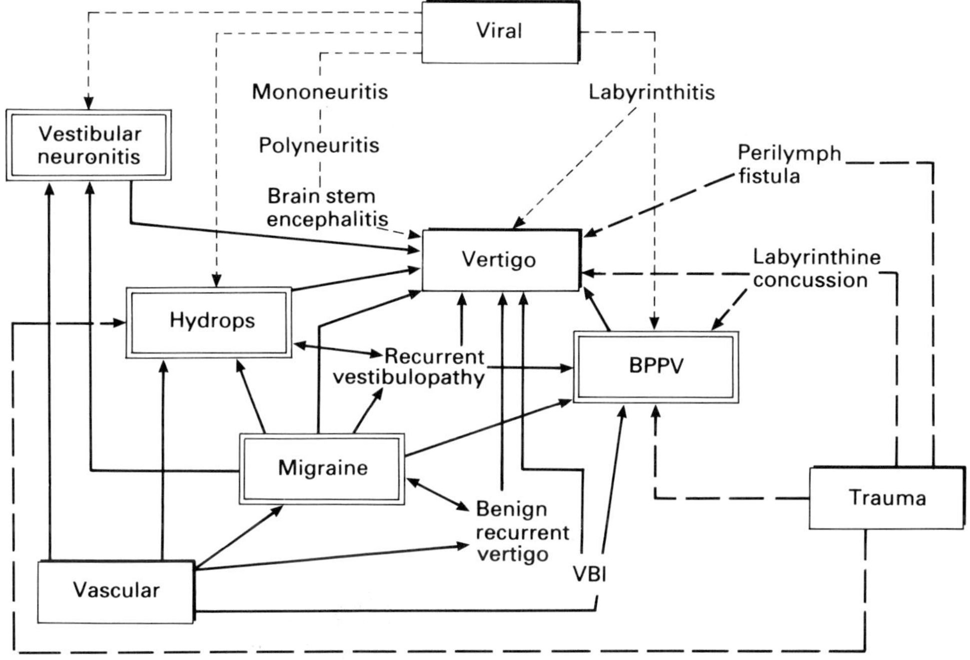

Fig. 6 Diagram to illustrate interrelationships of pathophysiological mechanisms and clinical vestibular syndromes. BPPV, Benign paroxysmal positional vertigo; VBI, vertebro-basilar insufficiency.

pathophysiological mechanisms compounds the diagnostic difficulty when the clinician is confronted by a patient with vertigo/dizziness (Fig. 6).

CLINICAL ASPECTS AND DIAGNOSTIC STRATEGY

The most systematic classification of dizziness is to divide the causes into those due to general medical, neurological and otological disorders (Table 1). The initial task for the clinician is to assess the area to which he should be directing his attention and to this end a working knowledge of the differential diagnosis of dizziness is of value.

The diagnosis of any medical condition relies upon a characteristic history, specific clinical signs, diagnostic findings on clinical investigations and specific pathological abnormalities.

History

An accurate and detailed history is essential, and certain basic points including the character and time course of dizziness, together with as-

Table 1 Causes of dizziness

General medical

- Haematological
  - Anaemia
  - Hyperviscosity
  - Miscellaneous
- Cardiovascular
  - Postural hypertension
  - Carotid sinus syndrome
  - Dysrhythmias, including
    - sick sinus syndrome
    - mitral leaflet prolapse syndrome
  - Mechanical dysfunction
    - ventricular hypokinesis
    - aortic stenosis
- Metabolic
  - Hypoglycaemia
  - Hyperventilation

Otological

- Ménière's syndrome
- Post-traumatic syndrome
- Positional nystagmus
- Vestibular neuronitis
- Infection
- Otosclerosis and Paget's disease
- Vascular accidents
- Tumours
- Autoimmune disorders
- Drug intoxication

Neurological

- Supratentorial
  - Epilepsy
  - Syncope
  - Psychogenic
- Infratentorial
  - Multiple sclerosis
  - Vertebrobasilar insufficiency
    - subclavian steal syndrome
    - Wallenberg's syndrome
    - anterior inferior cerebellar artery syndrome
  - Infective disorders
    - Ramsay Hunt
    - neurosyphilis
    - tuberculosis
  - Degenerative disorders, including neuropathy
  - Tumours, including acoustic neuroma
  - Foramen magnum abnormalities

Miscellaneous

- Ocular
- Odontogenic
- Orthopaedic, including cervical

sociated symptoms, will frequently narrow the differential diagnosis to two or three possible disorders (Fig. 7).

Character of dizziness

Dizziness is a vague non-specific symptom, while vertigo is defined as an 'hallucination of movement' and is a cardinal manifestation of disordered vestibular function. However, such semantic differences are volunteered rarely by the patient, who, frightened and confused by new and unfamiliar sensations of movement, will frequently describe symptoms such as light-headedness, swimminess, giddiness, 'confusion in the head' or 'difficulties with the legs'. For practical purposes, vertigo and dizziness

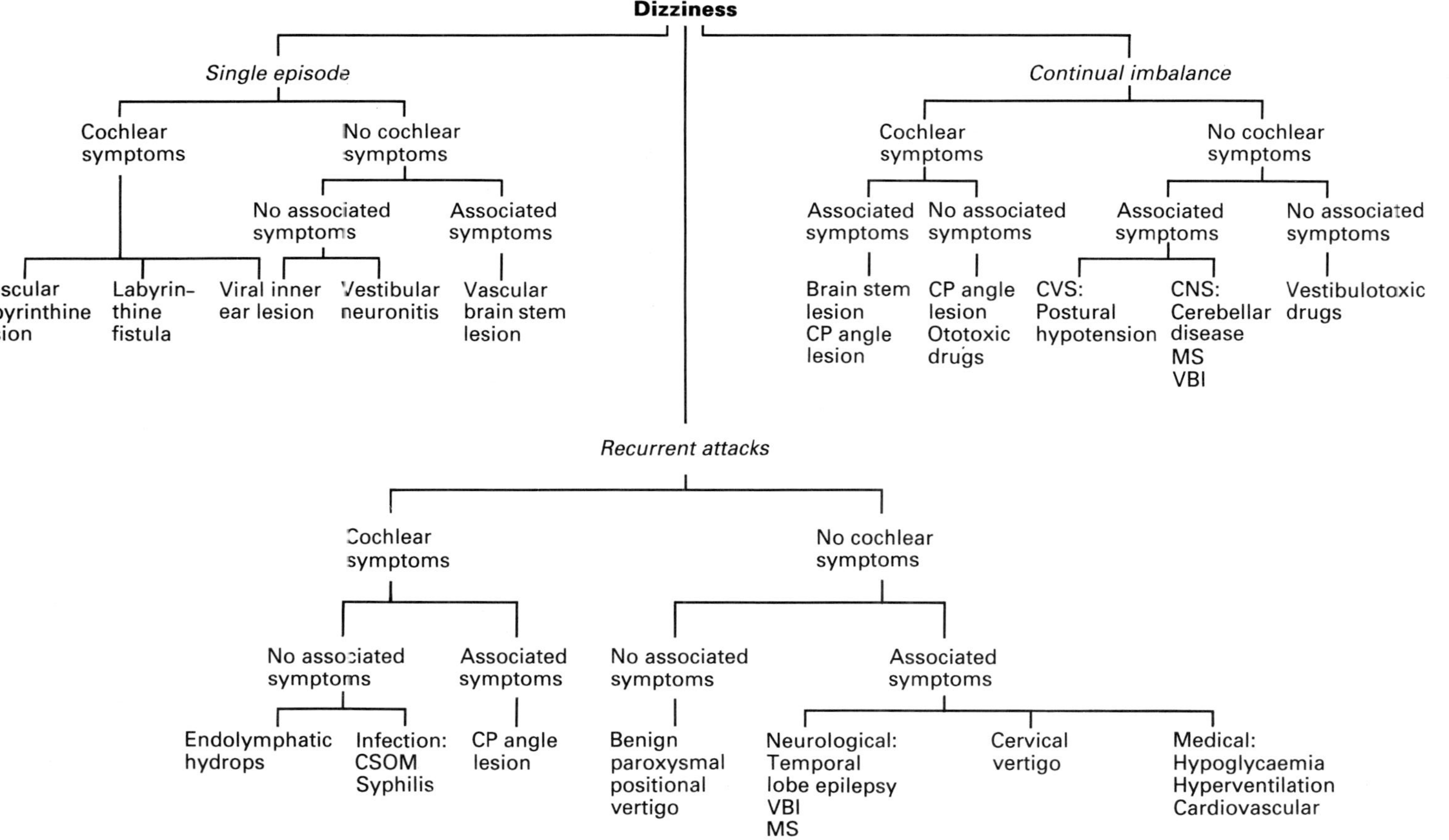

Fig. 7 Diagnostic tree in assessment of dizziness. CVS, Cardiovascular system; CNS, central nervous system; CP, cerebello-pontine; MS, multiple sclerosis; VBI, vertebrobasilar insufficiency; CSOM, chronic suppurative otitis media.

should therefore by considered to be synonymous terms in the investigation and management of disorders of balance.

Vertigo may be 'subjective', in that the patient experiences a sense of body movement, or may be 'objective', in that the subject perceives motion of his/her environment. The movement may be rotational, but frequently is described as a sense of rocking or of being at sea. Classically, the vertigo of peripheral labyrinthine origin presents as an acute, unprecipitated, short-lived attack of rotational movement of the environment, associated with nausea and vomiting, while the vertigo of central vestibular origin has a more insidious, protracted sense of instability. Whatever, a clear description of motion raises the suspicion of vestibular pathology, while symptoms of light-headedness, swimminess or faintness are more likely to be attributable to a general medical disorder.

Time course

A single episode of dizziness/vertigo may merely represent the first of recurrent attacks and it may take several months or longer for the full clinical picture of a chronic vertiginous state to evolve. For example, only 50% of Ménière's disease cases exhibit the triad of symptoms of tinnitus, fluctuating hearing loss and episodic vertigo within 6 months of the disorder [8]. Sudden unprecipitated episodes of rotational vertigo are usually ascribed to peripheral labyrinthine dysfunction, although they may occur in temporal lobe epilepsy and vertebrobasilar ischaemia. Repeated short episodes with complete recovery in between would suggest migraine, Ménière's disease or benign positional vertigo. Moreover, these disorders tend to occur in clusters, with episodes occurring over several months and then periods of freedom lasting months or even years. An acute episode, followed by a fluctuating course of improvement and worsening of symptoms, might suggest decompensation from a peripheral vestibular disorder.

Central vestibular dysfunction is classically associated with a gradual and insidious onset of continual imbalance, but patients with vestibular failure and anxious/depressed patients may also complain of this type of dysequilibrium. In this latter group special diagnostic care should be exercised, as there is evidence that psychological disorders are associated with vestibular dysfunction and may prolong recovery [9].

The duration of the individual attack is of considerable value in defining vestibular pathology. Episodes of benign positional vertigo of paroxysmal type may last only 30 or 40 seconds, whereas episodes of vertigo associated with endolymphatic hydrops or migraine can last up to 24 hours. The dizziness of an acute vestibular insult of vascular or viral origin may last for 7–10 days with a gradual recovery over a number of months.

Associated symptoms

Cochlear. Within the labyrinth and eighth cranial nerve the vestibular and cochlear elements are intimately related but, at the level of the brain stem, the auditory and vestibular pathways diverge. Hence, vestibular symptoms accompanied by hearing loss or tinnitus would suggest a more peripherally sited pathology, while imbalance associated with neurological symptoms and/or an eye movement disorder would point to neurological dysfunction. It must be emphasized that associated symptoms must be actively sought. For example, in the elderly population hearing loss and tinnitus are rarely reported as they are deemed by the patient to be 'normal'.

Fluctuating cochlear symptoms, in association with vertigo, are characteristic of Ménière's syndrome, whereas sudden, complete unilateral deafness and dizziness may occur with viral or vascular labyrinthitis. A progressive unilateral hearing loss and/or tinnitus raises the possibility of an underlying acoustic neurinoma.

Neurological symptoms. Neurological symptoms may also provide valuable clues as to site of lesion. The compact anatomical arrangement of the cranial nerve nuclei and long tracts within the small confines of the brain stem gives rise to a characteristic constellation of symptoms and signs, including vertigo, ataxia, diplopia, dysarthria, facial weakness, facial numbness and drop attacks in brain stem pathology. However, episodes of acute vertigo unassociated with brain stem symptoms and/or signs are unlikely to be due to vertebrobasilar ischaemia, a common but frequently erroneous diagnosis in the elderly vertiginous patient [10]. It should be emphasized that acute rotational vertigo with loss of consciousness, in the absence of neurological symptoms, should prompt a careful assessment of the cardiovascular system [11] while, in the presence of neurological symptoms or signs, detailed neurological investigation is required [12]. Episodes of loss of consciousness are rarely, if ever, associated with primary vestibular disorders. Vertigo may occur as part of an aura of temporal lobe epilepsy, together with the characteristic symptoms of disordered smell, taste, vision and *déjà vu* or *jamais vu*.

General medical disorders. Space prohibits a detailed discussion of all the general medical disorders which may be associated with dizziness but certain areas are numerically of such importance that they are worthy of mention. Any complaint of cardiovascular symptoms, particularly if associated with risk factors such as hyperlipidaemia, smoking, diabetes or a raised haematocrit, are of upmost importance. Both the peripheral and central vestibular system are supplied by the vertebrobasilar system and ischaemia in this territory frequently begins with vestibular symptoms, but it must be emphasized that dizziness alone, unaccompanied by other neurological symptoms and/or signs, is most unusual in this diagnosis [10]. Primary cardiac disease may give rise to dizziness consequent upon an occult dysrhythmia, hypotension or mechanical cardiac dysfunction.

Iatrogenic dizziness is extremely common, particularly in the elderly population in whom polypharmacy, poor drug compliance and altered pharmacodynamics predispose to a multiplicity of drug-induced symptoms [12]. The medicolegal consequences of vestibular failure due to inadequately monitored aminoglycoside antibiotics should not be overlooked. Recent reports of acute vestibular symptoms in association with a variety of autoimmune disorders are of importance, particularly in the group of patients in whom no obvious explanation can be found for a sudden vestibular and/or auditory loss [13–15].

Clinical examination

The points noted above re-emphasize the importance of a full general medical examination in the assessment of dizziness. On the basis of this and a comprehensive history, many neurological and general medical conditions will be excluded. The diagnosis of vestibular disorders is then based on a detailed neuro-otological examination which may be divided into:

1 an otological assessment of the external ear and tympanic membrane;
2 an assessment of visuo- and vestibulo-ocular function;
3 an assessment of vestibulo-spinal function.

Otological examination

In all patients with dizziness, otoscopy is imperative to exclude middle ear pathology and, in particular, active chronic middle ear disease with labyrinthine erosion. This is particularly important in the elderly, immigrant and debilitated population. A clinical assessment of auditory function, tuning fork tests and whisper tests is important to assess the need for detailed audiometry and the likelihood of labyrinthine and/or eighth cranial nerve pathology.

Vestibulo-ocular examination

A detailed account of vestibular and ocular physiology is beyond the scope of this text, but a clear understanding of the subject is essential, if an informed assessment of vestibular function and appropriate interpretation of vestibular examination and test procedures is to be made [4]. Importantly, before any assessment of vestibulo-ocular function, the full range of eye movements in the horizontal and vertical planes should be assessed to ensure that there is no tethering or gaze paresis which may lead to misinterpretation of a vestibular response. Moreover, smooth pursuit (following) and saccadic (rapid) eye movements should be assessed. Smooth pursuit eye movements are intimately related with the mechanisms for visual suppression of vestibular responses as outlined above and, in the presence of deranged pursuit, there will be failure of suppression of the vestibulo-ocular reflex indicating central vestibular dysfunction. Involuntary saccades constitute the fast phase of nystagmus and in the presence of dysfunction, a normal vestibular nystagmic response cannot be elicited despite normal vestibular function.

As outlined above, an asymmetry of vestibular information may arise within the labyrinth, eighth cranial nerve and/or central nervous system connections. Clinically, spontaneous nystagmus is the most valuable sign in the assessment of dizziness and should be sought in every patient. The eyes should be examined in the mid-position of gaze and with the eyes deviated 30° to the right and to the left. Care should be taken not to exceed this angle otherwise physiological end-point nystagmus may be observed and misinterpreted as pathological nystagmus.

For clinical purposes, the direction of nystagmus is defined by the fast phase. Thus, a right peripheral vestibular lesion gives rise to horizontal left beating nystagmus which obeys Alexander's law. This law states that nystagmus is greatest when the eyes are deviated in the direction of the fast phase of the nystagmus. Thus, first degree of spontaneous nystagmus to the right is of greater frequency, amplitude and velocity than second degree (eyes are in the mid-position of gaze) spontaneous nystagmus to the right which, in turn, is greater than third degree spontaneous nystagmus to the right, which is observed when the eyes are deviated to the left despite the nystagmus beating to the right (Fig. 8). Bidirectional nystagmus (e.g. first degree nystagmus beating to the right and first degree nystagmus beating to the left, when the eyes are deviated 30° to the right and left respectively), dysconjugate nystagmus (i.e. when the two eyes are beating in different directions), and vertical nystagmus (down and/or up beat) are never of peripheral labyrinthine origin and require further neurological investigation.

Additional diagnostic information is obtained by reassessing the pre-

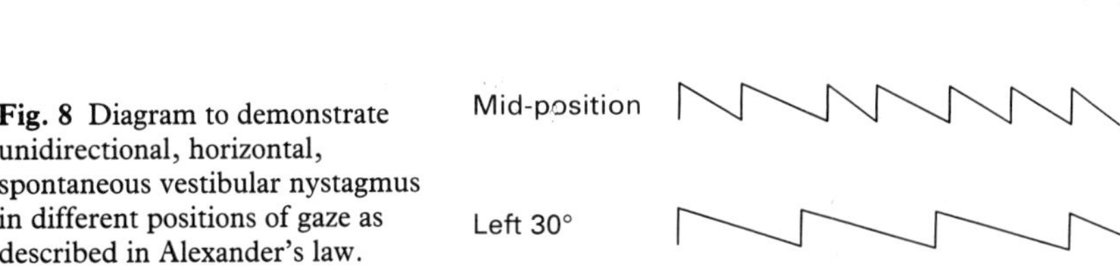

Fig. 8 Diagram to demonstrate unidirectional, horizontal, spontaneous vestibular nystagmus in different positions of gaze as described in Alexander's law.

Table 2 Features of peripheral and central spontaneous vestibular nystagmus

	Peripheral type	Central type
Duration	Temporary	Permanent
Direction	Unilateral	May be multidirectional
Character	Sawtooth	May be pendular
	Always conjugate	May be dysconjugate
Effect of removal of optic fixation	Enhances	Unchanged or inhibited

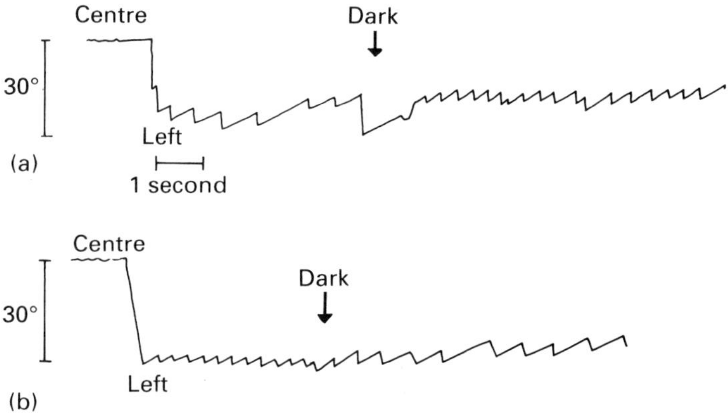

Fig. 9 Electronystagmographic tracings to illustrate the effect of the removal of optic fixation upon (a) peripheral vestibular nystagmus and (b) central vestibular nystagmus.

sence of a nystagmic response using Frenzl's glasses, which remove optic fixation. In the presence of optic fixation, visual input tends to suppress the presence of a vestibular-induced nystagmus and, by assessing the eyes in the absence of optic fixation, information regarding visuo-vestibular interaction within the central nervous system can be obtained (Table 2). In a peripheral lesion, it will be observed that any nystagmus present is enhanced in the absence of optic fixation, or nystagmus may only become manifest in the absence of optic fixation, while in a central vestibular lesion giving rise to nystagmus there will be little change with or without optic fixation (Fig. 9).

The presence of positional nystagmus is a valuable and frequently overlooked clinical sign. It is elicited by a briskly performed Hallpike manoeuvre (Fig. 10). The patient sits on the edge of a couch facing the examiner. The head is turned briskly 45° to the left and the patient is rapidly lowered, such that his head hangs over the edge of the couch. The eyes are observed for the development of positional nystagmus, which is observed until it disappears, or for 2 or 3 minutes, until it is apparent that the nystagmus is persisting. The patient is then returned to

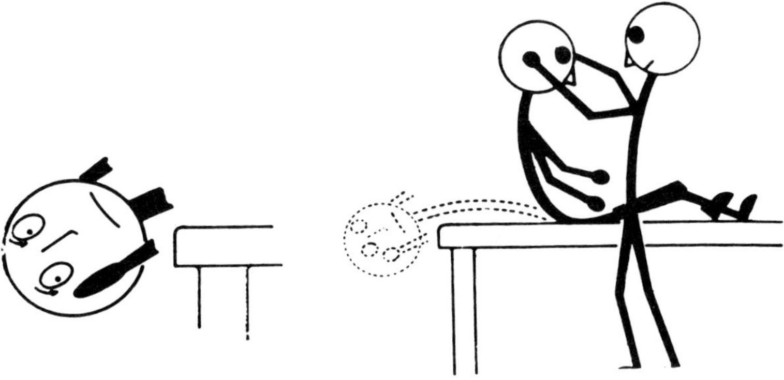

Fig. 10 Diagram to illustrate the Hallpike manoeuvre.

Table 3 Features of peripheral (benign positional) and central positional nystagmus

	Benign positional type	Central type
Latent period	2–20 seconds	None
Adaptation	Disappears in 50 seconds	Persists
Fatigability	Disappears on repetition	Persists
Vertigo	Always present	Variable
Nystagmus	Rotational to undermost ear	Any direction

the sitting position, with the eyes under continual observation to see if the nystagmus abates, reverses or a new form of nystagmus develops. This procedure is then repeated with the head turned to the right.

The nystagmus which may develop can be divided into two broad clinical types: benign positional nystagmus of paroxysmal type and central positional nystagmus. If all the characteristics in Table 3 are not identified the nystagmus should be deemed to be of central type and further neurological investigation is required. The importance of this test was underlined by Harrison and Ozsahinoglu [16] who found that 38% of patients with persistent positional nystagmus had central nervous pathology compared with only 4% of patients with benign paroxysmal positional nystagmus.

Optokinetic nystagmus is a reflex oscillation of the eyes induced by movement of areas in the visual surround. The common phenomenon of a train passenger's jerky eye movements, as he observes passing objects outside the train window, is familiar. The waveform of optokinetic nystagmus is identical to that of vestibular induced nystagmus with a slow phase followed by a rapid saccadic eye movement in the opposite direction. It would appear that there are two pathways subserving the optokinetic response: a cortical pathway, dependent upon foveal vision

Table 4 Abnormalities of optokinetic responses in 614 patients with pathology at different levels in the central nervous system. (From Yee *et al.* [17])

Anatomical site	Normal (%)	Abnormal (%)
Brain stem	41	59
Cerebellum	28	72
Basal ganglia	43	57
Parietal lobe	26	74
Labyrinth	99	1

and an intact cerebral cortex, and a subcortical non-pursuit pathway, dependent upon the peripheral visual field, the accessory optic tract and the brain stem [17].

The value of optokinetic nystagmus in the assessment of dizziness lies in the preservation of the optokinetic response in peripheral vestibular disorders, but the disruption of this response in central vestibular pathology (Table 4). Qualitative assessment of optokinetic nystagmus may be elicited by the bedside or in the outpatient department by asking the patient to observe a series of moving strips, either on a piece of material or a hand-held drum, while more precise qualitative measures may be obtained by recording eye movements, with a patient observing strips moving across the entire visual field, as for example when the patient is seated within a large revolving striped material drum.

Vestibulo-spinal assessment

Clinical tests of vestibular spinal function are non-specific and insensitive compared with tests of vestibulo-ocular function but they may provide an indication of the patient's disability. The Romberg test is performed by asking the patient to stand in the upright position, feet together, hands by the side and facing forward. When the patient feels balanced, he is asked to close the eyes and maintain his balance. A tendency to sway in one direction may indicate a peripheral or cerebellar lesion on that side while a tendency to fall backwards is usually associated with anxiety and psychological overlay.

Gait testing may be assessed by asking the patient to walk towards a fixed point in a normal manner with the eyes closed. Again a tendency to veer in one direction is most commonly observed with an ipsilateral peripheral vestibular disorder but a variety of gaits related to orthopaedic and/or neurological disorders may also be identified and may be of significance in terms of the patient's overall balance. Patients with bilateral vestibular failure may experience extreme difficulty in maintaining their balance while walking with eye closure, and if they are also deprived of proprioception, by walking over a soft mattress, they invariably tumble to the floor.

Investigations

Standard vestibular investigations include the caloric test and electronystagmographic recording of eye movements in the presence and absence of optic fixation, together with rotational stimuli, if the appropriate sophisticated equipment is available [18]. Such tests enable the distinction between lesions of the vestibular end organ and the eighth cranial nerve from pathology within the cerebello-pontine angle and central vestibular connections of the brain stem and cerebral cortex. However, the galvanic test is the only diagnostic procedure that allows the differentiation of an end-organ lesion from a lesion of the peripheral neurones [19]. As this test is not readily available, the distinction is usually made by associated auditory tests which allow the differentiation of cochlear from eighth nerve pathology.

The caloric test as described by Fitzgerald and Hallpike in 1942 [20] has stood the test of time and is the mainstay of vestibular assessment. In the majority of cases it enables the identification of a vestibular abnormality, together with the side of the lesion and the peripheral or central nature of pathology. The patient is placed in the supine position, with the head tilted 30° upwards such that the horizontal semicircular canals are brought into the vertical plane (Fig. 11). Water 7°C below and above body temperature is irrigated independently into each ear canal for a period of 40 seconds to produce a temperature gradient across the horizontal semicircular canals, which is believed to produce movement of the endolymph within the horizontal semicircular canal and thus cupular deflection. The result is an alteration of the vestibular neural activity on the stimulated side, generating a nystagmic response. This is observed and timed, while the patient fixates on a small light source above their head, or may be recorded electronystagmographically.

Three main derangements of the caloric response may be identified (Fig. 12).

1 A canal paresis in which responses obtained from one ear are reduced in comparison with the other ear. In general this abnormality is observed in lesions of the labyrinth or eighth nerve. Very rarely brain stem lesions may give rise to this configuration.

2 A directional preponderance of the nystagmic response in which the responses giving rise to nystagmus in one direction are more marked than those giving rise to nystagmus in the opposite direction. This may be seen in a lesion at any level in the vestibular apparatus and is merely a

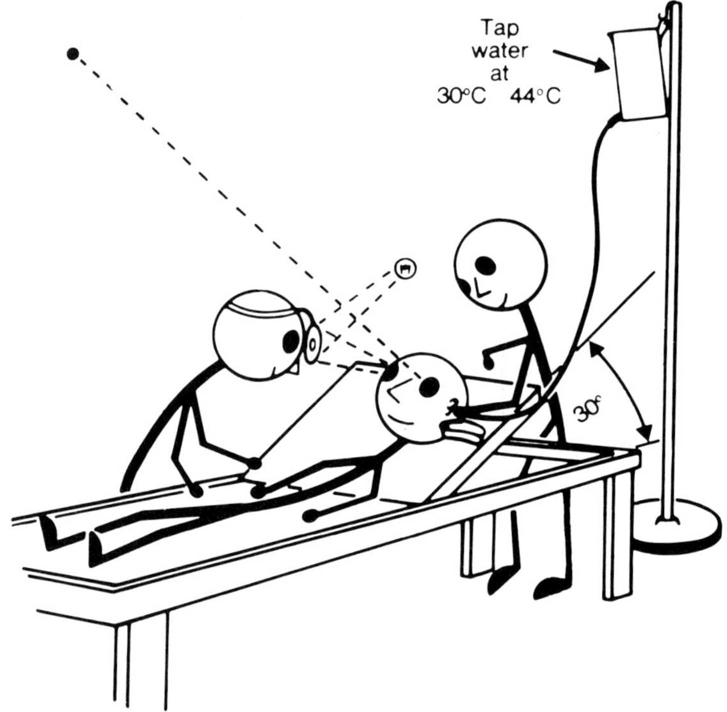

Fig. 11 Diagram of caloric test.

manifestation of an imbalance within the vestibular system which is not great enough to generate spontaneous vestibular nystagmus, but which may be revealed by inducing nystagmus using a vestibular stimulus.

3 A combination of these two characteristic patterns of response may be observed.

When the nystagmic response ceases, the eyes are observed in the absence of optic fixation in a darkened room, either with Frenzl's glasses or with an infrared viewer. This defines the effect of visual suppression upon the vestibular responses and thereby provides information about visuo-vestibular integrating activity within the central nervous system.

Clinically, rotational tests have not been widely used as part of the routine vestibular assessment, mainly because the sophisticated and expensive equipment required is not widely available. From a practical point of view, detailed analysis of rotational information can provide invaluable diagnostic data if the facility is available, although a major disadvantage of this technique is that both labyrinths are stimulated simultaneously and in the presence of one normal labyrinth, vestibular

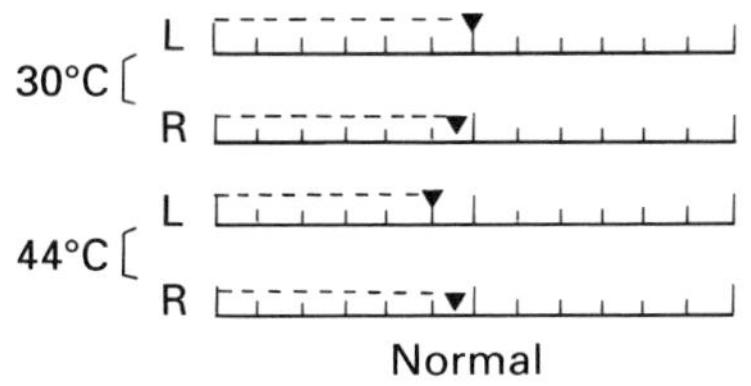

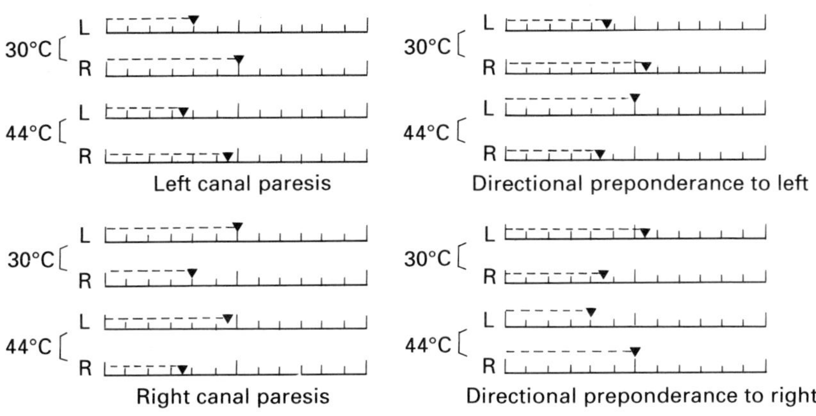

Fig. 12 Diagram to illustrate caloric pattern abnormalities.

abnormalities may be difficult to identify without extremely sophisticated computerized analysis. Nonetheless, rotational stimuli are particularly valuable in threshold studies of vestibular activity, e.g. in monitoring vestibular function during ototoxic drug administration. For this purpose caloric testing is too insensitive [21].

Posturography is the most recent test procedure in the assessment of dysequilibrium, but it must be emphasized that it is not simply a test of vestibular dysfunction but an overall assessment of balance which is dependent upon the complex sensory-motor mechanisms outlined earlier. Posturography is used:

1 to determine the presence and degree of imbalance;

2 to study the effect of various sensory and electric stimuli on balance;

3 to assess the progression of a balance disorder;

4 to assess the efficacy of treatment for balance disorder;

5 for research purposes to distinguish vestibular, visual, proprioceptive and central nervous system involvement in balance disorders.

Body sway is generally recorded by means of a force platform, which monitors vertical, horizontal and transverse forces applied to the plate by various strain gauge techniques. Although postural sway is found to be pathologically increased in a variety of conditions, posturographic patterns are not sufficiently defined to enable a pathological diagnosis to

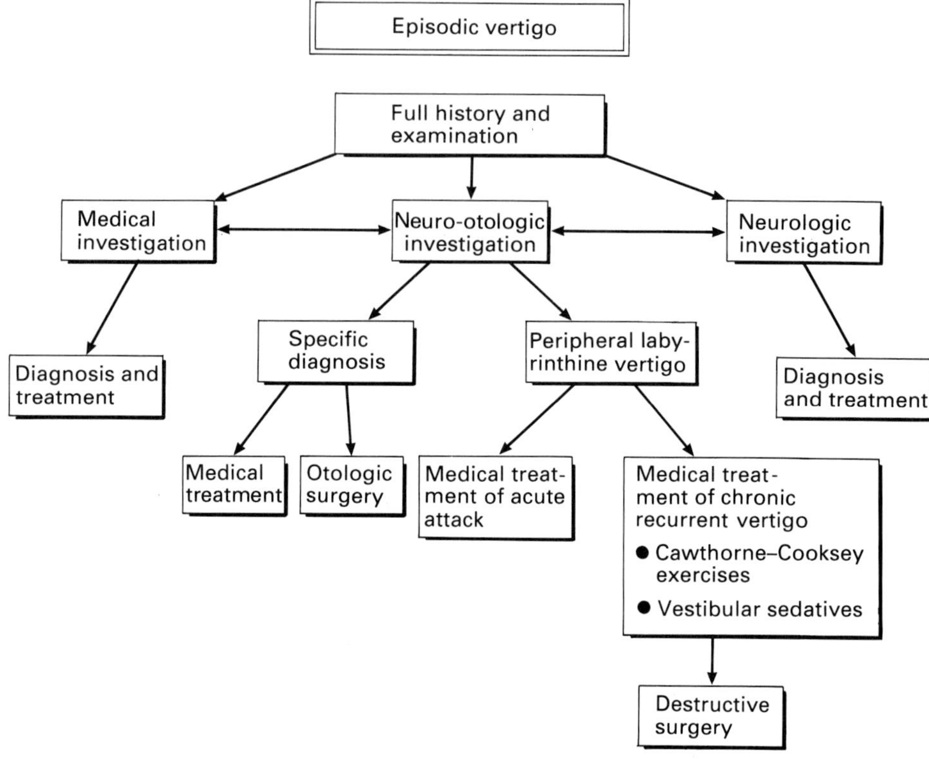

Fig. 13 Flow diagram to illustrate the assessment and subsequent management of dizziness/vertigo. (By permission from Luxon [22].)

be made. Indeed a recent panel of experts on posturography convened by the American Academy of Neurology concluded that there was no convincing evidence that posturography is useful in localizing the site of lesion, or in making a specific diagnosis. It is a method to obtain an objective quantified measure of balance, but should not be considered as primarily a vestibular test procedure.

In conclusion, a detailed history with the relevant points clearly defined, a thorough general and neuro-otological examination, together with the caloric test, will enable the vast majority of patients with dizziness to be given a diagnosis and appropriate management to be commenced (Fig. 13). Specific therapy for many general medical and neurological conditions is available, while for patients with peripheral vestibular disorder a clear explanation of the underlying aetiology of frightening and unfamiliar symptoms of disorientation is of the utmost importance. Many patients will benefit from a physical exercise regime (the Cawthorne–Cooksey exercises) and in a small number of patients vestibular sedatives may be the appropriate management course. Central vestibular disorders are notoriously difficult to treat but clonazepam, carbamazepine, cinnarizine and baclofen may each have a role in specific conditions. Psychological sequelae associated with vestibular disorders are well documented and behavioural therapy and/or psychiatric support may be required. The importance of a clear approach to the assessment of dizziness and the ability to make a correct diagnosis cannot be overstressed as patients with relatively minor vestibular disorders may become vestibular invalids terrified to leave the house and unable to work for fear of losing their balance and being thought drunk. Moreover, many of the plethora of conditions giving rise to this symptom are eminently treatable.

REFERENCES

1 Roydhouse N. Vertigo and its treatment. *Drugs* 1974;7:297–309.

2 Sheldon JH. Physical state of old people living at home. II Local symptoms. In: Shelton JH, ed. *The Social Medicine of Old Age*. London: Oxford University Press, 1948:46–106.

3 Luxon LM. The anatomy and physiology of the vestibular system. In: Dix MR, Hood JD, eds. *Vertigo*. Chicheser: John Wiley & Sons, 1984.

4 Luxon LM. Physiology of equilibrium and its application in the giddy patient. In: Kerr AG, Wright D, eds. *Diseases of the Ear, Nose and Throat*, Vol. 1. 5th edn. Basic Sciences. London: Butterworths, 1987:105–137.

5 Frenzel H. *Spontan-und-Provokations-Nystagmus als Krankheitssymptom*. Berlin/Gottingen/Heidelberg: Springer, 1955.

6 Wersall J, Gleisner L, Lundquist PG. *Symposium on Myotatic, Kinaesthetic and Vestibular Mechanisms*. London: J A Churchill, 1987.

7 Rudge P. *Clinical Neuro-otology*. London: Churchill Livingstone, 1983.

8 Morrison AW. Endolymphatic hydrops. In *Management of Sensorineural Deafness*. London: Butterworths, 1975:145–174.

9 Eagger S, Luxon LM, Davies RA, *et al*. Psychiatric morbidity in patients with peripheral vestibular disorder: a clinical and neuro-otological study. *J Neurol Neurosurg Psychiatry* 1980;55:383–387.

10 Luxon LM. Signs and symptoms of vertebrobasilar insufficiency. In: Hofferberth B, ed. *Vascular Brain Stem Diseases*. Basel: Karger, 1990:93–111.

11 Luxon LM, Crowther A, Harrison MJG, Coltart DJ. Controlled study of 24-hour ambulatory electrocardiographic monitoring in patients with transient neurological symptoms. *J Neurol Neurosurg Psychiatry* 1980;43:37–41.

12 Luxon LM. Causes of balance disorders. In: Kerr AG, Stephens SDG, eds. *Diseases of the Ear, Nose and Throat*, Vol. 9. 5th edn. Adult Audiology. London: Butterworths, 1987:157–202.

13 Stephens SDG, Luxon LM, Hinchcliffe R. Auditory lesions in immunological disorders. *Audiology* 1982;21:128–148.

14 Row-Jones JM, Macallan DC, Sorooshian M. Polyarteritis nodosa presenting as bilateral sudden onset cochleo-vestibular failure in a young woman. *J Laryngol Otol* 1990;104:562–564.

15 Vyse T, Luxon LM, Walport MJ. Audio-vestibular manifestations of the antiphospholipid syndrome. *J Laryngol Otol* 1994;108:57–59.

16 Harrison MS, Ozsahinoglu C. Positional vertigo: aetiology and clinical significance. *Brain* 1972;95:369–372.

17 Yee RD, Baloh RW, Hornrubia V, Jenkins HA. Pathophysiology of optokinetic nystagmus. In: Honrubia V, Brazier M, eds. *Nystagmus and Vertigo, Clinical Approaches to the Patient with Dizziness*. New York: Academic Press, 1982:251–296.

18 Luxon LM. Diseases of the eighth cranial nerve. In: Dyck P, Thomas PH, eds. *Peripheral Neuropathy*, 3rd edn. Philadelphia: WB Saunders, 1992:837–868.

19 Pfaltz CR. The diagnostic importance of galvanic test in neuro-otology. *Practica Oto-Rhino-Laryngol* 1969;31:193–203.
20 Fitzgerald G, Hallpike CS. Studies in human vestibular function. 1. Observations on the directional preponderance (Nystagmusbereitschaft) of caloric nystagmus resulting from cerebral lesions. *Brain* 1942;65:115–137.
21 Kayan A. Diagnostic tests of balance. In: Kerr AG, Wright D, eds. *Diseases of the Ear, Nose and Throat*, Vol. 1. 5th edn. Basic Sciences. London: Butterworths, 1987:304–367.
22 Luxon LM. Episodic vertigo. In: Rakel RB, ed. *Conn's Current Therapy*. Philadelphia: WB Saunders, 1990.

PART 4
GASTROENTEROLOGY

Nutritional support for general medical patients

J. E. LENNARD-JONES

INTRODUCTION

The message of this paper is simple: look for malnutrition and you will find it, treat it and you will be gratified by the results. Faced with a wasted patient, doctors tend not to notice tissue loss but concentrate on recognizable disease. They forget that food can be a treatment, and can be the most important treatment.

Thought associations are often learned and many of us were not taught clinical nutrition. Our immediate reaction to wasting or weakness should be to enquire about food. Is energy and protein intake adequate to meet losses, energy needs and tissue replacement or growth?

THE RECOGNITION AND ANTICIPATION OF MALNUTRITION

The wheel has come full circle. A simple 'subjective global assessment' performed by medical or paramedical staff correlates reasonably well with the most sophisticated anthropometric or laboratory measurements [1,2].

Malnutrition as reflected in body composition can be defined in quantitative terms. Probably the most useful single measure is the body mass index (weight in kilograms/height in metres^2, normal range 19–25), provided there is no oedema. Measurements of skinfold thickness and arm muscle circumference require skill in performance; normal ranges are wide and do not always correspond with the population under study. Serum protein measurements are affected by the acute phase reaction to inflammation and thus do not only mirror nutritional status. Measurement of electrical bio-impedance may become useful as a measure of body water. Isotopic determinations of body water, nitrogen or potassium are not suitable for routine clinical use and are subject to changes in body composition [1].

The clinical assessment which is appropriate for everyday use [2] relies on a history of recent weight loss, the magnitude of the loss, and qualitative observation of loss of subcutaneous fat (over the triceps and lower ribs in the mid-axillary line) and muscle bulk (deltoid and quadriceps). Account is taken of the rapidity and continuation of weight loss and the presence of oedema or ascites. Warning features in the history which suggest the possibility of malnutrition are decrease in food intake, and gastrointestinal losses (Table 1). Patients can be divided into those with normal nutritional state, moderately malnourished (loss of 5–10% body weight, no obvious tissue loss) and severely malnourished (greater than 10% body weight, obvious tissue loss). Taking account of the likely outcome of the illness and the present nutritional state, patients can also be divided into those with a normal, low or high risk of developing malnutrition.

A good example of those at high risk are patients with motor neurone disease. When their energy intake falls to less than 1.5 times their basal energy expenditure they begin to lose weight. Prompt action can then be taken to reverse the trend [3].

Are we good at recognizing malnutrition?

Surveys in British hospitals show that the most elementary nutritional assessment is rarely undertaken. In two medical and surgical wards in a district general hospital, only 11 of 72 patients had been weighed and only 14 of 32 severely malnourished patients were detected by ward staff [4]. In a London teaching hospital, a survey of 470 patients in two

Table 1 'Subjective global assessment' of nutritional status adapted from Detsky *et al.* [2]. The most important features are marked with an asterisk. Severe malnutrition is regarded as continued weight loss amounting to more than 10% of normal body weight with obvious loss of muscle bulk and subcutaneous fat assessed by observation and qualitative palpation. Assessment of weight change is qualified by the presence of oedema or ascites

History
*Weight change
Past 6 months
Past 2 weeks
Food intake
Gastrointestinal symptoms (appetite, losses)
Functional capacity (loss of strength, etc.)
Examination
*Body weight
*Subcutaneous fat (triceps, chest)
*Muscle wasting (quadriceps, deltoid)
Oedema/ascites
Categorize
Well nourished
Moderately malnourished
Severely malnourished

medical, two surgical and two wards for the elderly showed that one-third of patients were at severe risk of malnutrition as judged by their nutritional state and the outlook of their illness; only 42% of these patients were referred to a dietitian. Of the patients whose notes mentioned weight loss, only 3% were weighed. Overall only 29% of all patients were found to have a record of weight in medical or nursing notes [5].

The provision of weighing scales in hospital wards is often lamentable. Occasional wards have no scales, others often have inadequate or poorly calibrated instruments.

Recommendation about nutritional assessment

A good case can be made for insisting that all medical and nursing admission notes should contain a reference to nutritional state and that every ambulant patient admitted should be weighed on a reliable machine [6]. Furthermore, patients should be weighed at weekly intervals as long as they are in hospital and each result should be compared with previous values. There is ample evidence that medical patients admitted to hospital [7,8], including the elderly [9,10], tend to lose weight progressively as time passes. Ideally every patient's height should also be measured once in general practice or hospital. Our paediatric colleagues have much to teach those of us who look after adults about attention to weight and height; they note growth, we must watch for wasting.

WHY MALNUTRITION IS IMPORTANT

Physiological and psychological consequences of malnutrition

It is now rare for a patient to die of malnutrition, though before the development of modern means of nutritional support this happened. The tragic experience of a hunger strike shows that healthy young men lose around 35% of their body weight over about 8 weeks and by this stage one-third of them die [3]. The clinical situation is more closely mirrored by the experiment in which healthy young men took only 20% of their energy needs over 6 months [11]. They lost about 20% of their body weight, mainly fat but also some protein. More important, they also lost muscle strength and they became depressed and unsociable, preferring to be alone and not mix with others [12]. Similar changes were noted in prisoners of war deprived of adequate food; they lost a sense of well being, developed progressive mental and physical lethargy, needed more sleep than usual, became slow in thought and speech and failed to maintain personal cleanliness [12].

Objective studies in obese subjects using electrical stimulation of striated muscle have shown a reduction in the force and endurance of contraction in response to stimulation after 2 weeks on a 400 kcal diet followed by 2 weeks starvation. All abnormalities returned to normal within 2 weeks of refeeding [13]. These changes in muscle function, which can also be demonstrated by grip strength and respiratory function tests [14,15], recover rapidly on refeeding before there is major restoration of lean body mass [14]. Experimentally, semi-starvation also induces insensitivity of the respiratory centre to anoxia [16]. Malnutrition can also lead to defective conservation of body heat in the elderly [17] which in turn may contribute to hypothermia and falls. There is evidence that chronic malnutrition diminishes cellular immunity [18] and may reduce the rate of tissue healing.

The clinical and economic consequences of malnutrition

Clinical malnutrition itself may not kill but it increases the risk of complications during illness (Fig. 1). Loss of muscle power reduces mobility and the ability to cough. Impaired cellular immunity may increase liability to infection. Depression, apathy, loss of sociability and an increased desire for sleep all impair motivation for recovery and activity. Loss of strength and appetite further decrease food intake (Fig. 2). Asher has graphically listed the dangers for a patient of lying long in bed [19]. 'The blood clotting in his veins, the lime draining from his bones, . . . the

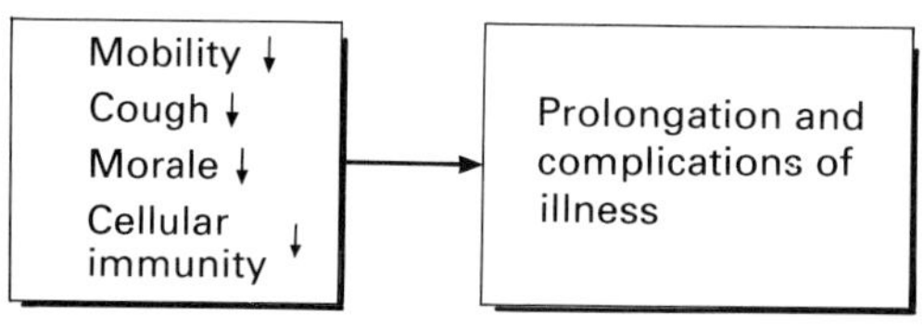

Fig. 1 Clinical consequences of malnutrition. The functional complications of malnutrition increase the liability to complications from the underlying illness.

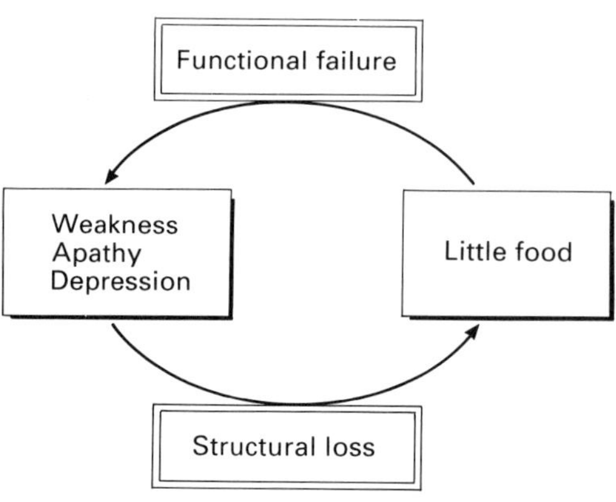

Fig. 2 Malnutrition leads not only to structural changes measured as loss of body tissue but also to functional changes of muscle weakness, apathy and depression. These physiological and psychological factors perpetuate poor food intake so that self-improvement does not occur.

flesh rotting from his seat, . . . and the spirit evaporating from his soul.'

It is difficult to demonstrate the clinical effects of malnutrition in medical patients. Correlations suggest a positive correlation between poor nutritional status on admission, length of hospital stay, complications and mortality in both a general medical service [20] and a geriatric rehabilitation unit [21]. However, the severity of the underlying illness must be a confounding factor. A controlled trial among 435 elderly inpatients has shown that a dietary supplement given in addition to meals reduced mortality over 6 months whether or not there was evidence of malnutrition at the time of admission [10].

Much evidence is available from surgical studies since patients with differing nutritional status undergo operations involving definable trauma. In an elegant study of this type two groups of patients were distinguished before operation, one with a normal and the other with a depleted total body protein as judged by isotopic whole-body nitrogen measurements. Respiratory function tests showed that those with depleted body protein had a lower vital capacity and peak expiratory flow rate. These patients suffered significantly more frequent episodes of postoperative pneumonia from which two died, and a third died from thromboembolism; there were no fatal instances of postoperative pneumonia among those with normal body protein before operation [22].

Classic studies have shown positive correlation between malnutrition, mortality and slow mobilization among patients with fractured hip [17,23,24]. Controlled trials showed that provision of a dietary supplement decreased mortality, improved the rate of mobilization and decreased the length of hospital stay among survivors [23,24].

In America where episodes of illness are timed and costed, malnutrition is a co-morbidity factor used to allow for a greater duration of hospital stay and greater cost of admission than average for a given Diagnosis Related Group. A study among 100 consecutive patients admitted to a general medical unit showed that the 40 who were malnourished stayed on average 5 days longer than those who were normally nourished, and their admission cost more than twice as much because of both longer stay and more intensive treatment [25]. Data with the same trends have been published for patients admitted to medical wards with pneumonia or inflammatory bowel disease [20]. Even if malnutrition in many cases was a manifestation of the severity of illness, it still proved to be a valid clinical indicator of prognosis.

FREQUENCY AND CAUSES OF MALNUTRITION AMONG MEDICAL PATIENTS

There are no published surveys on the incidence of malnutrition among patients in general medical wards in this country. Unpublished series suggest that the incidence of malnutrition judged on subjective global assessment or anthropometric data is of the order 20–40% [4,5]. Body weight, triceps skinfold and arm muscle circumference were below the fifth percentile of the normal range for active elderly women in 30–60% of 91 women admitted to acute or long-stay wards for the elderly [26].

It is likely that the commonest cause of malnutrition among medical patients is a product of age, continued disability and social deprivation. Inability to swallow for a neurological or obstructive reason is another obvious risk factor. Malabsorption is an uncommon cause. Eating disorders, alcoholism and cancer are among the many other possible causes that come to mind.

Illness may be associated not only with decreased food intake but with increased energy expenditure or an inflammatory response. Inflammation leads to an increased rate of weight loss and a failure to respond to nutritional replacement therapy, a problem noted in patients with HIV infection. Increased energy expenditure of about 30% over that expected has been demonstrated in elderly patients with a chest infection [27]. Malnutrition is a feature of the late stages of chronic obstructive airways disease, probably due to a combination of factors including decreased food intake and the increased work of breathing [28]. The nutritional problems of patients with a variety of respiratory disorders have recently been reviewed [29]. Increased muscle tone and the involuntary movements of Parkinson's disease are associated with increased energy expenditure [30]. Even ordinary activities such as walking are associated with greater energy cost in elderly patients than in younger subjects [31].

PREVENTION AND TREATMENT

Appreciation and action

If malnutrition is unrecognized it remains untreated. It is therefore incumbent on all medical and nursing staff to be alert to the possibility of malnutrition, to plan treatment when needed and to monitor the outcome. The nursing care plan is an obvious way of identifying the problem and maintaining concern. A Nutritional Standards Working Party of the South-East Thames Region recommends that a named nurse on each ward should be given responsibility for coordination of all aspects of patient feeding [32]. This suggestion is similar to the 'Nutrition Link Nurse' system operating in Nottingham [3] in which one or two nurses on each ward develop a special interest in nutrition and meet regularly as a club to discuss programmes of care and special projects, and to exchange information.

Naturally, communication with catering staff and referral to a dietitian are often appropriate. At present the Code of Practice for dietitians states that all referrals must be through a doctor. The Working Party suggests that consultants can help by authorizing 'blanket referral' to a dietitian by the ward staff whenever it is considered necessary.

Food is the first line of treatment

Ordinary food is the first and main means of nutritional support. Its effectiveness depends not only on its nutritional content but on its provision at the right time, in appropriate quantity and in a palatable form. The Working Party mentioned above has produced excellent guidelines in Part I of its Report on menu planning in hospital. The importance of providing and identifying an energy dense choice is recognized, as well as the need to meet specific cultural and medical diets. Part II of its Report introduces the useful concept of a 'food chain' from supplier, through preparation and distribution, to consumption [32]. Stress is placed on the importance of creating as pleasant an environment as possible during meal-times, on the need to prepare the position of immobile patients so that they can eat easily and to assist some patients with eating. Doctors can help by avoiding ward rounds, investigative procedures or other distractions during meal-times. Hospital meals should be regarded as part of clinical care for many patients and not simply as an element of the 'hotel service'.

Adjustments of diet, snacks and supplements

Some patients need special types of food, others need alterations to its consistency or texture. A patient with a sore mouth or difficulty in swallowing may need a blenderized semi-liquid, or even a liquid diet. To increase energy intake, patients may need high energy snacks between meals and at bed time. Relatives may be able to provide welcome food supplements though these should be discussed with nursing staff and may present a problem if storage is needed due to increasingly strict food hygiene regulations. Lastly, several palatable commercially available supplements, either liquids or semi-solids, are available in convenient sterile containers holding a single portion. Nursing staff need a stock of such supplements to use at their discretion.

Monitoring food intake

Having made every effort to achieve adequate food intake, usefully described as 'assertive feeding', failure to eat should be monitored by noting food left on plates and unconsumed snacks. A dietitian can be asked to assess dietary intake. User friendly computer systems have been devised based on the hospital menu and portion sizes [33,34] to estimate nutritional intake. Data can be entered by patients or by nurses based on proportions of hospital food portions eaten or household measures. The results corresponded with weighed food analyses within the limits necessary for clinical assessment.

Sip feeds

Several commercially prepared sip feeds with sweet or savoury flavours are available in convenient sterile containers. They can be used as supplements or as a complete nutritionally balanced diet. In general, liquid feeds are not now prepared in diet kitchens because of the danger of bacterial contamination and proliferation before the last portion of the feed is consumed.

Tube feeds

A tube feed requires no effort on the part of the patient and is independent of appetite. It allows provision of nutrients by day and/or night so that more food can be given than usual.

The simplest and safest tube feed is via a fine-bore nasogastric tube. A small electric pump controls the rate of infusion and ensures that all the feed prescribed is given. Using a polyurethane or silicone rubber tube, nasal discomfort is unusual and feeding can be maintained for many weeks without changing the tube.

A recent survey of the whole Cambridge Health District over a year [35] showed that the commonest reason for a tube feed was neurological dysphagia after a stroke or head injury; at the onset 45% of patients were unconscious or confused. Of all post-neonatal patients, 14.5% were treated in medical wards. One-third of the 291 patients suffered a chest infection but pulmonary aspiration was attributed to the feed in only 4.5% of patients. Other complications attributed to the feed were diarrhoea, shown in another study often to be due to concurrent use of antibiotics [36], and less commonly constipation.

Placement of a gastrostomy tube as an endoscopic or radiological procedure is being increasingly used for long-term feeding. This technique avoids the annoyance, possible discomfort, and embarrassment of a tube around the face. A controlled trial showed that patients preferred a gastrostomy to a nasogastric tube for these reasons [37]. Complications, particularly infections, do occur at the entry site but in general the technique is well tolerated and is particularly suited to treatment at home.

Domiciliary tube feeds

The survey for Cambridge showed that though only 19 of 291 patients given a tube feed were treated at home, in terms of patient days of treatment, these patients accounted for over one-third of the total because of the long duration of their treatment [35]. Home treatment with either a nasogastric or gastrostomy tube is especially useful for patients with neurological feeding difficulties. Care is needed in the tuition of all carers and liaison with the community health care team is also important.

Parenteral feeding

Parenteral feeding is needed only if absorption of sufficient nourishment from the small intestine is impossible and this is uncommon in medical patients. Such a situation may arise due to 'mucositis' during cytotoxic drug therapy or after bone marrow transplantation. Unusual needs are small intestinal neuropathy or myopathy, and after resection of all but 50–100 cm of jejunum. Most parenteral nutrition in adults is needed in surgical and intensive care wards.

Infusion of nutrients via a peripheral vein is increasingly used for relatively short-term parenteral nutrition. Slow infusion controlled by a pump through very fine silicone rubber cannulas, and the use of a lipid emulsion as the major energy source to reduce osmolarity of the nutrient solution, minimize the risk of venous thrombosis. This technique avoids the potential hazards of a central indwelling venous cannula, though a central line is still needed for long-term use.

Parenteral nutrition is potentially dangerous, as well as expensive. The complications can be greatly reduced if the procedure is organized and supervised by a well-trained nutrition team consisting of a specialist nurse, clinician with a special interest, pharmacist and dietitian with good backing from a consultant biochemist and microbiologist. Such a team greatly reduces the incidence of dangerous and expensive complications, especially septicaemia [6].

ORGANIZATION OF NUTRITIONAL SUPPORT

Efficient nutritional support is as much a question of organization as of supply. A hospital nutritional policy group which includes representatives of the catering staff, dietitians, nurses, clinicians and managers can define overall organizational and financial strategy. One or more nutrition teams, to include not only general wards but also intensive care and paediatric wards, can greatly improve the effectiveness and safety of enteral tube feeds and parenteral nutrition.

CONCLUSION

Nutritional support has been a neglected aspect of clinical care. Recognition and anticipation of malnutrition should lead to more effective use of ordinary food for the majority of patients who need support. Monitoring of progress by assessing input and regular measurements of body weight are needed. For the minority of patients who need enteral tube or parenteral feeding, new techniques make them available for long-term use both in hospital and at home. The efficiency and safety of all types of tube feed are greatly improved by the integration of different skills in a nutrition team.

REFERENCES

1 Jeejeebhoy KN, Baker JP, Wolman SL, *et al.* Critical evaluation of the role of clinical assessment and body composition studies in patients with malnutrition and after total parenteral nutrition. *Am J Clin Nutr* 1982;35:1117–1127.
2 Detsky AS, McLaughlin JR, Baker JP, *et al.* What is subjective global assessment of nutritional status? *J Parent Ent Nutr* 1987;11:8–13.
3 Allison SP. The uses and limitations of nutritional support. *Clin Nutr* 1992;11:319–330.
4 Burnham WR. The role of nutrition support teams. In: Payne-James J, Grimble G, Silk DA, eds. *Nutrition Support in Clinical Practice.* London: Edward Arnold, 1993.
5 Hayes S, Bryant K, Wilson R. Nutritional risk assessment: a survey of hospitalized patients. *J Hum Nutr Dietet* 1994 (submitted).
6 Lennard-Jones, ed. *A Positive Approach to Nutrition as Treatment.* London: Kings Fund Centre, 1992.
7 Pinchcofsky GD, Kaminski MV. Increasing malnutrition during hospitalization: Documentation by a nutritional screening program. *J Am Coll Nutr* 1985;4:471–479.
8 Weinsier RL, Hunker EM, Krumdieck CL, Butterworth CE, Jr. A prospective evaluation of general medical patients during the course of hospitalization. *Am J Clin Nutr* 1979;32:418–426.
9 Thomas AJ, Bunker VW, Hinks LJ, *et al.* Energy, protein, zinc and copper status of twenty-one elderly inpatients: analysed dietary intake and biochemical indices. *Br J Nutr* 1988;59:181–191.
10 Larsson J, Unosson M, Ek A-C, *et al.* Effect of dietary supplement on nutritional status and clinical outcome in 501 geriatric patients – a randomised study. *Clin Nutr* 1990;9: 179–184.
11 Keys A, Brozek J, Henschel A, *et al.* (eds). In: *The Biology of Human Starvation.* Minneapolis MN: University of Minnesota Press, 1950.
12 Brozek J. Effects of generalised malnutrition on personality. *Nutrition* 1990;6:389–395.
13 Russell DMcR, Leiter LA, Whitwell J, *et al.* Skeletal muscle function during hypocaloric diets and fasting: a comparison with standard nutritional assessment parameters. *Am J Clin Nutr* 1983;37:133–138.
14 Christie PM, Hill GL. Effect of intravenous nutrition on nutrition and function in acute attacks of inflammatory bowel disease. *Gastroenterology* 1990;99:730–736.
15 Arora NS, Rochester DF. Respiratory muscle strength and maximal voluntary ventilation in undernourished patients. *Am Rev Respir Dis* 1982;126:5–8.
16 Doekel RC, Zwillich CW, Scoggin CH, *et al.* Clinical semi-starvation: depression of hypoxic ventilatory response. *N Engl J Med* 1976;295:358–361.
17 Bastow MD, Rawlings J, Allison SP. Undernutrition, hypothermia, and injury in elderly women with fractured femur: an injury response to altered metabolism? *Lancet* 1983;i:143–145.
18 Chandra RK. Nutrition, immunity, and infection: present knowledge and future directions. *Lancet* 1983;i:688–691.

19 Asher RAJ. The dangers of going to bed. *Br Med J* 1947;ii:967–968.
20 Reilly JJ, Hull SF, Albert N, *et al.* Economic impact of malnutrition: A model system for hospitalized patients. *J Parent Ent Nutr* 1988;12:371–376.
21 Sullivan DH, Patch GA, Walls RC, Lipschitz DA. Impact of nutrition status on morbidity and mortality in a select population of geriatric rehabilitation patients. *Am J Clin Nutr* 1990;51:749–758.
22 Windsor JA, Hill GL. Risk factors for post-operative pneumonia: the importance of protein depletion. *Ann Surg* 1988;208:209–214.
23 Bastow MD, Rawlings J, Allison SP. Benefits of supplementary tube feeding after fractured neck of femur: a randomised controlled trial. *Br Med J* 1983;287:1589–1592.
24 Delmi M, Rapin C-H, Bengoa J-M, *et al.* Dietary supplementation in elderly patients with fractured neck of the femur. *Lancet* 1990;335:1013–1016.
25 Robinson G, Goldstein M, Levine GM. Impact of nutritional status on DRG length of stay. *J Parent Ent Nutr* 1987;11:49–51.
26 Morgan DB, Newton HMV, Schorah CJ, *et al.* Abnormal indices of nutrition in the elderly: a study of different clinical groups. *Age Ageing* 1986;15:65–76.
27 Hodkinson HM, Cox M, Lugon M, *et al.* Energy cost of chest infections in the elderly. *J Clin Exp Gerontol* 1990;12:241–246.
28 Hunter AMB, Carey MA, Larsh HW. The nutritional status of patients with chronic obstructive pulmonary disease. *Am Rev Respir Dis* 1981;124:376–381.
29 Poole S. A requirement not to be overlooked: nutritional aspects of respiratory disease. *Prof Nurse* 1993;1:252–256.
30 Levi S, Cox M, Lugon M, *et al.* Increased energy expenditure in Parkinson's disease. *Br Med J* 1990;301:1256–1257.
31 Department of Health. *Report on Health and Social Subjects. No. 43. The Nutrition of Elderly People*. London: HMSO, 1992:10–16.
32 Nutritional standards working party. *Nutritional Guidelines. 1. Menu Planning. 2. The food chain.* London: South East Thames Regional Health Authority, 1993.
33 McIntyre AS, Ibbotson M, Duthie J, *et al.* Computer aided analysis of dietary nutrient and fibre intakes in gastroenterology. In: Vicary FR, ed. *Computers in Gastroenterology*. Springer-Verlag, 1988.
34 Levine JA, Madden AM, Morgan MY. Validation of a computer based system for assessing dietary intake. *Br Med J* 1987;295:369–372.
35 Wilcock H, Armstrong J, Cottee S, *et al.* Artificial nutrition support for patients in the Cambridge health district. *Health Trends* 1991;23:93–100.
36 Keohane PP, Attrill H, Love M, *et al.* Relation between osmolality of diet and gastrointestinal side effects in enteral nutrition. *Br Med J* 1984;288:678–680.
37 Park RHR, Allison MC, Lang J, *et al.* Randomised comparison of percutaneous endoscopic gastrostomy and nasogastric tube feeding in patients with persisting neurological dysphagia. *Br Med J* 1992;304:1406–1409.

Gastro-oesophageal reflux disease: some aspects of its epidemiology, natural history and cause

J. R. BENNETT

Dyspepsia is extremely common in the community. There have been studies carried out in Britain and other countries in recent years indicating that up to a third of the population report dyspepsia over a 6 month period [1]. Much of this is mild, two-thirds of it self-treated, but it causes considerable loss of work.

HEARTBURN

Of all the symptoms making up dyspepsia, heartburn is a feature in two-thirds of the subjects [1]. Heartburn may be a symptom of peptic ulcer, or of functional dyspepsia, but predominantly it indicates gastro-oesophageal reflux, and is the main discriminatory symptom for that diagnosis [2].

OTHER SYMPTOMS OF GASTRO-OESOPHAGEAL REFLUX DISEASE (GORD) [3]

Oesophageal pain

The oesophagus may give rise to pain other than heartburn, probably by motor changes ('spasm'). This may be of any character, but is often described as 'gripping' or 'knife-like'. These pains are usually central–sternal in origin, but may radiate widely to abdomen, back, neck and arms. The pain may be severe. The character, radiation and severity may cause diagnostic difficulty, readily simulating cardiac, biliary or duodenal pain. As many as one-third of patients admitted to hospital with a provisional diagnosis of cardiac pain may turn out to have only oesophageal disease.

Sometimes oesophageal pain is experienced entirely in the epigastrium, when it may mimic peptic ulceration.

Regurgitation and vomiting

Fluid may be regurgitated into the mouth when the patient lies down, bends or strains, and may even wake him at night. The fluid may taste bitter (bile) or sour (acid). There may be vomiting, and in some patients with gastro-oesophageal reflux the predominant symptom is frequent, effortless vomiting.

Odynophagia

This term describes a transitory discomfort, usually of burning character, felt behind the sternum when food or fluid (usually hot or alcoholic drinks, but also citrus fruit juices) is swallowed. It is characteristic and diagnostic of reflux oesophagitis.

Dysphagia

A sensation of delay at the lower end of the sternum as food is swallowed may be experienced in reflux oesophagitis. If it is more than mild and occasional it suggests that a stricture is present or that there is an associated motor abnormality.

Haemorrhage

Overt bleeding from reflux oesophagitis accounts for about 4% of all gastrointestinal (GI) haemorrhage. Occult bleeding is also uncommon. Identification of the oesophagus as the sole site of haemorrhage can only be achieved by GI endoscopy. 'Hiatal hernia' diagnosed radiologically is not a satisfactory explanation for overt or occult GI bleeding, and endoscopic confirmation of a site of bleeding is essential; if there is no visible abnormality the remaining GI tract must be investigated.

Oesophageal ulcers or gastric ulcers in the intrathoracic portion of a herniated stomach bleed more often than uncomplicated oesophagitis.

Respiratory symptoms

Some individuals with chronic bronchitis, recurrent pneumonia or asthma may be shown to have gastro-oesophageal reflux, and in some of these radio-opaque contrast medium swallowed at night has been demonstrated in the lung next morning.

The frequency with which reflux causes respiratory problems is uncertain; sometimes the conditions must be coincidental, and the intrathoracic pressure changes caused by respiratory disease may predispose to gastro-oesophageal reflux. However, reflux is worth searching for in any patient with a recurrent pulmonary problem where there is no other likely causative factor; if there is free reflux the patient may benefit from antireflux surgery, though at present no preoperative test offers a satisfactory prediction of outcome.

DIAGNOSIS

Characteristic GORD is sufficiently obvious that diagnostic tests are not essential, and a trial of therapy is sufficient confirmation. If symptoms are recurrent, severe, or atypical, or occur for the first time over 45 years (when malignancy starts to be a problem) then some test is desirable.

GI endoscopy [4]

Endoscopy has two purposes. It will demonstrate (or exclude) alternative diagnoses, such as peptic ulcer or malignancy; and it may confirm the diagosis by showing changes of erosive oesophagitis. However, up to 50% of patients considered to have GORD (by other criteria) will show no endoscopic abnormality. 'Grades' of oesophagitis may be misleading; they are open to observer variation and have only a modest correlation with the degree of acid reflux, and even less with symptoms.

Barium meal

This must now be considered a second-rate investigation in suspected GORD. It will usually demonstrate alternative pathology if present, but its positive discriminating value in the diagnosis is low [5].

Scintiscanning

γ-camera measurement of the reflux of isotopes swallowed and instilled into the stomach can be used to test for reflux with reasonable accuracy, but has never become popular because it is cumbersome and not easy to perform accurately [6].

Intra-oesophageal pH monitoring

This is the most accurate way to measure the frequency and duration of acid reflux into the oesophagus. The methodology is now fairly standardized, though different sorts of pH records, pH electrodes and analytical programmes are available. It has to be done carefully if reproducible results are to be obtained; a particular problem is that of siting the electrode accurately (usually 5 cm above the gastro-oesophageal sphincter) which can only be done manometrically, though careful placement by 'dead-reckoning' (based on patient height and endoscopic measurement) may suffice [7].

Everyone refluxes acid at some time during the day; determining the level of reflux which is pathological requires establishment of a normal range: not easy because of variation in age, habitus, meals, exercise [8]. Ideally, 'abnormal' is defined as above the ninety-fifth centile, or by the construction of receiver operator characteristic analysis. Many units have no real opportunity to do so, and take an arbitrary level of 5% of 24 hours below pH 4 as the upper limit of normal.

NATURAL HISTORY

The normal course of GORD is unclear, and has been confused by claims attached to different therapies. For powerful drugs or surgery there has been an inclination to portray GORD as a progressive disease with the likelihood of complications.

Data are hard to interpret: unfortunately, no good information exists as to the course of GORD with simple antacid therapy alone; all recent studies inevitably have patients with a variety of therapy.

A study of 701 patients in Lausanne [9] (treated with various regimens) showed only 23% pursuing a progressive course (i.e. worsening oesophagitis with about 9% developing an ulcer or stricture), 31% remaining static or improving, and 46% having a single isolated episode. The annual relapse rate was 14–18%, but in 5 years 43% relapsed. This is consonant with Schindlbeck's study of 105 patients [10] where only 24 needed regular therapy, and 41 received no therapy at all.

Conversely, 80–90% of patients with complications have no previously known oesophagitis, though they often have a history of GORD symptoms.

AETIOLOGY

The production of symptoms, oesophagitis and its complications, is the end result of a sequence of abnormalities of gastro-oesophageal function and structure.

Gastro-oesophageal reflux

The normal barrier to reflux (which is never complete) is made up of the anatomical arrangement of the gastro-oesophageal functional area, diaphragmatic 'squeeze' and the action of the gastro-oesophageal sphincter. Incompetence, leading to abnormally frequent reflux, results from changes in anatomy, weakness of the sphincter [11], or (most frequently) transient relaxation of the sphincter for unknown reasons – possibly triggered by gastric distension or other vagal stimulation [12].

Obesity increases reflux: smoking, alcohol, caffeine and various drugs diminish sphincter tone.

Stomach abnormalities

Gastric emptying is slow in some GORD patients, and gastric distension may trigger inappropriate sphincter relaxation [13].

Gastric juice

The refluxed juice is injurious mainly because of its acid–pepsin content. Acid secretion is not obviously abnormal in most GORD patients, but some may have a higher than normal basal acid output [14].

Bile and duodenal juices are damaging, but it is doubtful whether they play any part in GORD with an intact (unoperated) stomach [13].

Ineffective oesophageal defences

Peristalsis

Peristalsis empties most refluxed material from the oesophagus, but becomes increasingly ineffective as the degree of oesophagitis increases [15].

Saliva

The high bicarbonate content of saliva can neutralize small volumes of acid juice remaining after peristalsis has cleared the majority of the refluxate [16]. Salivation may become less effective in other patients.

Mucosa

The mucosa is protected by a thin layer of mucus (predominantly from saliva), the mechanical resistance of the squamous cells (and their hydrogen ion/potassium ion adenosine triphosphatase), and blood flow, which maintains nutrition and scavenges injurious agents. Integrity of the defences is damaged by smoking and by drugs, especially non-steroidal anti-inflammatory agents [17].

REFERENCES

1 Jones R, Lydeard S. Prevalence of symptoms of dyspepsia in the community. *Br Med J* 1989;298:30–32.

2 Klauser AG, Schindlbeck NE, Muller-Lissner SA. Symptoms in gastro-oesophageal reflux disease. *Lancet* 1990;335:205–208.

3 Bennett JR. Symptoms of gastro-oesophageal reflux. In: Bouchier IAD, Allan RN, Hodgson HJF, Keighley MRB, eds. *Textbook of Gastroenterology*, London: Baillière Tindall, 1984:42–43.

4 Armstrong D, Monnier P, Nicolet M, *et al.* Endoscopic assessment of oesophagitis. *Gullet* 1991;1:63–67.

5 Ott DJ, Wu WC, Gelfand DW. Reflux esophagitis revisited: prospective analysis of radiologic accuracy. *Gastroenterol Radiol* 1981;6:1–7.

6 Isaacs PET, Martins JCR, Edwards S, *et al.* Assessment of gastro-oesophageal reflux disease: comparison of reflux scintigraphy with endoscopy, biopsy and oesophageal pH monitoring. *Hepatol Gastroenterol* 1990;37:198–200.

7 Bennett JR. pH measurement in the oesophagus. *Baillière's Clin Gastroenterol* 1987; 1:747–767.

8 Schindlbeck NE, Heinrick C, Konig A, *et al.* Optimal threshold, sensitivity and specificity of long-term pH monitoring for the detection of gastro-oesophageal reflux. *Gastroenterology* 1987;93:85–90.

9 Ollyo JB, Monnier P, Fontolhet C, Savary M. The natural history, prevalence and incidence of reflux oesophagitis. *Gullet* 1993;3(Suppl):3–10.

10 Schindlbeck NE, Klauser AG, Berglassmer G, Muller-Lissner SA. Three year follow-up of patients with gastro-oesophageal reflux. *Eur J Gastroenterol Hepatol* 1991;3:1.

11 Mittal RK, Fisher M, McCallum RW, *et al.* Human lower esophageal sphincter pressure response to increased intra-abdominal pressures. *Am J Physiol* 1990;258:G624–G630.

12 Dent J, Halloway RH, Toouli J, Dodds JW. Mechanisms of lower oesophageal sphincter incompetence in patients with symptomatic gastro-oesophageal reflux. *Gut* 1988;29: 1020–1028.

13 Ferrarini F, Longanesi A, Baldi F. Pathophysiology and pathogenesis of reflux oesophagitis. *Gullet* 1993;3(Suppl):11–20.

14 Collen MJ, Lewis JH, Benjamin SB. Gastro hypersecretion in refractory gastroesopageal reflux disease. *Gastroenterology* 1990;98:654–661.

15 Kahrilas PJ, Dodds WJ, Hogan WJ, *et al.* Esophageal peristaltic dysfunction in peptic esophagitis. *Gastroenterology* 1986;91:897–904.

16 Helm JF, Dodds WJ, Hogan WJ. Salivary response to esophageal acid in normal subjects and in patients with reflux esophagitis. *Gastroenterology* 1987;93:1393–1397.

17 Orlando RC. Esophageal epithelial resistance. *J Clin Gastroenterol* 1986;8(Suppl):12–16.

Duodenal ulceration

R. POUNDER

Duodenal ulceration has been transformed in the last 17 years by a succession of innovations that have had direct effects on clinical practice. The widespread introduction of fibreoptic endoscopy allowed diagnostic precision and accurate assessment of ulcer healing; the introduction of gastric acid antisecretory drugs provided the opportunity to speed peptic ulcer healing; the discovery of *Helicobacter pylori* raised the prospect of a medical 'cure' for duodenal ulceration; finally, the prospect of laparoscopic surgery offers the potential for day case elective surgery.

FIBREOPTIC ENDOSCOPY

Basil Hirschowitz, the father of fibreoptic endoscopy, has recently written a historical review of the development and early application of flexible fibreoptic endoscopes [1]. Modern endoscopy means that every district general hospital now has the opportunity for the precise diagnosis of active duodenal ulceration. Within the framework of clinical trials, fibreoptic endoscopy allows accurate documentation of ulcer healing. Finally, the endoscopist can identify those patients at risk of recurrent haemorrhage from a duodenal ulcer and, using inexpensive sclerotherapy, may decrease the dangers of continuing or recurrent haemorrhage [2].

CONTROL OF GASTRIC ACID SECRETION

Histamine H_2-receptor antagonists

Control of intragastric acidity is related to the dose of the H_2-antagonist and frequency of dosing [3]. Hence, a small dose of an H_2-antagonist at bedtime results in a decrease of intragastric acidity lasting approximately 6–8 hours, whereas a four-times-a-day regimen (e.g. ranitidine 150 mg four times daily) will result in marked control of intragastric acidity that is exerted throughout the 24 hours. However, due to the phenomenon of tolerance, competitive H_2-receptor antagonists will never produce an unremitting, profound decrease of 24-hour intragastric acidity [4].

Duodenal ulcer healing under the influence of an H_2-receptor antagonist relates directly to the control of intragastric acidity [5]. The critical threshold appears to be a pH of 3 (1 mmol/l).

After 8 weeks of full-dose treatment with an H_2-receptor antagonist, approximately 95% of duodenal ulcers will be healed. Non-healing ulcers after 8 weeks of treatment are termed 'refractory' or 'intractable', i.e. not responding to conventional treatment [6]. Any duodenal ulcer patient with continuing dyspepsia after 8 weeks of treatment should be subjected to a further endoscopy – to assess whether there is active ulceration, to biopsy any ulceration, and also to perform an antral biopsy for *H. pylori*. The fasting plasma gastric concentration should also be measured, to exclude the rare patient with the Zollinger–Ellison syndrome. The biopsy of the duodenal ulcer will exclude rare causes of non-peptic ulceration in the duodenum, e.g. Crohn's disease, tuberculosis, lymphoma or carcinoma, or cytomegalovirus infection in the immunocompromised. Having excluded the rare causes of continuing duodenal ulceration, and confirmed continuing infection with *H. pylori*, patients with refractory duodenal ulceration should continue with an H_2-blocker, but also receive treatment to eradicate *H. pylori*.

Long-term treatment with a low dose of an H_2-antagonist should be offered to patients who either have a history of aggressive ulceration (e.g. past haemorrhage or perforation, or repeated relapse) or those duodenal ulcer patients who are elderly or who have other serious medical problems [7]. Such patients may also be eligible for attempted eradication of *H. pylori*, but otherwise they should be offered indefinite treatment with an H_2-receptor antagonist.

Inhibitors of the proton pump hydrogen ion/potassium ion adenosine triphosphatase, such as omeprazole [8] or lansoprazole, cause a profound decrease of 24-hour intragastric acidity and hence are associated with faster duodenal ulcer healing. Both drugs result in the healing of approximately 95% of ulcers after 4 weeks of full-dose treatment. However, the problem with the proton pump inhibitors is that they do not have a 'mild' dosing regimen. Hence, the long-term use of omeprazole has been restricted to patients with the Zollinger–Ellison syndrome, severe reflux oesophagitis, or those with complicated duodenal ulceration [9]. There are theoretical concerns about unremitting elimination of intragastric acidity, but paradoxically it has recently been reported that long-term recipients of omeprazole may develop gastric mucosal atrophy [10].

HELICOBACTER PYLORI

The identification of *H. pylori*, just 10 years ago, has produced a flurry of research activity [11]. However, the role of the organism in the pathogenesis of duodenal ulceration remains unclear.

H. pylori survives in the mucus of the gastric mucosa, extending into areas of gastric metaplasia in the duodenum. The organism may survive in the mouth, and it is possible that it is excreted in the faeces. There is no animal reservoir for this species, and it is not clear how the organism is transmitted from person to person. In the British population, approximately 20% of 20-year-olds are infected, and 60% of 60-year-olds. However, it is not certain whether only 20% of the present 20-year-olds will continue to carry the organism for the rest of their lives whilst the remaining 80% remain uninfected. Conversely, we do not know how long the present 60-year-olds have been infected. It seems quite likely that most people are infected in childhood, and that spontaneous loss of infection is rare. Active infection is associated with both humoral and cell-mediated immunity, but it is not clear whether this immunity provides against reinfection after eradication; this will prove an important point if a vaccination programme is to prove successful.

H. pylori is associated with active or acute gastritis; that is, inflammation of the gastric mucosa assessed by histological examination. The organism results in hypergastrinaemia and hyperpepsinogenaemia, both of which are reversed after eradication of the organism [12,13]. However, it does not have a direct effect on gastric acid secretion; so far, the only documented abnormality has been an augmentation of acid secretion when stimulated by gastrin releasing peptide.

Eradicating *H. pylori* from the gastric mucosa remains a major clinical challenge; a recent meta-analysis of clinical trials suggests that a combination of bismuth, metronidazole and oxytetracycline will provide the best results [14]. A suitable regimen might be tripotassium dicitrato bismuthate tab 1 four times daily, metronidazole 200 mg four times daily, and oxytetracycline 500 mg four times daily, all three drugs taken simultaneously for 2 weeks. This regimen will eradicate the organism from approximately 90% of subjects, with less success in populations where there is widespread clinical use of metronidazole. The management of metronidazole-resistant *H. pylori* remains problematical.

The strongest evidence that *H. pylori* is of importance to the duodenal ulcer patient is provided by studies which demonstrate that eradication of the organism is associated with decreased ulcer relapse [15]. The latest study, unlike almost all of its predecessors, involved a double-blind protocol, showing that the addition of antibiotics to ranitidine not only increased the rate of ulcer healing, but also provided long-term remission from relapse (Fig. 1) [16]. Omeprazole has been coprescribed with antibiotics, but most regimens have used extremely high doses of both omeprazole and amoxycillin, with implications for both cost and safety.

The widespread use of treatment to eradicate *H. pylori* is at the moment relatively unpopular. This is because the treatment regimens are

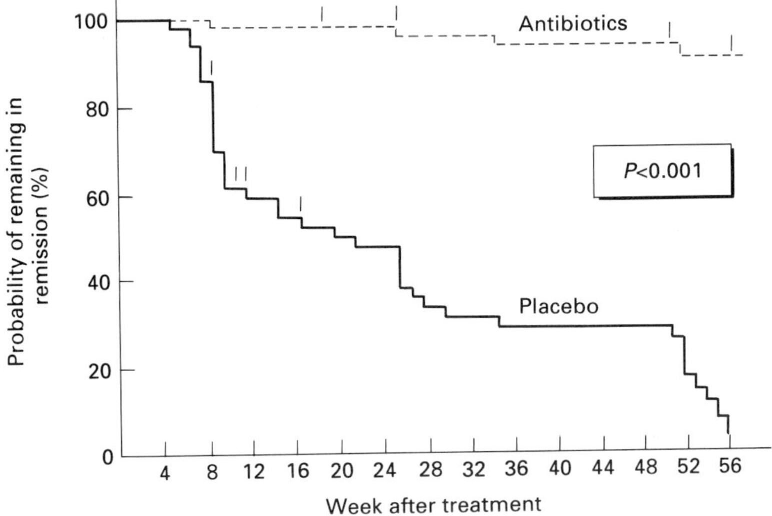

Fig. 1 Probability that a duodenal ulcer would remain in remission during one year of follow-up – after healing with either ranitidine and antibiotics (amoxycillin and metronidazole) or ranitidine plus placebo. (Reprinted, by permission of the *New England Journal of Medicine* [16].)

both complicated and relatively unreliable, and the existing clinical trials have rarely been double-blind, subject to external audit, or performed with large numbers of patients.

LAPAROSCOPIC SURGERY

The introduction of laparoscopic surgery in the last few years has raised the prospect that a highly selective vagotomy might be performed as a day case procedure [17]. There are few published studies or reports, but this type of manoeuvre might be helpful in the young patient with a metronidazole-resistant infection with *H. pylori*.

SUMMARY

Fibreoptic endoscopy is now the standard technique for the precise diagnosis of active duodenal ulceration. Most doctors choose to treat acute ulcer patients using a full dose of a histamine H_2-receptor antagonist at the time of ulcer relapse, selecting long-term maintenance treatment for those patients with either aggressive ulceration, old age or serious coincidental medical illnesses. *H. pylori* appears to be an important factor in the chronicity of duodenal ulceration, and those patients with difficult or aggressive ulceration may benefit from an attempt to eradicate the organism from the gastric mucosa. Finally, laparoscopic highly selective vagotomy is in the early stages of clinical assessment, but it is unlikely to have a widespread application.

REFERENCES

1 Hirschowitz BI. Development and application of endoscopy. *Gastroenterology* 1993; 104:337–342.
2 Swain CP. Upper gastrointestinal haemorrhage. In: Pounder RE, ed. *Recent Advances in Gastroenterology 9*. Edinburgh: Churchill Livingstone, 1992:135–150.
3 Burget DW, Chiverton SG, Hunt RH. Is there an optimal degree of acid suppression for healing of duodenal ulcers? A model of the relationship between ulcer healing and acid suppression. *Gastroenterology* 1990;99:345–351.
4 Smith JTL, Nwokolo CU, Gavey C, Pounder RE. Tolerance during eight days of high-dose H_2-blockade: placebo-controlled studies of 24 hour acidity and gastrin. *Aliment Pharmacol Ther* 1990;4S:47–63.
5 McIsaac RL, Dixon JS, Mills JG, Wood JR. Ranitidine in the treatment of duodenal ulcer disease: relationship between antisecretory effects and ulcer healing rate. *Aliment Pharmacol Ther* 1991;5:227–244.
6 Pounder RE. Duodenal ulcers that are difficult to heal. *Br Med J* 1988;297:1560–1561.
7 Penston JG, Wormsley KG. Review article: maintenance treatment with H_2-receptor antagonists for peptic ulcer disease. *Aliment Pharmacol Ther* 1992;6:3–29.
8 Maton PN. Omeprazole. *N Engl J Med* 1991;324:965–975.
9 Pounder RE. Degrees of acid suppression and ulcer healing: dosage considerations. *Aliment Pharmacol Ther* 1991:5(Suppl 1):5–14.
10 Solcia E, Fiocca R, Havu N, *et al.* Gastric endocrine cells and gastritis in patients receiving long-term omeprazole treatment. *Digestion* 1992;51(Suppl 1):82–92.
11 Pounder RE. *Helicobacter pylori* and duodenal ulceration. In: Summerfield J, Seymour CA, eds. *Horizons in Medicine, No 3*. Eastbourne: TransMedica Europe, 1991:370–376.
12 Prewett EJ, Smith JTL, Nwokolo CU, *et al.* Eradication of *Helicobacter pylori* abolishes 24-hour hypergastrinaemia: a prospective study in healthy subjects. *Aliment Pharmacol Ther* 1991;5:283–290.
13 Fraser AG, Prewett EJ, Pounder RE, Samloff IM. Twenty-four hour hyperpepsinogenaemia in *Helicobacter pylori*-positive subjects is abolished by eradication of the infection. *Aliment Pharmacol Ther* 1992;6:389–394.
14 Chiba N, Rao BV, Rademaker JW, Hunt RH. Meta-analysis of the efficacy of antibiotic therapy in eradicating *Helicobacter pylori*. *Am J Gastroenterol* 1992;12:1716–1724.
15 Rauws EAJ. Role of *Helicobacter pylori* in duodenal ulcer. *Drugs* 1992;44:921–927.
16 Hentschel E, Brandstatter G, Dragosics B, *et al.* Effect of ranitidine and amoxicillin plus metronidazole on the eradication of *Helicobacter pylori* and the recurrence of duodenal ulcer. *N Engl J Med* 1993;328:308–312.
17 Boyce HW. Laparoscopy. In: Cotton PB, Tytgat GNJ, Williams CB, eds. *Annual of Gastrointestinal Endoscopy*. London: Current Science, 1993:113–122.

Crohn's disease: recent advances in medical treatment

R. N. ALLAN

INTRODUCTION

Crohn's disease is not a single disease but comprises a wide variety of disorders masquerading under the same name. Each symptomatic patient requires careful individual evaluation, including review of previous resections, and clear definition of the site and extent of macroscopic disease. Metabolic problems such as anaemia and fluid or electrolyte depletion must be identified and corrected or excluded. Symptomatic patients may have local complications which are the province of the surgeon including stricture formation, abscess or enterocutaneous fistula. The possibility that abdominal pain may be due to associated disorders such as renal stones, gallstones or peptic ulcer must be considered. Prescription of specific medical treatment is thus only a small part of the physician's role in caring for patients with Crohn's disease.

DRUG THERAPY

Symptomatic patients with macroscopic Crohn's disease without complications (which are appropriately treated surgically) need to be considered for medical management. Several reports have summarized recent therapeutic advances [1–3].

This treatment includes:

1 symptomatic relief;
2 aminosalicylates (sulphasalazine and the new derivatives);
3 corticosteroids;
4 immunosuppressive therapy;
5 antibacterial agents including metronidazole;
6 inflammatory mediators;
7 dietary manipulation and enteral or parenteral feeding.

SYMPTOMATIC TREATMENT

Non-specific treatment with codeine phosphate and diphenoxylate or loperamide are well established for patients with mild diarrhoea associated with macroscopic disease or following colectomy. Double-blind crossover trials have shown that loperamide decreases stool frequency and weight in patients with Crohn's disease treated by ileocolonic resection or after colectomy and ileorectal anastomosis [4,5]. Loperamide and codeine phosphate both reduce ileostomy output in patients with Crohn's disease by 20–25% [6,7].

AMINOSALICYLATES

Sulphasalazine (Salazopyrin)

Sulphasalazine has been used for the medical treatment of active Crohn's disease for many years. It consists of a carrier, sulphapyridine, linked by a diazo-bond to the active component, 5-aminosalicylic acid (5-ASA). When taken orally most of the drug is delivered to the colon intact. A small amount is absorbed in the small intestine, undergoes enterohepatic circulation and is then excreted in the bile so that plasma concentrations are very low. The diazo-bond is split in the colon by bacterial action liberating sulphapyridine and the active component 5-ASA. Sulphapyridine is responsible for many of the side-effects of sulphasalazine such as headache, nausea, vomiting, skin rashes and impaired fertility in men [8].

The evidence for the beneficial effect of sulphasalazine is based on the American National Cooperative Crohn's Disease Trial Study (NCCDS) which showed that sulphasalazine given in a weight-related does of 2–5 g per day for a period of 17 weeks was superior to placebo in patients with ileocolonic and colonic Crohn's disease [9]. In the European studies patients with active disease treated for 6 weeks with sulphasalazine (3 g daily) showed responses at all sites, which were superior to those with placebo [10]. In a Swedish study, sulphasalazine (3 g daily over 4 months) was superior to placebo, but its benefit was more marked in colonic disease than in disease confined to the small intestine [11]. All these short-term studies (maximum 4 months) were consistent in demonstrating that sulphasalazine is superior to placebo in the treatment of active Crohn's disease.

The two studies in which treatment was continued beyond 4 months showed that any initial benefit had been lost within 2 years and by that time the outcome was no better than that obtained using placebo treatment.

The new salicylates

The new formulations eliminate the carrier sulphapyridine and have been designed to deliver 5-ASA to the small or large intestine [12].

Olsalazine (Dipentum) most closely resembles the parent molecule since two 5-ASA molecules are linked by the diazo-bond thus eliminating the carrier sulphapyridine and its associated side-effects. The 5-ASA is released by bacterial action, as for sulphasalazine [13]. The other preparations for delivery of 5-ASAs incorporate either a mechanical or pH dependent release. This increases the small intestinal delivery and reduces the colonic delivery of 5-ASA. For example, Asacol is 5-ASA coated with eudragit which dissolves at a pH over 7, so that 5-ASA is released into the distal small bowel and colon. The ethylcellulose coating of Pentasa granules dissolves gradually during the passage through the small bowel. Thus, with these preparations free 5-ASA is released in both the small bowel and colon.

At both sites 5-ASA is acetylated by the epithelium. In the small bowel this process can be overloaded by rapid release of 5-ASA which allows an appreciable amount of 5-ASA to be absorbed which, unlike acetylated 5-ASA, is nephrotoxic in experimental animals. Rapid release of 5-ASA is more likely in the small bowel with Asacol than with slow release Pentasa.

Other 5-ASA preparations include a slow release system achieved by compressing 5-ASA with sodium carbonate and glycerine and protecting this core with an enteric coating of eudragit L. 5-ASA is released from this preparation at a pH over 5.5. Other preparations include a core surrounded by an envelope of resin which dissolves at different pH levels predominantly in the terminal ileum and caecum (rauwolfia) [14].

Treatment of active Crohn's disease

Sulphasalazine is significantly superior to placebo for treatment of active Crohn's disease but is not effective as maintenance therapy. Since most of the newer 5-ASA compounds depending on the formulation are released in both the small bowel and the large bowel rather than the colon alone, it is reasonable to expect that salicylates might be useful in both the treatment of active Crohn's disease and maintenance of remission.

Active disease

In a study of slow release 5-ASA (Pentasa) in the treatment of 40 patients with active Crohn's disease allocated to receive either 5-ASA (1.5 g daily) or placebo for 6 weeks, there was no significant difference in clinical activity or laboratory indices. There were also no serious side-effects [15].

There was, however, a significant benefit compared with placebo in the treatment of active Crohn's disease when the dose of 5-ASA (Pentasa) was increased to 4 g daily, although the benefit was not dramatic [16].

Maintenance treatment for Crohn's disease

The role of 5-ASA in maintenance treatment has not yet been established but it may benefit certain groups of patients. In the management of Crohn's disease in remission, 5-ASA (0.5 g three times a day) was compared with placebo over 12 months. No major differences were found, except for a reduction in the ileal disease relapse rate in the patients taking 5-ASA [17].

In a series of 161 patients with inactive Crohn's disease Pentasa (2 g daily) was compared with placebo over 2 years. There was no overall benefit but a significant reduction of relapse rates was noted in patients with ileal disease treated early after induction of remission [18].

In a recent study [19], 44 patients were randomized in a double-blind manner to receive either 5-ASA (2 g per day) or placebo for 4 months. The groups were well matched in respect of site of disease and previous corticosteroid treatment. Overall there was no difference between the active treatment and placebo-treated groups but again there was a lower relapse rate in patients with ileal disease in the active treatment group [19].

Side-effects of 5-ASA

Serious renal complications following ingestion of 5-ASA compounds have been reported in nine patients in the UK [20]. The mechanism of the nephrotoxicity is unknown, but is probably related to absorption of 5-ASA from the small intestine. 5-ASA released in the large intestine from the parent compound, sulphasalazine, and olsalazine is readily acetylated and less likely to cause problems.

Olsalazine may cause watery diarrhoea in some patients, but this effect can be minimized using a low starting dose. The proportion of patients with intolerance to this preparation is similar overall to that with other aminosalicylates [13].

Summary

Sulphasalazine has been used for many years. Its safety profile and side-effects are well understood and it is cost-effective and is still appropriate therapy for most patients. For those with sulphasalazine intolerance, one of the newer preparations can be used. Of the available preparations olsalazine (Dipentum) is best for large bowel disease despite the occasional problem of watery diarrhoea, while the slow release preparations such as 5-aminosalicylic acid (Pentasa) may be particularly useful for small bowel disease. New preparations which are being tested include balsalazide (4-aminosalicylate linked to an inactive carrier). This might well prove to have all the benefits of the other salicylates but without their occasional disadvantages. Both the parent compound and the newer derivatives only have short-term benefit in active disease.

CORTICOSTEROIDS

The value of short-term corticosteroids in the treatment of active Crohn's disease is well established, but this has to be balanced with the well-known side-effects including depression of the hypothalamic–pituitary–adrenal axis, growth impairment in children and possible adverse long-term effects on the skeleton.

Acute disease

A controlled trial which included patients with Crohn's colitis showed that corticotrophin 40 U daily gave equivalent results to hydrocortisone 300 mg daily; however, both drugs were given intravenously [21].

Active disease

The NCCDS trial showed that prednisolone 0.25–0.75 mg per kg body weight, given as a maximum 60 mg daily over 4 months, was more effective than placebo (*P* less than 0.0006). These results were significant in patients with both ileal and ileocolonic disease, but the results in patients with colonic disease alone were not significant, probably due to small sample size [9].

In the European Co-operative Crohn's Disease Study a tapered 6 week course of oral 6-methylprednisolone (from 48 mg per day to 12 mg per day) was more effective than placebo (*P* less than 0.001), in small and large bowel disease alone and in small and large bowel disease together [10].

New developments

Locally acting corticosteroids which are metabolized during first pass through the liver might provide effective anti-inflammatory activity and minimize the side-effects.

Their benefit has been demonstrated in a controlled trial in patients with distal colitis using beclomethasone enemas which are rapidly metabolized by first pass through the liver, compared with systemically absorbed betamethasone. The outcome was similar in the two groups, but beclomethasone did not depress the hypothalamic–pituitary–adrenal axis [22].

Budesonide, which has similar properties, has been used for many years in the treatment of bronchial asthma. The patent on this drug has now expired, and a new carrier system to target budesonide in the distal ileum and colon is now under evaluation [23] and this drug could potentially provide effective local anti-inflammatory activity with minimum side-effects.

IMMUNOSUPPRESSIVE THERAPY

Azathioprine and 6-mercaptopurine

Azathioprine and its metabolite 6-mercaptopurine have both been used in the treatment of active Crohn's disease. The NCCDS trial found no significant benefit for azathioprine in the treatment of active Crohn's disease over a period of 17 weeks, or in the maintenance of remission over a period of 2 years [9].

Good evidence for its value was, however, documented in a study of 51 patients in remission after treatment with azathioprine, who were randomized to either continued treatment or changed to placebo. In the next 12 months 41% of patients on placebo relapsed compared with 5% of those continuing with azathioprine. The study did not, however, identify those patients who might respond well to azathioprine in the first place [24].

Side-effects from azathioprine are uncommon; of these pancreatitis (3.3%), bone marrow depression (2.2%), allergy (2%) and infection (7.4%) are the most frequent [25].

Summary

Azathioprine has a place in those patients with severe persistent disease, particularly extensive small bowel or extensive colonic disease, but there is no controlled evidence for its long-term benefit (more than 2 years).

Cyclosporin

The role of cyclosporin in severe active Crohn's disease has been evaluated in a placebo-controlled randomized trial with 3 months treatment of cyclosporin by mouth, 5.0–7.5 mg per kg per day. Of 37 patients treated with cyclosporin 59% improved over 3 months compared with 32% of 34 placebo treated patients – a significantly greater proportion [26].

However, the potential side-effects, particularly nephrotoxicity, have limited its use and the group who conducted the controlled trial now rarely use cyclosporin in clinical practice (V. Binder, personal communication).

In addition to side-effects, the fact that most patients relapse when the drug is withdrawn suggests that it will have very limited use in the treatment of patients with Crohn's disease.

METRONIDAZOLE

A small Swedish cross-over study compared metronidazole and sulphasalazine in active Crohn's disease over a period of 4 months. Metronidazole proved marginally superior to sulphasalazine using clinical laboratory indices for evaluation. In practice, metronidazole is particularly useful in treating secondary infection associated with perianal Crohn's disease [11].

INFLAMMATORY MEDIATORS

Induction of remission is associated with inhibition or reduction in the formation of inflammatory mediators. Active drugs in the treatment of Crohn's disease such as corticosteroids, sulphasalazine and 5-aminosalicylic acid affect most or all of these inflammatory mediators. Current efforts have been directed to the development of new drugs with selective inhibition or a receptor blockade of a single mediator involving, e.g. prostanoids, leukotrienes, platelet activating factors, cytokines or free oxygen radicals.

The raised leukotriene concentrations in rectal mucosa and rectal dialysates of patients with active inflammatory bowel disease suggested that selective 5-lipoxygenase inhibitors or leukotriene receptor antagonists may offer a new therapeutic approach. To date results of a double-blind study of an oral specific 5-lipoxygenase inhibitor in the treatment of ulcerative colitis are disappointing [27]. It is likely that only drugs which affect most or all of the agonists are likely to be of benefit, and those which affect one single mediator and/or block one single receptor are unlikely to be helpful [28].

The efficacy of fish oil containing 3-ω fatty acids, which are inhibitors of leukotriene synthesis, have been evaluated in a 7 month double-blind placebo-controlled crossover trial. There was limited morphological improvement, but the clinical benefits were small and confined to patients with ulcerative colitis [29].

DIET, ENTERAL FEEDING AND PARENTERAL NUTRITION

Diet

While patients and their families often have an intense interest in dietary factors, there is no evidence as yet that dietary measures have a major impact on the natural history of the disease. Initial studies suggested that a diet rich in unrefined carbohydrate and low in sugar might reduce the relapse rate in Crohn's disease [30]. However, an extensive national controlled study of patients with quiescent or mildly active Crohn's disease compared the two dietary regimes but found no significant difference between the two groups [31].

Enteral and elemental diets

The group who published the first study comparing enteral feeding and oral prednisolone have recently evaluated their long-term results. In those patients who could follow the diet successfully, 96/113 (85%) had a good response which was unrelated to age, gender and site or severity of disease. Most other studies suggest that patients with small bowel disease respond better than those with large intestinal disease. After discontinuing treatment, the relapse rate was 22% at 6 months, with an annual relapse rate of 8–10% thereafter. The outcome was very similar, whether remission was induced by elemental diet or oral prednisolone [32].

The European Co-operative Crohn's Disease Study Group has carried out a number of studies. In one study, a liquid formula diet was compared with 6-methylprednisolone (48 mg per day initially, reducing the dose weekly over 6 weeks to 12 mg daily), and sulphasalazine (3 g daily) in a 6 week randomized prospective multicentre trial of 95 patients with active Crohn's disease.

Of the 44 randomized to receive drug treatment, 32 showed improvement in the Crohn's disease activity index (CDAI), compared with 21 of 51 receiving an oral defined formula diet (*P* less than 0.05). The number of patients withdrawn was much higher in the formula diet group, usually because the liquid diet proved unpalatable. In those who completed the study, the formula diet and drug treatment were equally effective [33]. The same group compared enteral nutrition with 6-methylprednisolone and sulphasalazine in the treatment of active Crohn's disease, where the drug treatment proved to be superior [34].

The long-term outcome after completion of a course of elemental diet in the treatment of active Crohn's disease is of particular interest. Most patients with colonic disease (80%) relapsed within 6 months, while the relapse rate was much lower in patients with small bowel disease (27%). One-third of the patients had a prolonged remission of 12–36 months [35].

In the treatment of active Crohn's disease, oral prednisolone is simple and effective, but where corticosteroids are contraindicated, particularly in the younger patients, elemental or enteral nutrition are useful alternatives in those who can tolerate the regime. Response rates are particularly encouraging in small bowel disease.

Total parenteral nutrition

The pendulum has swung back against the short-term use of total parenteral nutrition since the benefits are limited and may even cause harm by inducing intestinal mucosal atrophy with breakdown of the normal gut mucosal barrier, thus allowing ingress of bacteria and endotoxins. Enteral or oral feeding provides energy sources for the intestinal epithelium and minimizes the risk of infection from bacteria and endotoxins [36].

The recent introduction of peripheral intravenous feeding with fine bore silicone catheters can maximize the benefits and minimize the hazards, but total parenteral nutrition is now only usually used for nutritional support in those few patients with severe complications of the disease and occasionally for postoperative complications.

MEDICAL VERSUS SURGICAL TREATMENT

Surgical treatment for Crohn's disease is often recommended when medical treatment has failed, but this would now be regarded as an outdated concept.

There are certain situations where surgical treatment is the treatment of choice including the relief of recurrent episodes of intestinal obstruction caused by fibrous stricture formation and complications such as abscess and enterocutaneous fistula formation.

While medical treatment is particularly appropriate for episodes of, e.g. acute Crohn's colitis when remission can be rapidly induced in the previously severely ill individual, there is no evidence that drug treatment modifies the natural history in the medium term (more than 2 years). Medical treatment may induce remission earlier than would have occurred without treatment, particularly in those patients with extensive Crohn's colitis, and may delay surgical intervention.

The medical team working closely with an experienced surgical team are likely to produce the best outcome in the interim, before the pathogenesis of Crohn's disease is unravelled.

REFERENCES

1 Allan RN. Medical management: its accomplishments in Crohn's disease and indication for surgery. *World J Surg* 1988;12:174–179.

2 Allan RN, Hodgson HJF. Inflammatory bowel disease. In: Pounder RE, ed. *Recent Advances in Gastroenterology 9*. Edinburgh: Churchill-Livingstone, 1992:1–25.

3 Lennard-Jones JE. Crohn's disease: medical treatment. In: Bouchier IAD, Allan RN, Hodgson HJF, Keighley MRB, eds. *Gastroenterology: Clinical Science and Practice*. London: Harcourt Brace Jovanovich, 1993.

4 Mainguet P, Fiasse R. Double blind placebo-controlled study of loperamide (Imodium) in chronic diarrhoea caused by ileocolonic disease or resection. *Gut* 1977;18:575–579.

5 Pelemans W, Vantrappen G. A double-blind crossover comparison of loperamide with diphenoxylate in the symptomatic treatment of chronic diarrhoea. *Gastroenterology* 1976;70:1030–1034.

6 Tytgat GN, Huibretse K. Loperamide and ileostomy output: Placebo-controlled double-blind crossover study. *Br Med J* 1975;ii:667.

7 Newton CR. Effect of codeine phosphate, Lomotil and Isogel on ileostomy function. *Gut* 1978;19:377–383.

8 Hayllar J, Bjarnasson I. Sulphasalazine in ulcerative colitis: in memoriam? *Gut* 1991; 32:462–463.

9 Summers RW, Switz DM, Sessions JT Jr, *et al*. National Co-operative Crohn's Disease Study: Results of drug treatment. *Gastroenterology* 1979;77:847–869.

10 Malchow H, Ewe K, Brandes JW, *et al*. European Co-operative Crohn's Disease Study: Results of drug treatment. *Gastroenterology* 1984;86:249–266.

11 Ursing B, Alm T, Barany F, *et al*. A comparative study of metronidazole and sulphasalazine for active Crohn's disease. *Gastroenterology* 1982;83:550–562.

12 Ireland A, Jewell DP. Mechanism of action of 5-aminosalicyclic acid and its derivatives. *Clin Sci* 1990;78:119–125.

13 Staerk Laursen L, Stokholm M, Bukhave K, *et al*. Disposition of 5-aminosalicylic acid by olsalazine and three mesalazine preparations in patients with ulcerative colitis: comparison of intraluminal colonic concentrations, serum values and urinary excretion. *Gut* 1990;31:1271–1276.

14 Jarnerot G. Newer 5-aminosalcylic acid based drugs in chronic inflammatory bowel disease. *Drugs* 1989;37:73–86.

15 Mahida YR, Jewell DP. Slow-release 5-aminosalicylic acid (Pentasa) for the treatment of active Crohn's disease. *Digestion* 1990;99:113–118.

16 Law R, Hanauer S, Rick G. Multicentre open label long-term cohort study of oral Pentasa in Crohn's disease. *Gastroenterology* 1990;98:A185.

17 Thomson ABR (on behalf of the International Mesalazine Study Group). Coated oral 5-aminosalicylic acid versus placebo in maintaining remission of inactive Crohn's disease. *Aliment Pharmacol Therap* 1990;4:55–64.

18 Gendie JP, Mary JY, Florent C. Does Pentasa prevent relapses in quiescent Crohn's disease? *Gastroenterology* 1990;98:A171.

19 Brignola C, Iannone P, Pasquati S, *et al*. Placebo controlled trial of oral 5-ASA in relapse prevention of Crohn's disease. *Dig Dis Sci* 1992;37:29–32.

20 Committee on Safety of Medicines. *Current Problems*. 30 December 1990.

21 Kaplan HP, Portnoy B, Binder HJ, *et al*. A controlled evaluation of intravenous adrenocorticotrophic hormone and hydrocortisone in the treatment of acute colitis. *Gastroenterology* 1975;69:91–95.

22 Halpern Z, Sold O, Baratz M, *et al*. A controlled trial of beclomethasone versus betamethasone enemas in distal ulcerarative colitis. *J Clin Gastroenterol* 1991;13:38–41.

23 Lofberg R, Danielsson A, Salde L. Oral budesonide in active ileo-cecal Crohn's disease – A pilot trial with a topically acting steroid. *Gastroenterology* 1991;100:A26.

24 O'Donoghue DP, Dawson AM, Powell-Tuck J, *et al*. Double blind withdrawal trial of azathioprine as maintenance treatment for Crohn's disease. *Lancet* 1978;ii:955–957.

25 Present DH, Meltzer SJ, Krumholz MP, *et al*. 6-Mercaptopurine in the management of

inflammatory bowel disease: short and long-term toxicity. *Ann Intern Med* 1989;111: 641–649.

26 Brynskov J, Freund L, Rasmussen SN, *et al.* A placebo-controlled, double blind, randomised trial of cyclosporine therapy in active chronic Crohn's disease. *N Engl J Med* 1989;321:845–850.

27 Stenson WF, Lauritsen K, Laursen LS, *et al.* A clinical trial of Zileuton, a specific inhibitor of 5-lipoxygenase in ulcerative colitis. *Gastroenterology* 1991;100:A253.

28 Rachmilewitz D. New forms of treatment for inflammatory bowel disease. *Gut* 1992;33: 1301–1302.

29 Lorenz R. Supplementation with n-3 fatty acids from fish oil in chronic inflammatory bowel disease. *J Intern Med* 1989;225(Suppl):225–232.

30 Heaton KW, Thornton JR, Emmett PM. Treatment of Crohn's disease with an unrefined carbohydrate, fibre rich diet. *Br Med J* 1979;ii:764–767.

31 Ritchie JK, Wadsworth J, Lennard-Jones JE, Rogers E. Controlled multicentre therapeutic trial of an unrefined carbohydrate, fibre rich diet in Crohn's disease. *Gut* 1986;27:A1278.

32 Teahon K, Bjarnason I, Pearson M, Levi AJ. Ten years' experience with an elemental diet in the management of Crohn's disease. *Gut* 1990;31:1133–1137.

33 Malchow H, Steinhardt HJ, Lorenz-Meyer H, *et al.* Feasibility and effectiveness of a defined-formula diet regimen in treating active Crohn's disease. European Co-operative Crohn's Disease Study III. *Scand J Gastroenterol* 1990;25:235–244.

34 Lochs H, Steinhardt HJ, Klaus-Wentz B, *et al.* Comparison of enteral nutrition and drug treatment in active Crohn's disease. Results of the European Co-operative Crohn's Disease Study IV. *Gastroenterology* 1991;101:881–888.

35 Giaffer MH, Cann P, Holdsworth CD. Long-term effects of elemental and exclusive diets for Crohn's disease. *Aliment Pharmacol Therap* 1991;5:115–126.

36 Maynard ND, Bihari DJ. Postoperative feeding. *Br Med J* 1991;303:1007–1008.

The gastrointestinal manifestations associated with human immunodeficiency virus infection

B. G. GAZZARD

The management of gastroenterological disease in HIV seropositive patients is markedly different from general gastroenterological practice. Symptoms often have multiple causes; thus, a quarter of all patients with diarrhoea have more than one pathogen responsible [1]. The majority of gastroenterological manifestations are due to infection; either virulent organisms which may have a more prolonged and relapsing course, or opportunistic infections causing no or self-limiting disease in the immunocompetent host. It follows that the investigation pathway of most gastroenterological symptoms in HIV seropositive individuals will be different from those with which most practising gastroenterologists are familiar.

OESOPHAGEAL DISEASE

Oesophageal manifestations account for about 10% of all AIDS diagnosis and occur in a further 10% of patients during the course of their illness. The commonest symptom is oesophagodynia which is accompanied by dysphagia in about two-thirds of patients. The symptoms are due to a variety of infections of the gullet, the commonest being *Candida* species followed by herpes viruses including cytomegalovirus and herpes simplex.

Barium swallow is a relatively insensitive guide to the diagnosis but the sensitivity and specificity of endoscopy with biopsy is excellent [2]. The appearances of *Candida* are typical and range from isolated plaques to confluent disease affecting the whole oesophagus (Plate 5, facing p. 210). Herpes simplex usually produces a distal oesophagitis although diagnostic discrete fluid-filled vesicles are often also present. Cytomegalovirus usually produces ulceration of the lower oesophagus with raised rolled edges reminiscent of cancer (Plate 6) although haemorrhagic oesophagitis is an alternative presentation. The risks of endoscopy in HIV seropositive patients are low and employing standard precautions there should be no risk to staff nor transmission of HIV or opportunistic infections to other individuals during subsequent procedures [3].

The majority of oesophageal infections can be diagnosed presumptively by careful inspection of the mouth where candidiasis or herpes simplex infection is often seen. If treatment without endoscopy is instigated multiple diagnoses present in 25% of patients will not be successfully treated initially.

Candidiasis of the oesophagus responds to a variety of azole compounds [4], ketoconazole being the cheapest but perhaps most likely to cause hepatic damage; fluconazole is effective as single-dose treatment but resistance can occur and this might be important in the subsequent treatment of cryptococcal meningitis. The symptoms of cytomegalovirus (CMV) infection improve with either intravenous ganciclovir or foscarnet [5]. Ganciclovir tends to produce bone marrow suppression particularly when azidothymidine (AZT) is administered as well. Although renal failure and hypocalcaemia are serious adverse events with foscarnet it does have anti-HIV activity and can be used in conjunction with AZT. A recent study of CMV retinitis suggested that the survival of patients who were able to tolerate foscarnet was longer than those treated with ganciclovir [6].

WEIGHT LOSS

Wasting producing more than 10% loss of ideal body weight is an AIDS diagnosis and is a common presenting feature of HIV disease. Wasting with no apparent cause (Slim disease) was common in Africa early in the epidemic [7], but subsequently cryptosporidiosis or oesophageal *Candida* has frequently been found as an underlying cause. In the developed world, wasting usually occurs as a result of opportunistic infections, particularly those which cause diarrhoea. Other patients have psychological or social problems which contribute to weight loss and only in a small minority is there no obvious cause. Most patients lose weight because of anorexia associated with infection leading to a reduced intake. Studies of basal metabolic rate in these individuals have been conflicting [8]; metabolic rate might be increased by cytokine release either from HIV infected immunocompetent cells or as a response to opportunistic organisms, but in most individuals this measurement has been normal.

Malabsorption may also contribute to weight loss in HIV infected individuals. Severe carbohydrate malabsorption has been shown to be common irrespective of the stage of disease or the presence or absence of diarrhoea [9]. The crypt hyperplasia and mild villus blunting which have been observed in jejunal biopsies taken from HIV infected patients [10] are not sufficiently severe to account for the functional abnormalities observed. These anatomical changes are not associated with symptoms and may be produced as a direct result of HIV infection, either of epithelial cells [11] or immunocompetent cells within the lamina propria.

DIARRHOEA

Diarrhoea occurs in nearly all patients at some stage of HIV infection.

Bacterial diarrhoea

A variety of bacterial infections cause acute diarrhoea. *Shigella*, which is venereally transmitted, tends to occur in the earlier stages of HIV infection. Unusual species of *Campylobacter* and *Salmonella* may cause symptoms in immunocompromised individuals resulting from ingestion of undercooked food. Although both infections are associated with relapse, this is commoner with *Salmonella* particularly in those with an initial septicaemic illness or in those with AIDS and profound immune suppression [12]. In contrast to *Salmonella* species which produce a more severe illness in the immunocompromised host, *Campylobacter* infection is often associated with less toxicity than that seen in general gastroenterological practice. Prolonged treatment of bacterial diarrhoea, particularly for *Salmonella* infection, is required to prevent relapse; ciprofloxacin remains the drug of choice despite a small number of resistant *Salmonella* infections.

Mycobacterium avium intracellulare (MAI)

This opportunistic mycobacterium, which is only common in very advanced immunosuppression, produces diarrhoea mainly in HIV infection rather than in those with immunosuppression due to other causes. MAI may colonize the gut without causing disease and so positive stool cultures are occasionally seen in asymptomatic individuals. The presence of macrophages containing numerous MAI organisms in the lamina propria of the small intestine may be more closely connected with the presence of diarrhoea. Although MAI within macrophages appears to cause no inflammatory reaction or structural damage, marked villus stunting is often apparent on jejunal biopsy. Treatment with the newer macrolide antibiotics, e.g. clarithromycin, produces considerable symptomatic improvement with resolution of temperature, anaemia and diarrhoea. Survival may also be increased although improvement in weight loss is usually modest.

Cryptosporidiosis

This is the commonest infection producing diarrhoea in HIV. It can be diagnosed in the majority of instances by stool analysis but about 10% of patients have evidence of infection on gut biopsy only. Cryptosporidial diarrhoea in patients with a T-helper-cell (OKT4) count above 200 per mm^3 resolves eventually but in those with lower OKT4 counts, it is usually continuous (Fig. 1). In a minority, large volume diarrhoea of greater than 2 litres a day leads rapidly to death [13].

Cryptosporidiosis is particularly difficult to treat as there are no animal models or culture techniques which allow *in vitro* testing of drug sensitivity. Additionally, *Cryptosporidium* is unusual amongst the sporozoa as immediately infective spores allow autoreinfection. Cryptosporidia reproduce in a relatively protected extracytosolic but intracellular position, being covered by a host cell membrane where non-absorbable drugs may not be effective. Thus it is not surprising there is no treatment which eradicates cryptosporidia from the gut. A wide variety of macrolide antibiotics have been shown to reduce the volume of diarrhoea (including paromomycin). However, similar results are obtained with a variety of antimotility agents [14], perhaps because the described ballooning degeneration of autonomic nerves in the rectal mucosa indicates a motility disorder [15].

Microsporidiosis

This is the second commonest cause of diarrhoea in people with marked immune suppression. One species, *Enterocytozoon bienusi*, appears to be

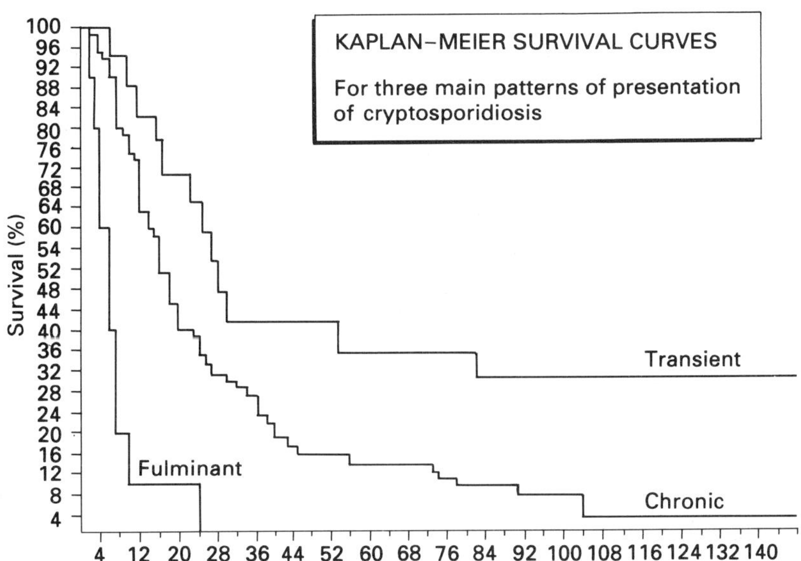

Fig. 1 The survival of patients with different patterns of cryptosporidial diarrhoea. Symptoms eventually resolve in those with transient diarrhoea while diarrhoea continued to death in those with chronic symptoms; and in those with fulminant diarrhoea there were more than 2 litres of stool per day.

unique to humans and affects the gut only, but other species including *Encephalitozoon cuniculi* and *Septata intestinalis* infect the intestine, the cornea and the sinuses. These species disseminate because they infect macrophages. They may occasionally cause renal failure and might be shown to be responsible for cases of myopathy or encephalopathy in the future.

Initially the diagnosis of microsporidial infection could only be made by electron microscopic examination of jejunal biopsy material; it is now recognized that light microscopic examination is equally successful (Plate 7) and in cases of sparse infection may even be more sensitive. More recently, it has become possible to identify spores in the stool using fluorescent stains and this is likely to become the preferred method of diagnosis. The disseminated forms of microsporidial infection can be diagnosed by routine examination of urine samples, lacrimal secretions or samples obtained following a sinus washout.

The role of albendazole therapy in the treatment of *E. bienusi* remains controversial; although there is some symptomatic improvement parasitic eradication is not achieved [16]. The situation is clearer with the disseminated species where rapid improvement in symptoms and parasite eradication are achieved with this drug.

Other protozoa

Giardia is a common parasite in homosexual males who may be asymptomatic carriers or have pronounced diarrhoea. Although cysts can be detected in stools, jejunal biopsy or staining of duodenal aspirate improves the diagnostic accuracy. *Isospora* is endemic in parts of southern America and appears to be commoner in HIV infected patients who respond to treatment with cotrimoxazole but often relapse. Again the diagnosis can be made on stool analysis but the parasite is also frequently seen on jejunal biopsy specimens.

Cytomegalovirus (CMV)

CMV infection can occur anywhere along the gut lining. However, before a pathogenic role in the causation of diarrhoea can be inferred, multiple inclusion bodies surrounded by dense inflammation must be seen in either jejunal or rectal biopsy material. It is not known whether this combination of biopsies will detect all cases of CMV infection as the largest American series suggests that disease on the right side of the colon, only detected by colonoscopic biopsies, occurs in up to a third of cases [17].

Adenovirus

This infection, for which there is no known treatment, is a common infection in children and iatrogenically immune suppressed individuals. It was thought to be rare in HIV infected patients but recently a number of cases have been described, usually in association with other potential pathogens [18]. This untreatable disease is diagnosed by gut biopsy, demonstrating abnormalities of the epithelial layer and by specific immunoperoxidase staining (Fig. 2).

Algorithm for investigation of diarrhoea

In those patients who are not severely immunosuppressed with an OKT4 count above 200 per mm^3, the diagnosis is usually made by stool analysis and blood culture [5], whereas in patients with a lower count, gut biopsy is also required. Small intestinal biopsy is particularly helpful as most protozoal infections occur at this site.

Therefore our patients routinely have three stools examined with a modified Ziehl–Neelsen stain for *Cryptosporidium* and standard culture techniques. Stools in those with a T4 count of less than 100 per mm^3 are also cultured for MAI. Following stool analysis patients undergo gastroscopy and sigmoidoscopy during which four duodenal pinch

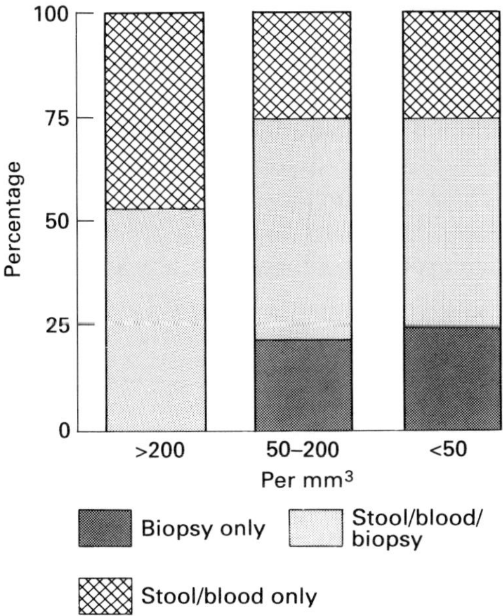

Fig. 2 Theoretical ways in which a cause of diarrhoea could have been uncovered in patients with different OKT4 counts.

biopsies and a rectal biopsy are obtained. This results in an accurate diagnosis in 85% of cases.

One of the major difficulties is deciding when diarrhoea in HIV seropositive individuals is truly pathogen negative. Those patients with marked weight loss (more than 5 kg), high stool volumes (greater than 500 cm^3 a day), macroscopically abnormal sigmoidoscopic appearances, or pronounced malabsorption of vitamin B_{12} should have investigations repeated as a pathogen responsible for diarrhoea is likely to be uncovered eventually [19].

Recently in a group of patients with repeated investigations who had no pathogen uncovered as a cause of their diarrhoea, symptoms resolved in about 50% over a period of 3 months. In a further 25% symptoms were easily controlled by opiates and in a small number, tumours of the gut were found on small bowel enteroscopy. Overall only 0.5% of all individuals investigated had unexplained large-volume diarrhoea which persisted for longer than 3 months.

TUMOURS ASSOCIATED WITH GASTROINTESTINAL DISEASE

Non-Hodgkin's lymphoma

Either the immunoblastic or Burkitt's type, the incidence of which is increased in HIV seropositive patients, may be caused by Epstein–Barr virus infection or by a loss of normal tumour surveillance mechanisms [20]. They often first present with non-lymph node manifestations and have a predilection for the gut, causing surgical emergencies with abdominal masses and obstruction, or weight loss, diarrhoea and recurrent fever. Treatment is critically dependent on the OKT4 count; in those with well-preserved counts initial response to standard therapy is good but relapse is likely, while in those with severe immune suppression standard chemotherapeutic regimens produce an unacceptably high incidence of opportunistic infection, and treatment is directed towards alleviation of symptoms.

Kaposi's sarcoma

Most patients with gut Kaposi's sarcoma also have cutaneous disease. Involvement of the palate (Plate 8) probably predicts disease elsewhere along the gastrointestinal tract. This is an unusual non-metastasizing tumour which is multicentric in origin. It is likely that products of HIV infection including the TAT protein and cytokines released as a result of HIV infection of immunocompetent cells both play a role in the proliferation of the vascular endothelial cells and the mesenchyme spindle

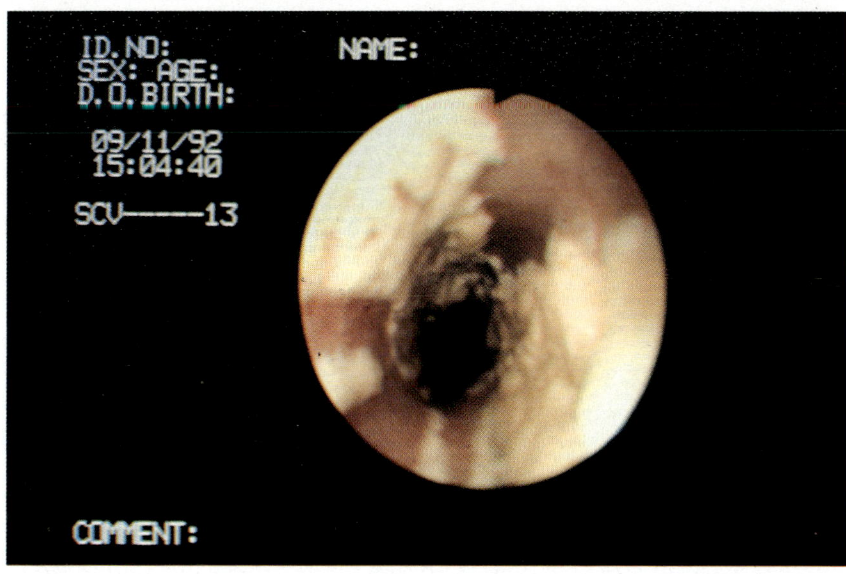

Plate 5 Extensive oesophageal candidiasis.

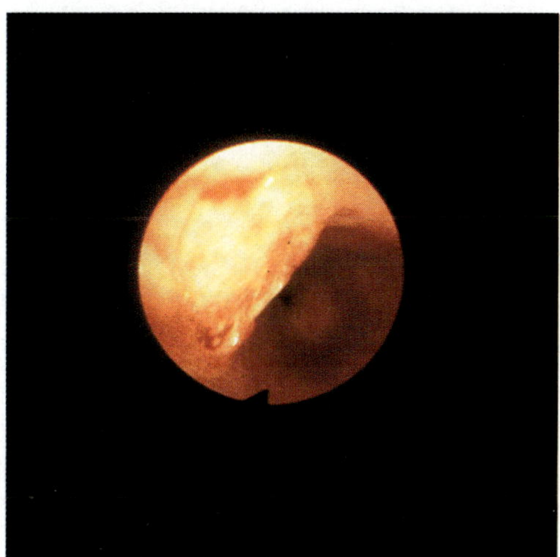

Plate 6 Ulcer in the lower oesophagus, found on biopsy to be associated with multiple CMV inclusions.

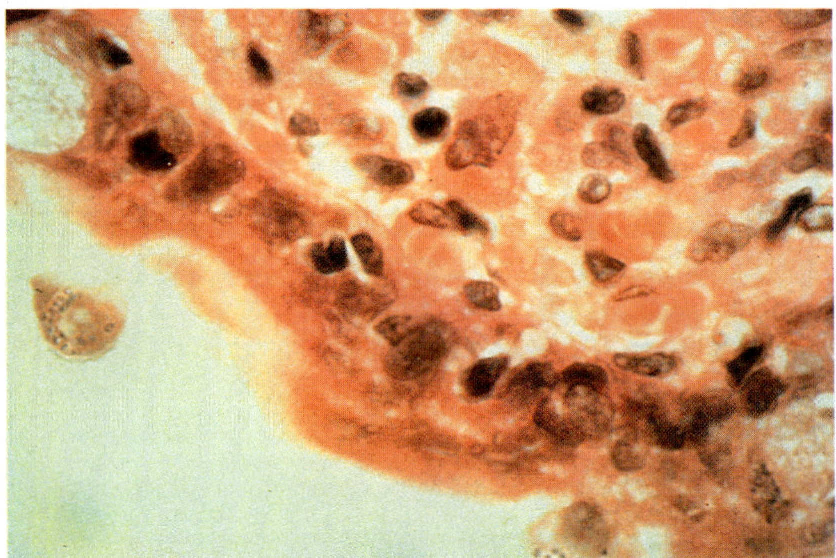

Plate 7 Microsporidial spores seen on light microscopy.

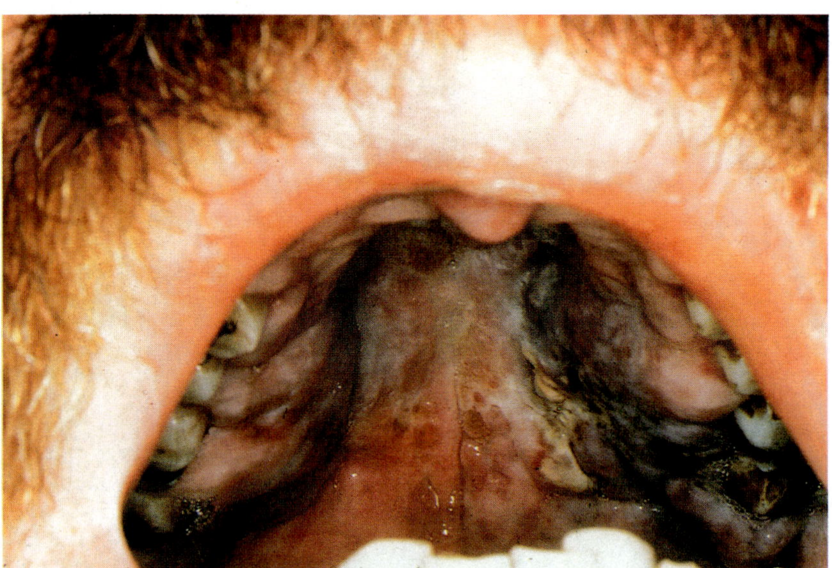

Plate 8 Extensive Kaposi's sarcoma involving the palate.

cells which are thought to be the neoplastic component [21]. Most commonly, Kaposi's sarcoma involvement of the gut produces no symptoms but occasionally obstruction, diarrhoea, gastrointestinal haemorrhage or protein-losing-enteropathy occur. Kaposi's sarcoma is sensitive to both chemical agents and radiotherapy, which may improve symptoms. However, no combination of regimens have been clearly shown to prolong life.

ABDOMINAL PAIN

Abdominal pain is a common feature of HIV seropositive individuals [22]. Lower abdominal pain is most frequently caused by severe constipation because of concomitant use of opiate analgesics. Appendicitis, which is relatively common, may be due to CMV. The commonest cause of diffuse abdominal pain often with signs of peritonism is CMV of the colon, which may be associated with toxic dilatation or perforation secondary to an arteritis. Toxic dilatation often responds to non-surgical treatment with antiviral agents.

The syndrome of right upper quadrant pain is most commonly associated with appearances on cholangiography of sclerosing cholangitis. AIDS-related sclerosing cholangitis is similar to the idiopathic sclerosing cholangitis seen in association with inflammatory bowel disease. Both intrahepatic and extrahepatic narrowing of the bile ducts may be seen

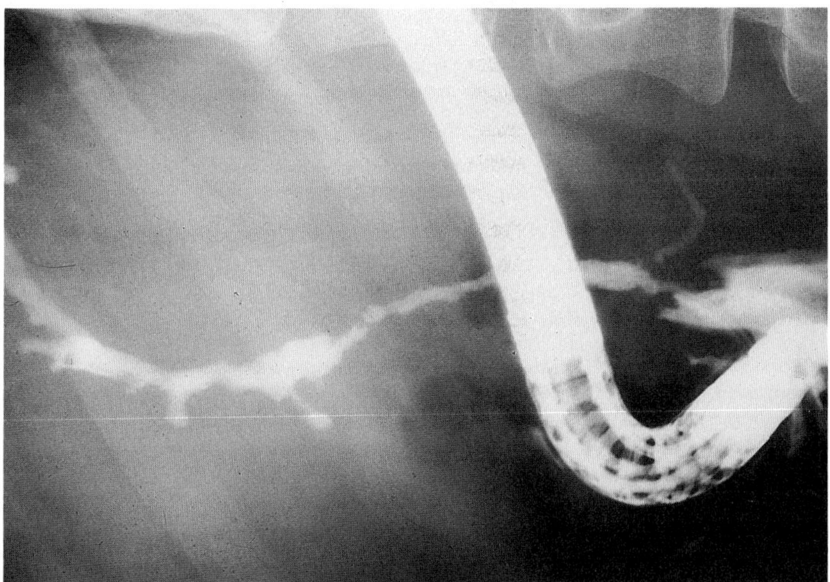

Fig. 3 AIDS-related sclerosing cholangitis seen on retrograde cholangiography.

(Fig. 3) although occasionally single strictures either of the ampulla or the extrahepatic ducts are the only sign of disease. In the majority of instances AIDS-related sclerosing cholangitis is associated with cryto-sporidiosis, CMV or microsporidial infection. Frequently patients have evidence of these infections elsewhere in the gut but occasionally the diagnosis can only be obtained by biopsy of the biliary system or analysis of bile.

It has been suggested that sphincterotomy in cases of ampullary stenosis relieve pain but the natural history of AIDS-related sclerosing cholangitis is not clearly understood [23]. In contrast to idiopathic sclerosing cholangitis, ascending infection, deepening jaundice and liver failure are uncommon. Abdominal pain is a persistent problem in a minority of patients only, the majority responding well to opiate analgesics. This condition tends to occur in those with very advanced immune suppression and the prognosis is limited to less than a year. Treatment of the associated opportunistic infections does not improve either the prognosis or the pain.

REFERENCES

1 Connolly GM, Shanson D, Hawkins DA, *et al.* Non-cryptosporidial diarrhoea in human immunodeficiency virus (HIV) infected patients. *Gut* 1989;30:195–200.

2 Connolly GM, Hawkins D, Harcourt-Webster JN, *et al.* Oesophageal symptoms, their causes, treatment and prognosis in patients with the acquired immunodeficiency syndrome. *Gut* 1989;30:1033–1039.

3 A Working Party of the British Society of Gastroenterology. Cleaning and disinfection of equipment for gastrointestinal flexible endoscopy: interim recommendations. *Gut* 1988;29:1134–1151.

4 Smith DE, Midgley J, Allan M, *et al.* Itraconazole versus ketoconazole in the treatment of oral and oesophageal candidiosis in patients infected with HIV. *AIDS* 1991;5: 1367–1371.

5 Nelson MR, Connolly GM, Hawkins DA, Gazzard BG. Foscarnet in the treatment of cytomegalovirus infection of the oesophagus and colon in patients with the acquired immunodeficiency syndrome. *Am J Gastroenterol* 1991;86:876–881.

6 Studies of ocular complications of AIDS research group, in collaboration with the AIDS clinical trials group. Mortality in patients with the acquired immunodeficiency syndrome treated with either foscarnet or ganciclovir for cytomegalovirus retinitis. *N Engl J Med* 1992;326:213–220.

7 Serwadda D, Mugerwa RD, Sewankambo NK, *et al.* Slim disease; a new disease in Uganda associated with HTLV-III infection. *Lancet* 1985;ii:849–852.

8 Grunfeld C, Feingold KR. Metabolic disturbances and wasting in the acquired immunodeficiency syndrome. *N Engl J Med* 1992;327:329–337.

9 Ehrenpreis ED, Gulino SP, Patterson BK, *et al.* Kinetics of D-xylose absorption in patients with human immunodeficiency virus enteropathy. *Clin Pharmacol Ther* 1991;49:632–640.

10 Ullrich R, Zeitz M, Heise W, *et al.* Small intestinal structure and function in patients infected with human immunodeficiency virus (HIV): evidence for HIV-induced enteropathy. *Ann Intern Med* 1989;111:15–21.

11 Nelson JA, Reynolds-Kohler C, Margaretten W, *et al.* Human immunodeficiency virus detected in bowel epithelium from patients with gastrointestinal symptoms. *Lancet* 1988;i:259–261.

12 Nelson MR, Shanson D, Hawkins DA, Gazzard BG. Salmonella, Campylobacter and Shigella in HIV seropositive patients. *AIDS* 1992;6:1495–1498.
13 Blanshard C, Jackson AM, Shanson DC, *et al.* Cryptosporidiosis in HIV-seropositive patients. *Q J Med* 1992;85:813–823.
14 Connolly GM, Dryden MS, Shanson DC, Gazzard BG. Cryptosporidial diarrhoea in AIDS and its treatment. *Gut* 1988;29:593–597.
15 Blanshard C, Ellis DS, Tovey DG, Gazzard BG. Electron microscopy of rectal biopsies in HIV-positive individuals. *J Pathol* 1993;169:79–87.
16 Blanshard C, Ellis DS, Tovey DG, *et al.* Treatment of intestinal microsporidiosis with albendazole in patients with AIDS. *AIDS* 1992;6:311–313.
17 Dietrich DT, Rahmin M. Cytomegalovirus colitis in AIDS: Presentation in 44 patients and a review of the literature. *J Acquired Immune Deficiency Syndromes* 1991;4(Suppl 1):S29–S35.
18 Maddox A, Francis N, Moss J, *et al.* Adenovirus infection of the large bowel in HIV positive patients. *J Clin Pathol* 1992;45:684–688.
19 Connolly GM, Forbes A, Gazzard BG, *et al.* The investigation of seemingly pathogen-negative diarrhoea in patients infected with HIV-I. *Gut* 1990;31:886–889.
20 Friedman SL. Kaposi's sarcoma and lymphoma of the gut in AIDS. *Baillière's Clin Gastroenterol* 1990;4:455–475.
21 Bovi PD, Curatola AM, Kern FG, *et al.* An oncogene isolated by transfection of Kaposi's sarcoma DNA encodes a growth factor that is a member of the FGF family. *Cell* 1987;50:729–737.
22 Thuluvath PJ, Connolly GM, Forbes A, Gazzard BG. Abdominal pain in HIV infection. *Q J Med* 1991;78:275–285.
23 Forbes A, Blanshard C, Gazzard B. The natural history of AIDS-related sclerosing cholangitis: a study of 20 cases. *Gut* 1993;34:116–121.

PART 5
MEDICAL MANAGEMENT

Computers in clinical management

T. A. HOWLETT

Few would deny that information technology is having an increasing impact in hospital practice, particularly in hospital management 'case-mix' and in medical audit systems. However, as yet, the direct use of personal computers in day-to-day clinical practice has been rare amongst hospital physicians. This is in contrast to general practice which has become increasing computerized in recent years, with some practices progressing to the fully-paperless medical record.

The presentation on which this paper is based was essentially a practical presentation of how readily-available personal computers can be used 'live' to enhance day-to-day clinical management. It is clearly not possible to reproduce the dynamic interaction with a computer user-interface in the printed word. I will therefore simply summarize the principles, and the practical progress now being made at local and at national level. In addition, I will make demonstration software available to any reader who wishes to learn more in practical terms.

THE BASIC REQUIREMENTS

If we accept that it is important to collect data on patients, whether for clinical reasons or for reasons of hospital management, then we must surely wish that these data should be accurate. However, the inaccuracies of the current central hospital returns are well recognized. One reason for these inaccuracies is that the data collected are dependent on the hospital coding-clerks' interpretation of the written medical record (which is itself frequently incomplete), yet these clerks are traditionally unrelated to the clinical team caring for the patient, both professionally and usually geographically. I would argue that only the clinicians caring for the patient are actually aware of the accurate 'main diagnosis' for an individual patient. If this is the case, then the data stored in information systems will only be accurate if they represent the clinically-relevant data which is *actually used* by the clinician in day-to-day practice. The inevitable logic of this is that data must be collected as close to the clinician–patient interface as possible, and ultimately entered and used directly by the clinician.

Previous generations of hospital computer software have not been designed for clinical use, and are usually slow, unfriendly and inflexible. If they are to be used by the clinician, then future information systems must display the following features.

- Systems must be user-friendly, intuitive and easily used with minimal training. I believe that this means the use of a graphical user interface now (windows, mouse, menus, icons, etc.), and in the relatively near future the use of voice and handwriting recognition.
- Clinician-users must be presented with simple choices in plain English when entering, reading and analyzing data stored in the information system.
- Data entry must be simplified to allow the use of abbreviations, 'keys' and clinically-relevant 'pick-lists' to find the terms required.
- Data must be coded, for central returns and for communication with other information systems, but this coding should occur automatically in the background during the use of the system and be 'transparent' to the user. Since the only system capable of coding clinical data in sufficient detail for clinical use is the Read Clinical Classification (RCC – 'Read Codes'), this should be universally adopted.
- Use of the information system must not be an additional chore for junior or senior staff – it must actually save the clinician time in performing day-to-day clinical activities, and provide additional information not normally available at the clinical interface. This can be achieved by including direct access to laboratory and imaging requests and results, by performing the word-processing functions necessary for clinical correspondence (and including the clinical data in that correspondence), by linking with the patient administration system (PAS) and case mix (for appointments, waiting lists, etc.), and by providing on-line access to medical journals, textbooks and guidelines.
- The technology must be made available at the clinical interface. Ultimately this must mean a computer on every desk in outpatients, and in every inpatient area, and/or the use of portable personal computers.

THE PRESENT

Most of the features discussed above are technically possible now, but are rarely provided – even as part of recently-installed 'case-mix' systems. My presentation at the conference was a practical demonstration of what is possible now (see Fig. 1 and final paragraph). I already use my own information system 'live' in my office, in the outpatient clinic and on my ward-rounds, and the data are shared over the hospital network by junior staff and secretaries in the production of routine correspondence, all resulting in the collection of valuable data for medical audit.

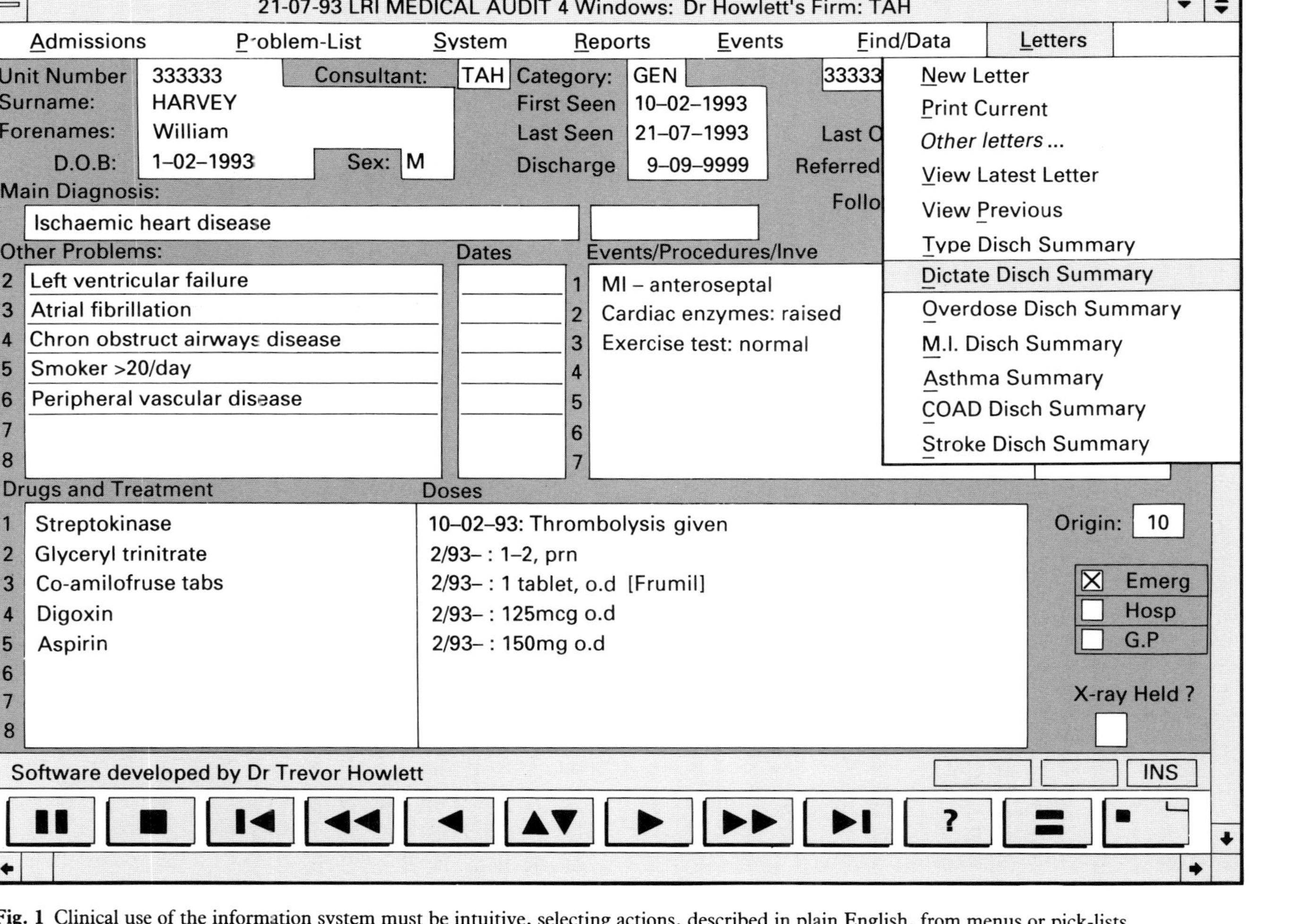

Fig. 1 Clinical use of the information system must be intuitive, selecting actions, described in plain English, from menus or pick-lists.

THE FUTURE

The NHS Management Executive, via its Information Management Group (NHS-IMG), in collaboration with the Conference of Royal Colleges and the Nursing Profession and Professions Allied to Medicine, have recognized the need to transform our hospital information systems along the lines outlined above. A number of joint projects between the professions and the NHS-IMG are currently underway or nearing completion.

Clinical Terms Project is developing a comprehensive electronic thesaurus of all 'clinical terms' or concepts currently commonly used in the written medical record, arranged into clinically-relevant 'display hierarchies' and 'pick-lists' for use by information systems. These terms will be coded and incorporated in Version 3 of the RCC due for release in 1994.

Integrated Clinical Workstation Project is defining the clinician-users' requirements for a computerized clinical workstation, researching the 'Human–Computer Interface', and developing software demonstrators to use the expanded RCC and demonstrate the feasibility of such systems.

Other infrastructure projects include work on more clinically-relevant iso-resource and iso-need groupings of clinical activity (HRGs and HNGs), a new unique NHS number for every patient and progress towards an electronic NHS network.

The results of these collaborative projects should allow the realization of information systems which can enhance the quality of medical care, and collect accurate data as a 'side-effect' of meaningful clinical activity. I hope that such systems will become a reality within the next decade, with subsequent progress being made towards fully-electronic medical record.

A fully-functional demonstration version of the author's current medical information system is available on request. The demonstration program will run on any PC-compatible with Microsoft Windows 3.1 installed. Please send a blank formatted 1.44 MByte, 3.5 inch disc and a self-addressed envelope to:

Dr T. A. Howlett
Consultant Physician
Leicester Royal Infirmary
Leicester LE1 5WW.

Developing a hospital information strategy: a clinician's perspective

C. BUNCH

Over the past few years, several profound changes have occurred within the National Health Service which highlight the need for a fresh look at information provision within hospitals. First, the Griffiths report on general management has emphasized the importance of involving clinicians in the management of their service, a theme that was reinforced by the Department of Health's Resource Management Initiative – which also stressed the need for better information on resource consumption and the ability to assess differences in case mix. These initiatives have brought clinicians and managers together and have helped to define common information requirements – centred around individual patients. The recent NHS reforms [1], and in particular the introduction of an internal market with contracts between purchasers and providers, has gone even further in demanding high quality information on clinical activity, and has raised the spectre of financial risk associated with poor information provision.

Unlike previous reforms in the NHS, the current changes, and especially the development of NHS Trusts, have dramatically changed the profile of the hospital into that of a 'business'. Concepts such as 'business planning' and 'business-led strategy' are now commonplace. Thus, to ensure effective use of information technology (IT), hospitals should first consider the nature of their business, how to develop their business to make the best of current and future opportunities, and how to organize it to achieve its goals effectively. Intelligent use of IT can help with all these aspects, and information strategies are most successful when they support clearly defined aims.

PRINCIPLES OF INFORMATION STRATEGY DEVELOPMENT

In developing an information strategy, certain basic principles must be followed. Many of these, such as good project management and adherence to accepted technical standards, should go without saying.

Some are perhaps less immediately obvious and are worth exploring in more detail.

Information systems should support rather than constrain

The most valuable information is that which helps one to achieve one's objectives. It follows that a successful information strategy cannot emerge unless objectives are clear, and the strategy supports rather than hinders any changes in organization that may be required to support those objectives. Information may be valuable for less critical purposes, but its provision will have a correspondingly lower priority.

This is not especially contentious, but the environment is changing and in a large organization such as the NHS, there are plenty of opportunities for objectives to conflict. The hospital service is currently experiencing the most far-reaching cultural and organizational changes since the inception of the NHS. These have been largely driven by pressure for greater accountability – both for the use of public funds but also to individual patients. The emphasis on accountability is driven on the one hand by spiralling healthcare costs, and on the other by a growth in patients' expectations coupled with a disturbing increase in their willingness to resort to litigation when these are not fulfilled.

In *structural* terms, the NHS is changing – at least on the ground – from a bureaucratic, administered organization, with strong but separate vertical administrative and professional hierarchies, to a more proactive, managed organization with a greater emphasis on flexibility and teamwork between doctors, nurses, managers and other healthcare professionals. This implies a flatter structure, and is illustrated by the development of clinical directorates and specialty management teams. In *process* terms, however, change has been slower and alterations in the flow of hospital funds, the separation of purchaser and provider, and the introduction of service agreements or contracts make it increasingly important that clinical teams plan their services and resource requirements in advance, rather than assuming everything will be 'all right on the night' (and complaining when it is not).

The implications of these trends for information strategy development are profound. Hospitals, and more especially their clinical or service teams, will need to produce realistic, costed service plans. For this, they will need accurate information about patient flows, the costs of investigations and treatment, etc. Assuming for the moment that they achieve the necessary funding through contracts, they must then be able *monitor* their activity and resource consumption in a timely fashion, so that they can take appropriate action if things don't go according to plan.

Our experience is that traditional NHS information systems have difficulty in providing this kind of information, and may thereby hinder the processes of service definition and planning. A fundamental change in the way in which hospital data is traditionally collected is required.

Whose data is it anyway?

Traditionally, hospitals have been required to collect data for transmission to their District Health Authority (DHA) and beyond. Existing systems (often manual) are not necessarily geared to providing information for internal consumption, and hospital management has often had to rely on digests of information being returned to them from their health authorities or the Department of Health at a later date. Not surprisingly, confidence in the accuracy and validity of this information is often low.

A local example may serve to illustrate the difficulty. Our hospital makes use of a remote patient administration system (PAS) which is located and managed at Regional headquarters and which covers all local hospitals. It tracks inpatient, outpatient and accident and emergency attendances. Data are input by medical records staff and admission clerks: there is no direct access from wards, who must telephone details of patient movements to a central office. Straightforward admissions and discharges are reasonably accurately recorded, but consultant-to-consultant and inter-hospital transfers are not. Diagnostic codes are added retrospectively by coders, working from 'diagnostic text strings': the accuracy in one recent internal validation exercise was as low as 38%.

The PAS cannot be interrogated: simple printouts are available to wards and consultants indicating which patients they currently have in the hospital (as if they didn't know already). Periodically, tapes are transferred to another computer running a relational model that seems to bear little relationship to the real world. This can be interrogated at DHA headquarters, but not by the hospital, and some 'reports' take many hours to run. The 'information' actually produced is highly dependent on how the query is formulated, and it is sometimes possible to obtain different answers to the same basic question.

This unhappy state of affairs leads us to another important principle: *where possible, those requiring the information should be responsible for collecting the data.* Clinical teams that are assuming responsibility for managing their service will be better served is they are able to capture the data they require themselves. It is far more likely to be accurate, and can more easily be validated before transmission to other interested parties. Which leads to another issue.

Does everyone really need to know everything?

There is a pervasive assumption that the advent of cheap and sophisticated IT will enable anyone to find out anything about anyone anywhere. Leaving aside for one moment issues such as confidentiality and personal feedom – which are extremely important nonetheless – do Regional Health Authorities (RHAs) *really* need on-line access to all their hospitals' information systems? What will they do with it? Is it sensible for purchasing DHAs to roam around inside their providers' systems? (This has actually been happening in our Region.)

One of the main reasons that large and complex organizations need to decentralize is simply to facilitate information management. In the 1960s it was predicted that computer technology would actually lead to *centralization*: management would have access to all the information required to make all the necessary decisions. The trouble is that the amount of information turns out to be too large to handle, and it becomes too difficult to see the wood for the trees. What is required in the NHS is for each part of the organization to be really clear about what it *needs* to know, and to obtain this information in the simplest way possible: a regular printed summary may often suffice. Electronic forms of communication may become indispensable in some areas, but should always be the servant, not the master.

Unfortunately, recent trends suggest that all will not be simple. The NHS Management Executive has issued plans for a national data highway, or network, across which any part of the NHS will be able to communicate with any other [2]. The expense will be considerable. The benefits may also be considerable, although little thought appears to have gone into what, precisely, will actually be communicated. Parallel moves towards a national administrative register (containing personal details of all NHS 'subjects' – effectively the entire population) and a unique identifier, paint a picture of Orwellian proportions [3].

Few would deny that the NHS needs improved communications. However, there seems here a real danger that confidentiality may be compromised. Britain has led the world in data protection legislation with its Data Protection Act, and the Data Protection Registrar has already shown disquiet over the apparent freedom with which personal information is already being exchanged [4,5].

The clinician's needs are important too

We are currently being encouraged to take a 'business' view of information systems and requirements. There is, however, a danger of taking the business-led approach too literally, concentrating on resource and financial information at the expense of clinical needs. Clinical activity is, after all, the main 'business' of most hospitals.

Clinicians need timely information to manage their patients effectively, and with decreasing lengths of hospital stay it becomes all the more important that patient management should not be hindered by lack of the necessary information. Also, whilst many clinicians are gradually accepting the need to become more involved in managing their services, few see the point of major investments in information systems that provide management information but do little to facilitate clinical activity. The application of information technology to clinical practice is poorly developed: simple office management technology is yet to reach many consultant practices, and the provision of clinical information by computer has often been eschewed in favour of financial and administrative needs.

The reasons for this are complex, but worth exploring. First, to be useful, information to support patient management has to be available to clinicians (doctors and nurses) more or less in real time, whilst information for service management and audit can be retrospective (though preferably not unduly historical). Real-time information systems are more complex to design and manage. Second, clinical practice and decision making is poorly understood by managers and information specialists, and there are few clinicians who are both managerially competent and computer literate. Clinical information has thus had low priority in most hospital IT implementations. A third reason is that historically most major NHS IT projects have been driven by the need to provide hospital activity information to *outside* organizations such as health authorities and central government, in keeping with a central, hierarchical administration. Even hospital departmental systems have had little to offer the clinician. Our hospital was one of the first in the country to install a laboratory computer, yet in most instances we still write requests by hand, and wait for results to be returned by the internal mail.

It is important that these deficiencies are not ignored. Many clinicians, aware from colleagues in North America what *could* be available, are acquiring sophisticated personal data management systems for their own practices, funded from soft money or from earmarked funding for audit. These initiatives fall outside the normal channels for developing hospital information systems, and can lead to problems with integration when clinicians want their systems linked into hospital systems, or require hospital staff to rekey data on their behalf. It would be far better if clinical needs could be satisfied as part of an overall hospital strategy.

The family silver

A reasonable principle must be to make the best possible use of existing investment in information systems. There is a limit, however, to how far this ideal can be pursued, and there will be many hospitals that are largely uncomputerized that may therefore have many more degrees of freedom than those that are saddled with out-of-date technology. A similar opportunity faced the major building societies, which in general computerized much later than the major banks.

Information strategy and organizational development should not be unduly constrained by previous IT investment, however large. Unlike the family silver, it may have little resale value. The changes in the NHS are profound enough to render many systems inadequate, and the costs of upgrading or modifying some must be carefully balanced against possible longer-term benefits of replacing them altogether.

DEVELOPING A STRATEGY IN PRACTICE

The John Radcliffe Hospital became a 'first wave' resource management (RM) site in 1989. Unlike many RM sites, which moved quickly to acquire case-mix management, nurse management and other systems, sometimes with little thought as to how they would fit in to an overall strategy, we concentrated first on service and organizational development. This involved identifying 60–70 service areas, or *service delivery units (SDUs)*; a typical SDU might be a specialty ward, a laboratory, the intensive therapy unit (ITU), theatres, etc. Each will typically be responsible for delivering a definable set of services to patients or to other SDUs, and will require various resources, some of which it will own and some of which it will obtain, by agreement, from other SDUs.

Each SDU is managed by a lead clinician (typically a consultant) and a nurse (or equivalent) manager. Together they are responsible for developing and managing the SDU service plan. SDUs with similar 'interests' are grouped into Service Centres, which are roughly analogous to clinical directorates. The Service Centre has a consultant (or equivalent) chairman and a full-time service manager: its role is to coordinate, support and monitor the activity of its constituent SDUs, and to provide an interface with senior management (finance, personnel, contracting, etc.). The Service Centre chairmen together with senior management meet monthly as the Hospital Board.

The organizational change is emphasized in some detail because it has major implications for information strategy, some of which have been covered above. Given that the information strategy should support objectives, it is clear that each level – Hospital Boards, Service Centres and SDUs – will have particular requirements, all of which need to be taken into account.

Steering the strategy

To develop an information strategy, the Hospital Board set up a standing committee – the *Information Strategy Steering Group* – comprising senior management, clinicians, and information technology specialists. The committee spawned a number of task groups, each responsible for working up a particular aspect of the overall strategy. In this way we have been able to involve a wide range of hospital staff and thus considerably increase commitment to the success of the strategy. Initial task groups were responsible for: (i) *information requirements definition*: working closely with pilot SDUs in developing service plans and determining what information they will need to monitor service delivery; (ii) *technical standards*: ensuring that systems conform as appropriate to national and local standards; (iii) *data standards*: defining data models and data sets, and providing consistency of widely-used data such as GP code lists; (iv) *information protection*: developing hospital policy, standards and procedures for compliance with the Data Protection Act as well as ensuring the safety of hospital information and data; (v) *training*: defining the skills required by key personnel and arranging the necessary training. More recently the Steering Group has taken responsibility for overseeing specific implementation projects.

Emerging concepts

It is clear that SDUs need simple processes for capturing activity data, and using this to monitor their service delivery. An initial step therefore was to provide a simple PC-based system to manage this as well as providing support for service planning; this was intended to ensure that accurate data are available for activities as diverse as contract management and clinical audit.

The next step is to provide a central 'patient data server' which will remove the need for SDU systems to store basic patient details locally. This will also maintain *spell* records (a spell is an instance of delivery of a particular service by an SDU: it could in future form a more rational 'currency' for service agreements than consultant episodes and similar measures that have little relevance to clinical practice), and *event* records (an event is an instance of consumption of a measurable resource; examples include bed days, outpatient visits, operations, laboratory tests, X-rays, etc.). The patient data server will in effect be the repository for the hospital's *public data*: data which may need to be accessible at a variety of levels. Individual SDU or service centre-based systems may retain *private data*: data that are only of interest to the individual service. This may include research or audit data, or operational data such as theatre scheduling or clinic booking.

The separation of global, public data from local, private data reflects the organizational model and makes it easier to shift the responsibility for data collection from central clerical staff to service delivery staff by ensuring that the latter have systems that *they* need whilst avoiding the need for rekeying basic data when the same patients encounter different services. A central data server will also provide consistent data for contract management, and will help the hospital fulfil its obligations to provide information to purchasers, RHAs and so on.

The service-based model of resource management – in which resource consumption is linked to instances of delivery of defined services – will, we believe, be superior to models based on case-mix analysis where case mix is primarily defined by diagnostic categories. In our model, case-mix analysis allows the examination of variances in resource consumption of individual services to promote improvements in efficiency as well as effectiveness. The analysis will encompass a wide range of criteria, including type of patient, diagnosis, severity of illness, complications, treatment protocol, etc.

Clinical workstations

A central concept to our strategy is to provide access to the central patient data server through integrated clinical workstations [6]. These have been successfully prototyped using a graphical user interface, and will be available throughout the hospital – in the wards, outpatient clinics, theatres – and on the desks of clinical staff and their secretaries. The concept aims to ensure accurate collection of data about clinical and related activity by appropriate professional and clerical staff in the course of their usual activity. This shifts the responsibility from clerical staff, situated apart from clinical areas, who have little vested interest in the quality of the data they collect. Where possible, we aim to make the data capture process simple. Indeed identical data are often collected by separate professional staff: in one survey we found that patient details were being scribbled down in six different places following admission to a ward. Where possible, we aim to capture the data just once and make the information available to all who need it.

At the same time, we aim to provide significant benefits to the users. Secretaries who register new patients, following receipt of a referral letter, can have standard letters sent to patient and general practitioner at the touch of a button. Clinical staff on the wards can have access to laboratory results and, in the near future, radiology and other reports, and will be able to request investigations on line.

During 1992 we undertook a major prototyping exercise in a large specialty which successfully proved many of the concepts outlined above. This also enabled us to achieve a high degree of commitment from all levels and types of staff. This is especially important, because a major cause of failure of many large and complex information systems is that the implementors have failed to bring the users with them.

THE PROBLEMS

It would be misleading to suggest that developing a hospital information strategy is a painless affair. The NHS reforms have made the hospital a volatile environment, and for a variety of reasons many staff still find themselves uncomfortable with some aspects of the reforms. In our experience, most are prepared to rise to the challenge and see potential benefits from being in a position to manage their own services, provided the resources are somewhere approaching adequate. One of the most important resources is information: without it we grope in the dark and have fair reason to blame the system when things go wrong; with it, we can begin to make rational decisions, develop a more effective service, and assume a greater degree of responsibility.

A curious aspect in which hospital information strategy development has been potentially constrained is the separation of funding for medical audit and resource management. Our belief is that the two go hand-in-hand, especially when clinical staff are being encouraged to take responsibility for managing their clinical services. Our experience in developing clinical management teams at the ward rather than directorate level suggests that this can lead to far better teamwork between doctors and nurses than might otherwise be the case. Since both professions are managing the same patients, this must be to the patients' advantage. Encouraging separate investment in medical audit and nurse management systems has not helped this, and seems set to perpetuate professional rivalries. Both professions currently capture similar patient data in their respective manual records, and both initiate separate care plans for the same patients – often without reference to each other. Perpetuating this division of labour in hardware and software makes little sense. It is therefore reassuring to see trends – at least locally – towards more multidisciplinary quality initiatives.

Perhaps the greatest problem is that although hospitals are being encouraged to develop their own strategies, their room for manoeuvre is limited. Guidelines – initially supportive in intent – become increasingly prescriptive and seemingly less relevant. Funding is earmarked for specific system developments, whether or not they eventually form part of a carefully-developed strategy. It is as though a great scientist, having initiated his/her experiment and impatient for the results, begins to write them up whilst turning a blind eye to the actual outcome. Although more recently the Department of Health appears to be moving away from 'earmarked' projects, public and parliamentary concern over misplaced large IT investments has introduced an air of extreme caution, with increasing regulation covering *how* IT should be procured. This is likely to introduce delays, frustration and perhaps planning blight. It remains to be seen whether the public interest will be better served.

A simple approach to an information strategy would be to ignore the clinical coalface, devolve hardly at all, and ensure that contract minimum data sets and other externally required information are delivered by installing central contract and case-mix systems fed by the traditional army of clerks. Boxes could be ticked, and paymasters kept happy – for a while. This would, however, be an extremely short-term view, and would do little to ensure the continuing goodwill and involvement of those who actually treat the patients.

ACKNOWLEDGEMENT

This is a revised version of a paper which was originally published in the *British Medical Journal* (1992;304:1033–1036) entitled 'Developing a hospital information strategy: a clinician's view'. We are grateful to the British Medical Association for permission to publish this version.

REFERENCES

1 *Working for Patients*. London: HMSO, January 1989.
2 National Health Service Management Executive. *An Information Management and Technology Strategy for the NHS in England*. London: HMSO, December 1992.
3 Editorial. No hiding place. *Economist* 1993:328(7823):7 August.
4 Cross M. Big brother. *Health Service Journal* 1993;103(5348):20–22.
5 The Office of the Data Protection Registrar. *NHS contract minimum data sets*. February 1993.
6 Nation Health Service Management Executive. *Report for the integrated clinical workstation programme. Review of existing initiatives*. October 1992.

Screening in the elderly

C. J. BULPITT & A. E. FLETCHER

DEFINITIONS

Traditionally, screening has been defined as population testing to identify early disease or precursors of disease in asymptomatic individuals. When considering the elderly, it is possible that we should screen not simply for disease but also for disability. Moreover the elderly see their primary care physicians so often that screening may be achieved by well organized case finding. Case finding may be defined as opportunistic identification of cases with disability or established disease not previously known to health care.

PRINCIPLES OF SCREENING

The principles of screening have been fully discussed by Wilson [1]. He was concerned with the detection of disease and thought that screening should be considered when the following are present: the disease is an important health problem, it has a well understood natural history and a recognizable early stage, when treatment at an early stage is of more benefit than treatment at a later stage, when there is a suitable test available, when the test is acceptable to the population, when there are adequate facilities for diagnosis and treatment of those who have the abnormality, when the necessary intervals between repeat screens is known, when any harm from screening is less than the benefit obtained and finally when costs may be balanced against benefits and judged not to be excessive.

Similar considerations lead us to consider the likelihood of benefit from screening to be related to the following: a high prevalence of the condition, a high severity of the condition, a high degree of acceptability of the test, a low false positive rate for the test, few adverse consequences of a false positive test, a low false negative rate, and few adverse consequences of such a false negative test, an effective treatment for the condition, a low cost of the test, and an acceptable burden on services affected by the screening programme [2].

DISEASE AND DISABILITY DETECTED BY SCREENING

Williamson *et al.* reported on the results of screening the elderly in 1964 [3]. They found that 'the amount of unmet need for general-practitioner care was high, as shown by the number of unknown disabilities'. Thomas *et al.* documented in 1968 that more than 10% of the elderly will be found to have hearing defects, problems with their feet, arthritis, varicose veins and a high blood pressure [4]. Cataracts were also a problem in 9% of the women they examined. These results were supported by Williams *et al.* in 1972 [5] who, like Williamson *et al.* [3], made the important distinction between previously known and newly discovered conditions. In this study, 9% were discovered to be deaf, 4% had cataracts, 2% had either hypertension or diabetes mellitus and 0.7% had carcinoma of the breast. A further 17% were already known to have cataracts, 4% to have diabetes and 2% to have carcinoma of the breast, but almost no-one had been previously recorded as deaf or having hypertension. A further important step in screening was when Freedman *et al.* screened patients and divided their conditions according to whether they were serious or not [6]. They also identified the actions and outcomes from screening. For example, although 6% had a local abnormality of the breast, only 20% of these proved to have cancer. Similarly, although 16% had hypertension, this was reduced to 3% for sustained hypertension, and of 15 patients with cataracts only 1 was referred to hospital. These authors considered that other screening abnormalities such as wax in the ear and obesity were not serious conditions.

SHOULD WE SCREEN FOR DISEASE OR DISABILITY (OR BOTH)?

Buckley and Williamson in 1988 [7] claimed that 'medical screening, especially that using multiple laboratory tests and measurements ("multiphasic screening") has been shown by controlled trials not to reduce morbidity and mortality and not to improve use of services'. Moreover 'emphasis in prevention . . . should not be on earlier detection of disease but rather on assessing loss of function'. The evidence for the failure of screening for diseases to have any benefit was reported to come from two trials. One of these was a trial in middle age [8] and the other considered all adults over the age of 18 [9]. The latter trial reported that 14% of subjects had abnormal haematology, 8% abnormal audiometry, 8% abnormal blood glucose, 5% abnormal thyroid function tests and 4% abnormal lipids. However, there appeared to be no benefits over one year, although there was a tendency for improvement in quality of life as measured by a health status index.

Most studies of screening have looked for both disease and disability, based on the reasonable hypothesis that disease will lead to disability. Nevertheless, the concept that we should only look for disability is important as it places emphasis on rehabilitation and not on the cure and prevention of further disease and disability. In the next section we will review the results of randomized controlled trials of screening in the elderly.

RESULTS OF THE TRIALS

Table 1 considers five trials. Tulloch and Moore reported in 1979 [10] on the results of screening in 295 patients over the age of 70 who had regular sociomedical assessments. They noticed that the screened group had fewer days in hospital but were more often referred to other agencies. They did not notice a reduction in medical problems and Harris has recently supported the notion that we should screen for disability [11]. In 1984, Hendriksen *et al.* [12] reported on the results of screening of subjects over age 75 living in Denmark. The screened group showed a 25% reduction in days in hospital, a 19% reduction in hospital admissions and most importantly a 15% reduction in mortality. Although a report in 1991 [13] showed that this mortality advantage had not been maintained over 7 years, the finding is still important as we would expect, in the very elderly, that the benefit would decrease with death and time. This study was particularly important as it looked at the expenditure on salaries for the screening personnel, office costs, increased use of home helps, modifications to the home and increased costs of pensions of those that stayed alive. It also compared these with financial gains from reductions of days in hospital and in nursing homes, and a reduction in the use of the emergency services. The financial savings were large and remarkable.

In 1984, Vetter *et al.* [14] randomly allocated 1310 patients over the

Table 1 Results in five randomized trials of screening in the elderly

	Reduction			Increase
Reference	Mortality	Bed days	Institutional care	Quality of life
Tulloch and Moore [10]	—	↓↓	—	—
Hendriksen *et al.* [12]	↓↓	↓↓	↓↓	—
Vetter *et al.* [14]	↓ (urban)	—	0	↑ (urban)
Carpenter and Demopoulos [15]	0	↑↑	↓	—
Pathy *et al.* [16]	↓↓	↓ (age $<$ 75)	↓ (age $>$ 75)	↑

↓↓, Definite reduction; ↑↑, definite increase; ↓, reduction in a subgroup or not significant; ↑, increase in a subgroup or not significant; 0, no difference; –, not assessable.

age of 70 to regular sociomedical assessments or not. There was one general practice in an urban area and one in a rural area. Deaths over 2 years were reduced from 20% to 12% in the urban area but were unaffected in the rural area. Furthermore, in the urban area, home help provision and district nursing were increased in the intervention group. These changes were not observed in the rural district. There was a tendency for an increased satisfaction with life in the screened group. It is obviously difficult to say whether the differences between the areas were due to the differences in location or due to the differences in staff employed on the intervention programmes.

Carpenter and Demopoulos reported in 1990 [15] a study that concentrated on screening for disability and needs. This led to fewer days in institutional care and to more patients attending day hospitals and being admitted to hospital. In 1992 Pathy *et al.* [16] described a trial of home visiting by a health visitor for subjects over the age of 65 who responded positively to problems on a questionnaire. In the control group 24% died, compared to 18% in the intervention group. Hospital admission, attendance at day hospital, and institutionalization were statistically not significantly different between the two groups. Twenty per cent of the control group received domiciliary consultations from consultant physicians as against only 7% in the intervention group. Quality of life, as measured by the Nottingham Health Profile or the Townsend or Life Satisfaction scores, did not differ between the groups but a self-rated health measure did differ in favour of the intervention group. A small trial in general practice demonstrated that routine assessment of the elderly was associated with a significant improvement in the Philadelphia Morale Scale, and the social and emotional dimensions of the Nottingham Health Profile [17].

From these studies, it would appear reasonable to suggest that screening may reduce hospital admissions, increase the use of services, improve quality of life, and even reduce mortality (Table 1). Screening for disability without attention to underlying diseases could reduce hospital admissions and improve quality of life, but may be less likely to reduce mortality. Nevertheless, it is possible that screening for disability could reduce total mortality. What to screen for, and how to screen for it, remain important open questions. It would appear unwise at the present time to be categorical as to whether or not we should concentrate on disability or disease.

THE SITUATION IN 1993

The UK general practice contract states that general practitioners should offer to screen the over 75s every year for problems with mobility and functioning, difficulty with their senses, problems of physical health, problems of mental health, social aspects of their life, and medication use. In 1992 Brown *et al.* [18] reported that 15% of practices were not performing any checks and over 50% did not follow non-responders to their invitations. However, 55% of the elderly population were seen and 43% of these were found to have a new problem which resulted in 7% receiving drug treatment, 7% occupational therapy and 7% chiropody. Tremellen [19] stated that doctors saw no merit in the contract, although patients found it worthwhile and 52% of nurses thought the assessment was important. Nurses were much better at picking up new problems than the doctors.

THE FUTURE

The disadvantages of screening are that cases discovered may have a longer period of morbidity when prognosis is not affected by screening, questionable abnormalities may be over-treated, the screening and subsequent treatment may be very expensive, false negatives lead to false reassurance and false positives to considerable and unnecessary anxiety and, lastly, the tests may themselves be hazardous. For this reason, many would agree that screening programmes for specific conditions should not be implemented unless there is evidence of more benefit than harm from randomized controlled trials.

Table 2 gives the conditions thought to be theoretically worth screening for, according to criteria set out by us [2], and also those conditions thought worth screening for by the US Preventive Services Task Force (USPSTF) [20]. Both sets of investigators thought that it was worth screening for hearing loss, visual impairment and also for hypertension. We also thought it was worth screening for hypothyroidism, anaemia, diabetes mellitus, foot problems requiring chiropody, and severe varicose veins and ulceration. The USPSTF considered that height and weight should be measured and that mammography was worthwhile up to the age of 75 and cervical smears up to the age of 65. They also suggested

Table 2 Conditions that may be worth screening for in the elderly on various theoretical grounds [2,20]

1 Hearing loss
2 Visual impairment
3 Hypertension
4 Hypothyroidism
5 Anaemia
6 Diabetes mellitus
7 Severe varicose veins and ulceration
8 Mammography up to age 75
9 Bacteriuria, haematuria and proteinuria

that Mantoux testing should be performed in residents of nursing homes, that bacteriuria, haematuria and proteinuria were worth looking for and that, when relevant, risk factors should be assessed for abnormal grieving. These included being alone, having an abnormal mental state and abusing alcohol. Both groups thought that it was not worth screening for cognitive impairment and cancer of the colon. In addition, the Task Force did not recommend screening for the following: blood cholesterol, electrocardiography, testing for carotid stenoses, testing for peripheral arterial disease, tests for prostate cancer, chest radiology, skin examination for cancer, ovarian cancer screening, pancreatic cancer, plasma glucose, thyroid function (although may be prudent in older persons, especially women), anaemia, osteoporosis, depression and physical abuse.

CONCLUSIONS

Much research has been done on the benefits, and otherwise, of screening in the elderly but much remains to be done. The high priority now is for trials which are large enough to assess outcome in terms of mortality, morbidity, quality of life, use of resources and cost effectiveness. Such trials should examine

1 the benefits that accrue from different methods of screening (different methods of contact, different personnel etc.);
2 the benefits of screening for different conditions, diseases or disability;
3 different methods of evaluating the subjects who have abnormalities on their screen.

We are optimistic that screening for certain conditions will prove cost effective with well-defined methods and well-defined processes of evaluation and care.

REFERENCES

1 Wilson JMG. The worth of detecting occult disease. In: Sharp CLEH, Keen H, eds. *Presymptomatic Detection and Early Diagnosis*. London: Pitman Medical, 1968.
2 Bulpitt CJ, Benos AS, Nicholl CG, Fletcher AE. Should medical screening of the elderly population be promoted? *Gerontology* 1990;36:230–245.
3 Williamson J, Stokoe IH, Gray S, *et al*. Old people at home. Their unreported needs. *Lancet* 1964;i:1117–1120.
4 Thomas P. Experiences of two preventive clinics for the elderly. *Br Med J* 1968;ii: 357–360.
5 Williams E, Bennett FM, Nixon JV, *et al*. Sociological study of patients over 75 in general practice. *Br Med J* 1972;ii:445–448.
6 Freedman GR, Charlewood JE, Dodds PA. Screening the aged in general practice. *J Roy Coll Gen Pract* 1978;28:421–425.
7 Buckley EG, Williamson J. What sort of 'health checks' for older people? *Br Med J* 1988;296:1144–1145.
8 The South East London Screening Study Group. A controlled trial of multiphasic

screening in middle-age: Results of the South-East London Screening Study. *Int J Epidemiol* 1988;6:357–363.

9 Olsen DM, Kane RL, Proctor PH. A controlled trial of multiphasic screening. *N Engl J Med* 1976;1294:925–930.

10 Tulloch AJ, Moore V. A randomized controlled trial of geriatric screening and surveillance in general practice. *J Roy Coll Gen Pract* 1979;29:733–742.

11 Harris A. Health checks for people over 75. The doubts persist. *Br Med J* 1992;305: 599–600.

12 Hendriksen C, Lund E, Stromgard E. Consequences of assessment and intervention among elderly people: a three year randomised controlled trial. *Br Med J* 1984;289: 1522–1524.

13 Hendriksen C. Consequences of prophylactic home visits to elderly people. A follow up investigation seven years after the conclusion of an intervention procedure. *Geriatrica Gerontol* 1991;26(Suppl 1):295.

14 Vetter NJ, Jones DA, Victor CR. Effect of health visitors working with elderly patients in general practice: a randomised controlled trial. *Br Med J* 1984;288:369–372.

15 Carpenter GI, Demopoulos GR. Screening the elderly in the community: controlled trial of dependency surveillance using a questionnaire administered by volunteers. *Br Med J* 1990;300:1253–1256.

16 Pathy MSJ, Bayer A, Harding K, Dibble A. Randomised trial of case finding and surveillance of elderly people at home. *Lancet* 1992;340:890–893.

17 McEwan RT, Davison N, Forster DP, *et al.* Screening elderly people in primary care: a randomised controlled trial. *Br J Gen* Pract 1990;40:94–97.

18 Brown KB, Idris Williams E, Groom L. Health checks on patients 75 years and over in Nottinghamshire after the new GP contract. *Br Med J* 1992;305:619–621.

19 Tremellen J. Assessment of patients aged over 75 in general practice. *Br Med J* 1992;305:621–624.

20 Woolf SH, Kamerow DB, Lawrence RS, *et al.* The periodic health examination of older adults: The recommendations of the US Preventive Services Task Force. Part II. Screening tests. *J Am Geriatr Soc* 1990;38:933–942.

Medical audit

P. BECK

In the midst of all the fascinating and high-flown science of this conference on Advanced Medicine, to be asked to discuss medical audit may be considered, if not a poisoned chalice, at least a bed of nails. I think that as recently as 5 years ago such a title would have attracted more incomprehension than distaste or disinterest. Apart from a few islands of activity, led by individual enthusiasts, the concept of medical audit was little understood and even less practised. Despite this, some forms of assessment of the practice of the medical profession have occurred sporadically for centuries and the standards set by current 'experts' have often formed the yardstick against which the standards of other doctors have been measured. Indeed this College in its Charter of 1518 took seriously its role in maintaining standards of practice of its Fellows 'both for their own honour and in the name of public benefit'.

In more recent years the enormously rapid increase in the technological possibilities of medical interventions, together with their demands on scarce resources, has led to a much greater tendency for governments, and the public at large, to question the efficacy, efficiency and appropriateness of medical care. Some national schemes aimed at assessing aspects of the quality of medical care have in fact been in place for many years. The Confidential Enquiries into Maternal Deaths began in 1952 and the National Quality Control Scheme for Pathology Laboratories in 1969. In the Professorial Department of Medicine in Birmingham regular review of the adequacy of case notes has occurred since 1978 and reviews of deaths have been similarly undertaken in Stoke-on-Trent since 1979.

Nevertheless, despite these oases of activity, the widespread pursuit of regular review of clinical activity remained firmly in the desert. The very phrase 'audit' was commonly perceived as threatening and inherently fiscally based. The Concise Oxford Dictionary defines audit as: 'Official examination of accounts, searching examination, especially Day of Judgment; (Audit ale – of special quality, formerly brewed in English Colleges, originally for use on day of audit).' A publication from my own health authority on the role and objectives of audit defined it as 'An independent appraisal function within an organisation for the review of activities as a service to all levels of management. It is a managerial control which measures, evaluates and reports upon the effectiveness of internal control and the efficient use of resources.' Chilling stuff to clinicians' ears: little wonder perhaps that appended – by whom I know not – to the document was an appraisal of the basic qualities of an auditor:

> The typical auditor is a man past middle age, spare, wrinkled, intelligent, cold, passive, non-committal, with eyes like a cod fish, polite in contact but at the same time un-responsive, cold and damnably composed as a concrete post or a plaster of paris cast; a human petrification with a heart of feldspar and without the charm of the friendly germ, minus bowels, passion or sense of humour. Happily they never reproduce and all of them go to hell.

Against this background and in the space of merely 2 or 3 years, the whole picture has changed. The *Report of a Confidential Enquiry into Perioperative Deaths (CEPOD)* in 1987 [1] was followed in 1989 by the Royal College of Physicians' first report of its working party on medical audit [2] and by the Government's White Paper, *Working for Patients, Working Paper No. 6*, on medical audit [3]. To marshall the contemporary clichés, 'at a stroke' medical audit seemed to have become not merely 'flavour of the month' but also 'politically correct'. *Working Paper No. 6* of *Working for Patients* also produced a useful definition of medical audit which has been widely adopted: 'The systematic critical analysis of the quality of medical care, including the procedures used for diagnosis and treatment, the use of resources and the resulting outcome and quality of life for the patient', making the point that this would provide quality assurance to doctors, patients and managers.

The College report, and another useful publication in 1989 from Dr Charles Shaw of the King's Fund Centre on *Medical Audit: a Hospital Handbook* [4], were both widely read and not only helped to explain the culture of medical audit to doubting doctors but also gave some practical advice on how to do it. Both of these publications emphasized that the traditional 'grand round' or case presentation was not an adequate method of appraisal as the cases discussed were self-selected, often atypical and inherently individual with no generalization of any lessons learned.

Medical audit should be seen as a systematic approach to peer review, whose primary objective is to improve the quality of care doctors provide for their patients [5]. In addition, it has an important educational role by promoting discussion among colleagues about good medical practice and should serve to identify ways of improving the efficiency of clinical care. Medical audit is not an end in itself; it is essentially a component or tool of the quality assurance of health care, where quality assurance is defined as a system by which provision or performance is measured against expectation with the declared intention of minimizing deficiencies [5].

Medical audit is therefore essentially a primarily clinical and educational exercise rather than a managerial one.

The College's First Report defined (after Donabedian [6]) the main categories of medical care to be evaluated as *structure*, *process* and *outcome*, stressing their inter-relations. Structure relates to the quantity and type of resources available and while this is often easy to measure, and even to change, it rarely alone provides a good indicator of the quality of care. Process is what is done to the patient and therefore includes investigations, drug therapy, operations, etc. and can include assessments of adequacy of case notes, adherence to drug formularies or management protocols for specific conditions. In many situations measures of process may be the only ones available, despite the (perhaps obvious) view that the most relevant indicator of the quality of patient care is outcome. The problem is that outcome is often difficult to assess in a timely fashion, in medicine perhaps more than in surgery, as the final outcome may be only apparent many years into the future. Measures of process are often therefore used as proxies for outcome, where the activity under review has been shown by credible research to result in a beneficial and acceptable outcome. Although mortality is a readily defined and measurable outcome, in medical conditions which are often complex and chronic it has a limited role in evaluating the quality of care.

Such assessments of the standards of care in terms of structure, process and outcome will, however, be of little use in improving the quality of care unless some *action*, to remedy detected defects, results. The whole purpose of medical audit must be to produce change and because this is often uncomfortable and threatening to long established practices, resistance is common. Audit does not consist merely of doing surveys, or observing current practice and making comments about it; its role is as a systematic and scientific process to determine the extent to which an action or set of actions was successful in achieving a set of predetermined objectives. Thus, in its *intention*, audit is distinct from research and other related activities. It is a formal sequence, based on a prior view of desirable standards (which themselves may well be research based), which measures practice against these standards, analyses the results to assess compliance and takes action to remedy any deficiencies. This remedial action will itself need to be monitored, thus 'closing the loop' of the audit cycle.

When choosing a suitable topic for audit it is worthwhile considering some desirable features of the proposed activity. It is crucial to ask whether the activity is amenable to change, because if it is not then doing an audit will be a waste of time. Questions such as: 'Does the activity occur commonly?' 'Can the activity be easily defined and examined?' and 'Can a standard of practice be easily defined and agreed?' are all pertinent when selecting an audit topic.

Once selected, it is reasonable to pass, as part of a pre-audit exercise, to an initially fairly unstructured look, an 'informal review' of the activity, to answer the question of 'Where does my standard of practice stand at present?' This can then be refined (still in a pre-audit exercise) to ask: 'Where am I precisely at present in relation to practice in relation to the chosen topic?' The real audit question is: 'Have I arrived at where I want to be?' and this has inherent in it a *prior* view, unlike research, for which the question is: 'Where should I be?' Research involves the collection or acquisition of new knowledge, entailing a *future* dimension, as compared to audit which is firmly based in the present.

If audit is designed to assess whether the quality of care has reached a defined standard, then clearly considerable care must be given at the outset to defining such standards. Standards of care can encompass a spectrum from general guidelines to very specific algorithms and it is important to avoid standards that are so vague as to make measurement difficult or so precise that they are not achievable. *Criteria* of good quality care should be defined which comprise a measurable aspect of care and include a yardstick of quality. Good criteria clearly need to have clinical validity (e.g. a defined length of hospital stay; specific diagnostic tests, etc.), to be defined precisely, to be capable of being measured objectively and to be relevant to the audit question and topic chosen. If such criteria are well chosen they should ease the practical burdens of conducting the audit by being potentially capable of being collected by non-medical personnel, such as audit assistants, and by being computer compatible and reproducible over time.

Such criteria can be used in conjunction with the Donabedian categories of medical care. Structure, process and outcome and standards of practice can be specified according to agreed criteria within each of these categories. The agreed standards may be expressed as requiring 100% compliance with the criteria, with agreed clinical or social exceptions. For example, 100% of patients with myocardial infarction (diagnostic criteria agreed) should leave the coronary care unit within 48 hours, except when they have heart failure, heart block or are continuing to experience pain. Alternatively, a set percentage should comply with the criteria: standards between 0% and 100% can be set according to clinical experience or research findings; they are useful for monitoring and can be used to act as a threshold for further investigations. Summarizing the setting of standards, the requirement is to define a measurable aspect of care and a yardstick of quality to provide the audit criteria, to which the percentage compliance desired is agreed by the participants in the audit exercise.

Once a suitable topic has been chosen and the standards and criteria set, the collection of data needs careful planning. What data, on which set of patients, where the data should be sought and how it should be collected are all aspects which must be addressed. The data items must be readily definable and valid, or, put another way, really related to the topic of interest and relevant to the agreed criteria. Adding data items merely because they are easy to collect or 'just in case' should be avoided. Ideally data items would be those which are generally recorded already and be readily accessible from the case notes – if these are themselves available! Decisions must be made about the sample population, with inclusion and exclusion criteria agreed to make the sample representative of the set of people required. The size of the sample should be agreed – not too large nor too small, although sample size is not so important from the statistical view point in audit as it is in research.

It is generally helpful if the sources of data are those which are already collected, for example patient administration system (PAS), hospital activity analysis (HAA) or Health Service 'performance indicators'. The hospital case record will often be a data source and giving some thought to retrieval of medical records will often pay dividends in terms of eventual data retrieval. Such retrospective data collection is often faster and cheaper than trying to arrange for prospective collection, but the data obviously need to be present, accessible and as complete and accurate as possible. This is not always readily achievable and if so, a prospective data collection may be the only option. This option may sometimes be preferentially selected if it is desirable to use the immediacy of the findings to effect change.

The decision about who should collect the data is often a difficult one. Should it be the busy clinician or a non-clinical reviewer or audit assistant? If the latter is chosen then explicit standard setting or data sets are essential which can sort out, for example, positive indications for selecting case notes for the clinician to review. This is necessary to take account of situations where there may well be, for example, good clinical reasons for being outwith an indicator standard, such as length of stay in hospital.

After addressing all these considerations – choosing a suitable topic, agreeing standards and criteria and how the data are to be collected – it should be possible to undertake a specific medical audit. The concept is quite straightforward but the real problems arise when the results show that the agreed standards are not being met. The process will be of value only if change occurs to remedy the situation, and this can lead to behavioural, professional and organizational problems. If changes can be agreed to attempt to redress any deficiencies discovered, then a re-audit must be planned to see whether the changes have achieved the desired result. The whole process is therefore an ongoing and dynamic one, and must also take account of changes in medical practice due to new discoveries, technological advances, results of controlled trials, etc. There is a danger that agreed standards or guidelines might become 'fossilized' in a certain time frame unless they are themselves regularly reviewed. If properly performed, therefore, medical audit is not a finite activity nor a passing fad, but should be a rolling programme of continuing quality assurance in health care.

Prior to the College's first report on medical audit (1989), the Working Party contacted the College tutors in all the health districts in England and Wales to enquire about audit activity in their respective hospitals. Apart from neonatal death surveys, the level of activity was very low. Charles Shaw, in 1989 [4], wrote 'Although little is known about the prevalence of formal audit throughout Britain, it appears that at the moment only a minority of doctors are involved.' Following the White Paper *Working for Patients* and the College report there has been an enormous increase in audit activity. Dr Anthony Hopkins, the Director of the Royal College of Physicians' Research Unit, and I have recently completed a second report on medical audit for the College [7]. As part of the preparation for this, the views of the Regional Advisers were sought on the status of audit activity in 1992 and we found that, with very few exceptions, almost all hospitals are now undertaking regular medical audit. It is apparent that programmes for medical audit meetings are usually planned and publicized well in advance, that all levels of staff attend and that attendance records and minutes of the meetings are generally being kept. The authors and the College Advisory Committee on medical audit have prepared model minutes for these medical audit meetings which have been approved by the Conference of Medical Royal Colleges and their Faculties in the UK and which have been published [8]. It is equally clear that although there has been this huge increase in audit activities over these 3 years, much of the activity remains based in case record review or surveys of practice, but increasing numbers of topic-based audits centred on agreed standards or practice guidelines are also being undertaken.

I have chosen to address primarily the desirability and techniques involved in performing adequate and useful medical audit on the quality of the medical care which we give to our patients. I am aware of many other specific issues related to audit which are still causes for concern or debate, but space precludes detailed examination of these. Such problems include confidentiality [9], both for the patients whose records are being audited and for the clinicians involved, the legal status of clinical guidelines and whether doctors could be sued for not following them, the relation of information technology and audit – cart or horse, and the interface between medical audit and medical education. These and many other related topics will continue to be debated and discussed. It is, however, quite clear that the government and the recipients of health care expect the profession to continue its activities in medical audit. As in many other walks of life, those charged with professional responsibility are now required to be more accountable to their client groups. I believe that the proper practice of medical audit will enable us to improve, and continue to improve, the care we give to our patients, which surely must be an aim which both doctors and their patients can share.

REFERENCES

1 Buck N, Devlin HB, Lunn JN. *Report of a Confidential Enquiry into Perioperative Deaths (CEPOD)*. London: Nuffield Provincial Hospitals Trust/King's Fund, 1987.

2 Royal College of Physicians of London. *Medical Audit. A First Report: What, Why and How?* A working party report. London: RCP Publications, 1989.

3 Department of Health. *Working for Patients: Working Paper No. 6. Medical Audit*. Command 555. London: HMSO, 1989.

4 Shaw C. *Medical Audit: a Hospital Handbook*. London: King's Fund, 1989.

5 Standing Medical Advisory Committee. *The Quality of Medical Care*. London: HMSO, 1990;1:6.

6 Donabedian A. *Evaluating the Quality of Medical Care*. Millbank Memorial Federation of Quality, No. 3. 1966:166–203.

7 Royal College of Physicians of London. *Medical Audit: A Second Report*. London: RCP Publications, 1993.

8 Conference of Medical Royal Colleges and their Faculties in the United Kingdom. Model Minutes for Medical Audit Meetings. *Br Med J* 1991;303:1525.

9 Conference of Medical Royal Colleges and their Faculties in the United Kingdom. Interim Guidelines on Confidentiality and Medical Audit. *Br Med J* 1991;303:1525.

Models of medical manpower planning

G. H. HALL

Medical manpower planning is often spoken of disparagingly as a mere numbers game. Although numbers are certainly involved, it is not a game, except for the elements of hazard, and the clash of competing interests. As de Tocqueville pointed out, the only factor in human endeavours which can consistently be relied on is the desire for self advantage. In this field, the aspiration and objectives of the main protagonists – the employers (Department of Health), the educational authorities (universities and colleges) and the work force (British Medical Association) may be widely disparate. The negotiations, concessions and agreements (often more apparent than real) which take place between the bodies do require a framework of theory and assumptions, which may be provided by various models. These are designed to depict an existing state of affairs, to indicate the various influences which have brought this state of affairs into existence, and to predict how changes in these factors, or the introduction of new ones, will affect them. Such an understanding may enable desirable changes to be brought into effect.

Bartholomew [1] has summarized the matter thus:

> At the national level, manpower planning aims to make the best use of the nation's human resources. This involves the attempt to forecast the demand and supply for people with various skills and qualifications and bring them into balance. A major area of activity here is the planning of the educational system – its inputs and outputs. At the level of the firm, manpower planning deals with the problems of recruitment, wastage, retention, promotion and transfer of people with the firm and in relation to the environment. . . . The basic uncertainties of the situation mean than an adequate analysis of manpower problems must be conducted in probabilistic terms.

Not mentioned are the need for accurate data (head counting), the ability effectively to regulate the system at all levels, and the implicit belief that targets are correct and achievable. For example, planned economies have not fared very well in comparison with free market economies. Nevertheless, with our NHS, manpower planning is likely to

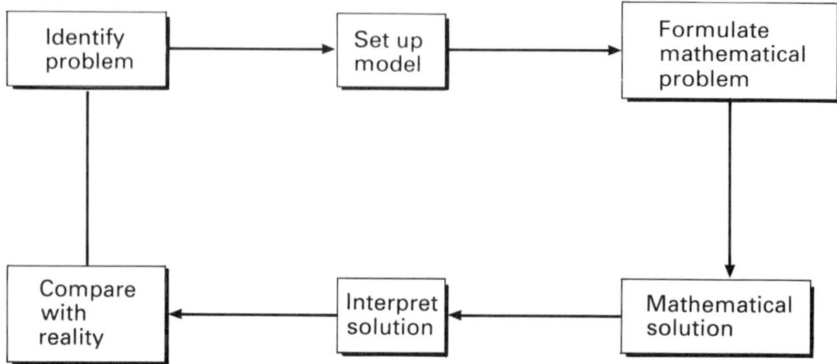

Fig. 1 A model of modelling.

remain an important feature of our professional life. Its success or failure deserves careful scrutiny because of its influence on our own careers and the careers of future doctors. A brief look at some of its methods is therefore worthwhile.

The standard model of 'modelling' is shown in Fig. 1. It bears some resemblance to the now familiar audit model and as frequently, the cycle is seldom completed or repeated. The models described here are mathematical, though they could be mechanical (like an orrery for the solar system), hydraulic (as in the notorious model of the economy produced in the 1960s) or indeed in any form which could be said plausibly to represent and reproduce in some way what is going on. A moment's reflection on what is going on 'out there' with doctors moving on through their career and through different jobs will indicate how deficient any model will be. With this reservation very much in mind, we will consider two particular examples of modelling in manpower problems.

Although there is little evidence that they actually did so, suppose the officials responsible for increasing the medical student output in the 1970s wished to predict the changed requirements in posts for the NHS. The problem might be more precisely defined as how many extra jobs would be required in each grade, and when. To keep matters simple, a

1 Consider one career path only
House Officer – Senior House Officer – Registrar – Senior Registrar – Consultant
2 Pre-existing steady state, i.e. no wastage or growth beforehand
3 Constant duration in grades
4 No subsequent wastage
5 Promotions increased to accommodate expansion

Fig. 2 Effect on expansion of input conditions.

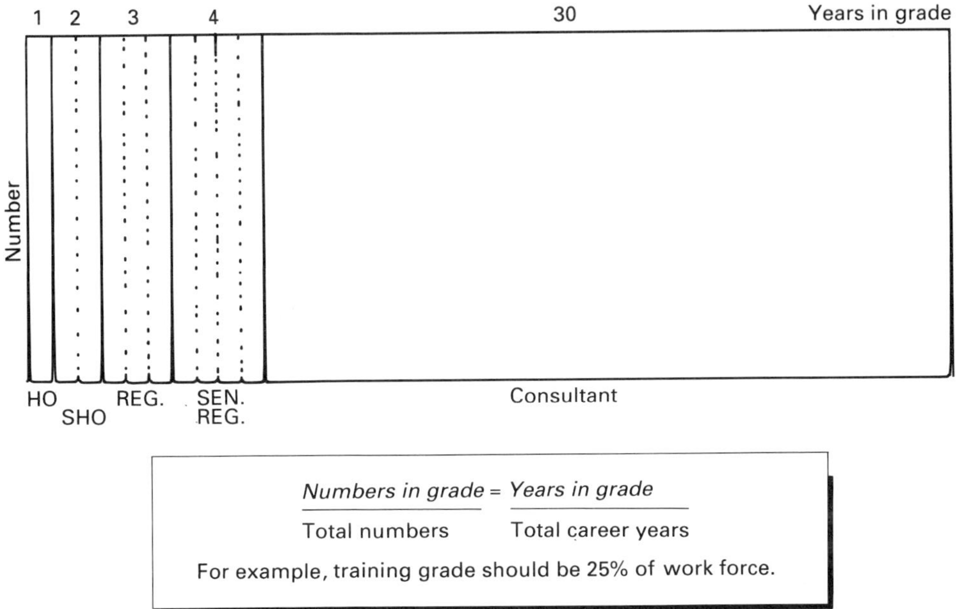

Fig. 3 Effect of duration in grade on total number of posts. HO, House Officer; SHO, Senior House Officer; REG., Registrar; SEN. REG., Senior Registrar.

number of explicit assumptions or conditions will have to be defined (Fig. 2). A graphic representation of the second condition (Fig. 3) provides a useful insight – namely, that in a steady state there is a relation between the numbers in each grade and its expected duration. Indeed, it is the perceived distortion of this relationship which caused concern in the House of Commons Select Committee Report in 1982. Also, unless condition 5 is met, bottlenecks and stagnation would lead to delays in training grade promotion, and this of course did happen. With an unperturbed implementation of the plan, an imaginary population would evolve in the way shown in Fig. 4. This demonstrates clearly that the increased numbers of posts required for each grade are proportional to the times spent in the grades, and that the requirements are postponed according to the number of years after graduation. One useful interpretation might be that there would be no point in expanding consultant numbers, and then only in a progressive way, until 10 years had elapsed from the beginning of the increased output from medical schools.

Some planners might prefer to have an algebraic representation of the process, to be able to answer the question:

> What number of posts (y) will we require in grade (j) at year (n) after expansion began?

The specification of the desired algorithm is shown in Fig. 5.

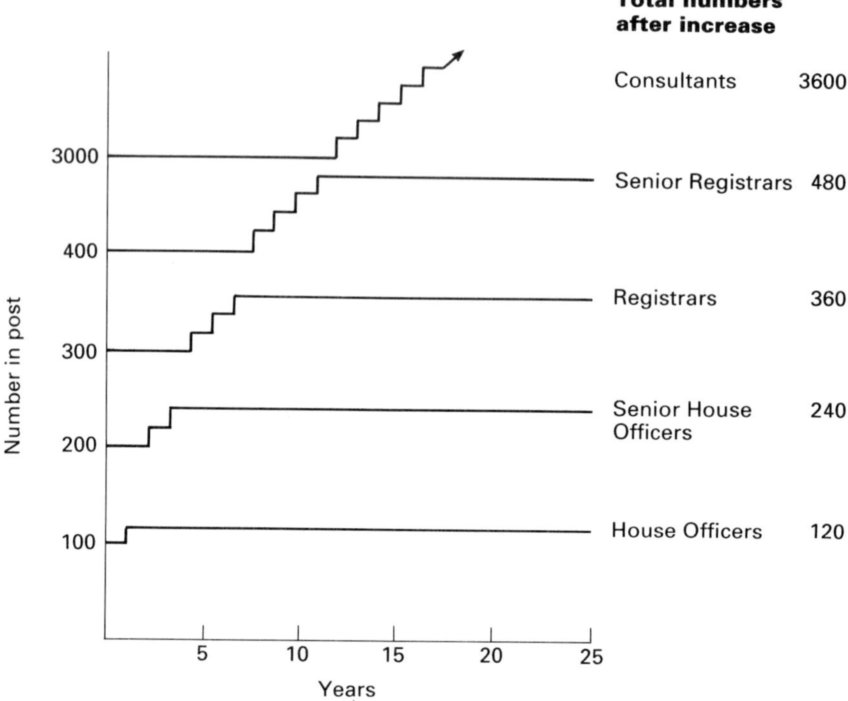

Fig. 4 Effect of increasing a small number of house officer posts on other grades in an imaginary population.

We want to know

Number (y) in grade (j) at year (n) after expansion began $= y_{jn}$

y_{j0} = original number in grade j at year 0

m_j = usual number of years spent in grades below j

z_j = usual number of years spent in grade j

i_{jn} = number of years spent in grade j at year n, where

$i_{jn} = 0,\ n < m_j$

$i_{jn} = z_j,\ n > m_j + z_j$

$i_{jn} = n - m_j$ otherwise

e = number added per annum by expansion

Then, $y_{jn} = y_{j0} + y_{jn}e$

e.g. Senior Registrar (j) at n = year 8 after expansion per annum by 20, $m = 6$

so $i = 8 - 6 = 2$

$y_{j8} = 400 + 2 \times 20 = 440$

Fig. 5 Algebraic representation of effects of expansion of input.

The overall interpretation of the model would include these points:

1 there will be a linear increase in the total numbers until 40 years have elapsed (i.e. the ordinary duration of the career);

2 the delay in the required increase in each grade will be proportional to the seniority of the grade;

3 the largest absolute increases in numbers will be observed in the grades of longest duration;
4 unrealistic assumptions have been made about the phenomena of wastage, promotion, participation rates and migration (in and out).

Twenty years on from the changes effected we should be able to assess the accuracy of our model or any improved models devised to approximate more closely our views of the reality of career activity and employment. Monitoring developments is a vital component of manpower planning. Regrettably, inaccuracies (e.g. non-return of honorary registrar posts, delays) and changes in the methods of data collection have undermined confidence in such assessments. Sometimes, misconceptions about how things happen are responsible for faulty prophecies. We have seen how an increased input into the system leads to a linear increase in career numbers, yet disappointment is frequently expressed at a failure to increase consultant numbers in a geometric (compound) fashion; consideration of our model would help avoid this error.

One of the most notorious medical manpower modelling formulas has been that derived for the use of the Joint Planning Advisory Committee (JPAC) in determining the requisite number of training posts at registrar and senior registrar levels. This states, quite reasonably, that the total number of posts required depends on the number of annual opportunities for promotion to the next appropriate grade, and the recommended duration of the grade, with an allowance made for wastage (i.e. movement out of that career pathway for whatever reason).

Number of posts required = annual promotion opportunities × duration in grade + wastage.

Here we shall confine ourselves to considering certain aspects of the vexed question of wastage, with particular reference to the situation of the medical registrar grade. JPAC takes the view that if, say, 50% of registrars leave for other specialties, then the requisite number of posts (promotions × duration) should be increased by 50%. The situation is, however, rather complex (Fig. 6). Much depends on when the 'wasters' leave. For an estimated 10% wastage in 300 required posts, the corrected numbers range between 330 when the loss occurs in the first year, to 360 when it occurs in the last of a 3 year average appointment.

A general formula to handle the problem is presented in Fig. 7. Although the formula itself appears a little forbidding, it is useful when specific calculations are needed. An additional problem develops if promotion can occur sooner or later than the 3 year deadline. If some lucky incumbents were promoted early, then only 315 posts might be needed, while delayed promotion might demand 365 posts. Clearly a better understanding of the behaviour of a cohort of registrars is required. Unfortunately, the technical difficulties of identifying such a cohort, and following it even if there were full cooperation, would make such a study

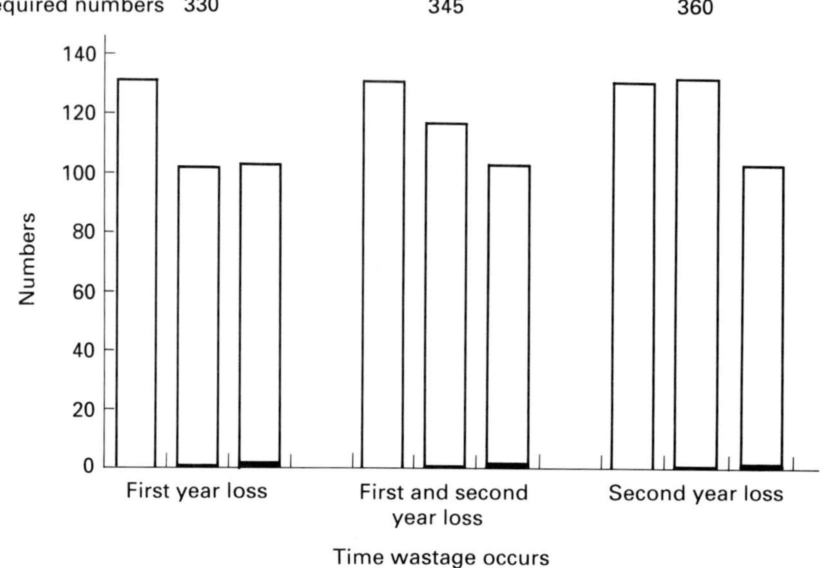

Fig. 6 Effect of time at which post loss (wastage) occurs on required number of posts.

x_i = number in ith year

Total in grade $= x_1 + x_2 \ldots + x_n$

$$= \sum_{i=1}^{n} x_i$$

w_i = wastage in ith year

Then, $x_2 = x_1 - w_1$, $x_3 = x_2 - w_2 = x_1 - w_1 - w_2$, etc.

So, total in grade $= x_1 + (x_1 - w_1) + (x_1 - w_1 - w_2) \ldots$

$$= nx_1 - [w_1(n-1) + w_2(n-2) \ldots + w_{n-1}]$$

$$= nx_1 - \sum_{i=1}^{n=1} w_1(n-i)$$

Because of the multiplier $(n - i)$, total required is less if wastage occurs early in the grade

Example:	**Early loss**	**Late loss**
	30 in first year	30 in second year
Total required	$= 3 \times 130 - (30 \times 2)$	$= 3 \times 130 - (30 \times 1)$
	$= 330$	$= 360$

Fig. 7 Algebraic representation of the effect of time of wastage on required numbers in the grade.

quite impracticable. The best that can be (and has been) done is a cross-sectional study of the medical registrars at a certain time – the census day in 1990 (Fig. 8). How much can be inferred from this histogram? It refers to NHS appointments only. There are approximately 1700 medical registrars. With an expected 200 opportunities available per year for promotion to the senior registrar grade, and an advised duration in the

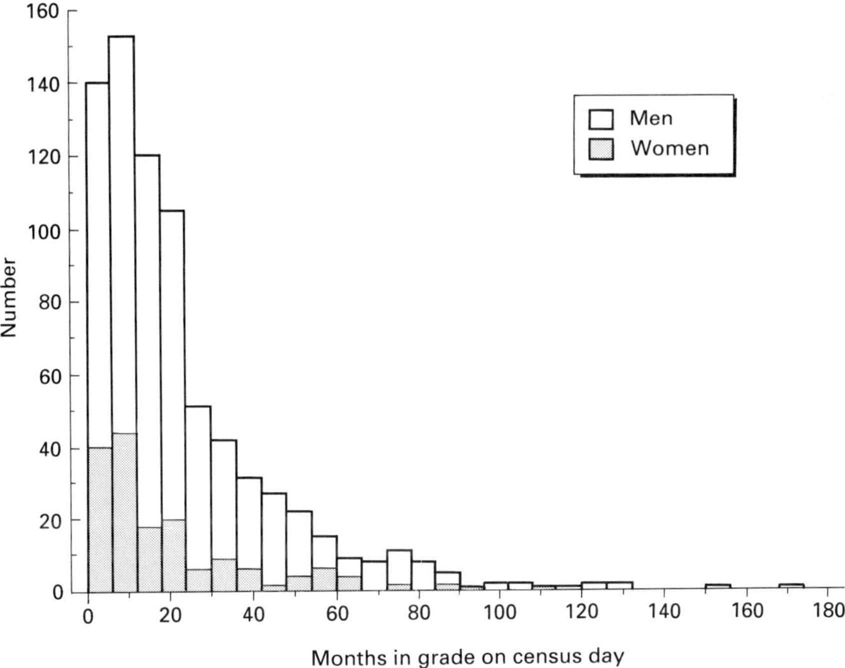

Fig. 8 Cross-sectional survey of medical registrars in 1990 showing duration in grade.

grade of 3 years, it is clear that there must be considerable wastage to other career paths. The following questions might be asked.

1 How long do registrars stay in the grade on average?
2 How much variation in stay is there?
3 Are different streams discernible?

First, the numbers appear to fall off with time in a roughly exponential fashion. Second, the numbers in the second half year exceed those in the first. This must mean either incomplete ascertainment of those in the first period, or that recruitment to the grade fell off during that period, which would certainly indicate that a steady state did not obtain. It is possible, however, to estimate the mean duration of stay (X) and its variance (V), without defining the type of probability distribution that the random variable 'duration of stay in the grade' has. For our data $X = 23.17$ months and $V(X) = 986$ (months) with sample SD = 31 months.

Next we wish to determine which probability distribution would best correspond to the data. The two most likely candidates are the normal distribution and the exponential distribution (derived from the Poisson distribution). Both of these will provide estimates of the probability of the duration of registrars attaining or exceeding a certain value. The initial numbers entering the grade would decline according to the characteristics of those distributions, and the estimates may be compared with the actual decline observed.

Goodness of fit can be assessed by the χ^2 distribution, and the best choice of distribution made (Fig. 9). Another way of testing which distribution is best is to use a probability plot (Fig. 10). It can be seen immediately that in both cases there is a satisfactory linear relationship. The possibility that two decay lines could be fitted to the data, as suggested by the semilog plot of the raw data (Fig. 11), is not borne out. Thus, a fairly simple analysis has provided useful information about the constitution and 'life' of the medical registrar population. It will be observed that these inferences have been drawn from a cross-sectional study and not a longitudinal (or cohort) study. The validity of equating the random variables of duration in grade for a population over several years, estimated in these different ways, is clearly open to question, and is an interesting question in its own right.

A salaried profession is really a contradiction in terms achieved only by the British capacity for compromise and fudging the issues. Traditionally, professions jealously guard and control their numbers to maintain scarcity value. Such a monopoly – or conspiracy against the laity – can be shattered by determined government action, which happened in Sweden in the 1970s when the government rapidly expanded medical student intake. Here in the UK, health economists are examining the inexplicable variations in work done by doctors of the same specialty in different

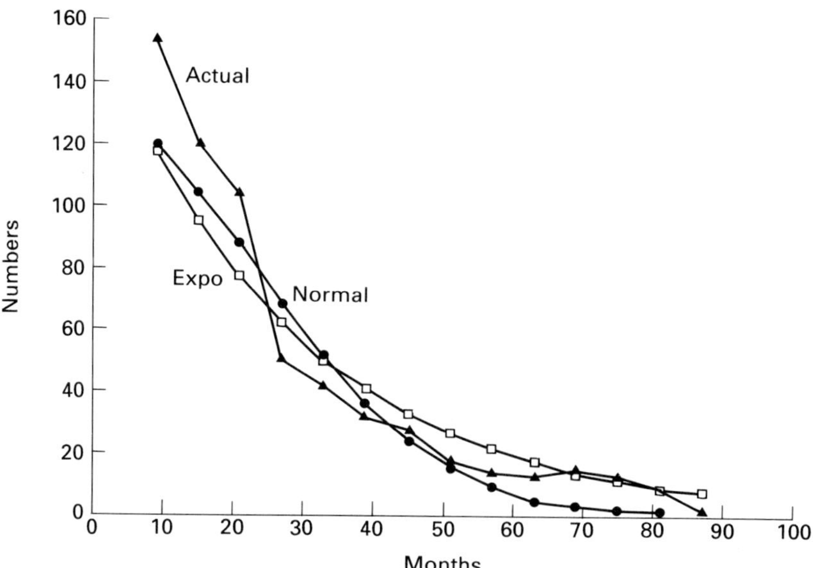

Fig. 9 Goodness of fit curves for duration of medical registrar posts. Expo, Exponential distribution.

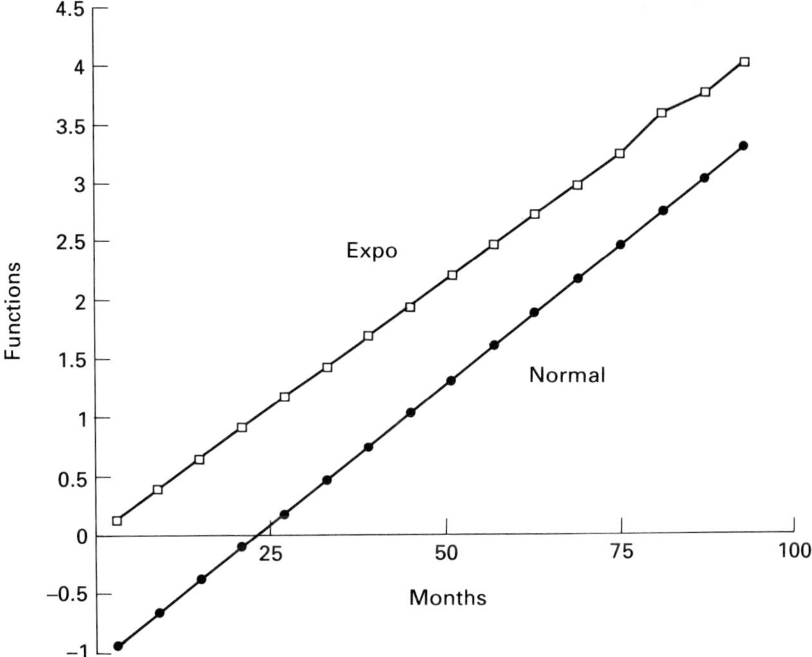

Fig. 10 Probability plot of duration of medical registrar posts. Expo, Exponential distribution.

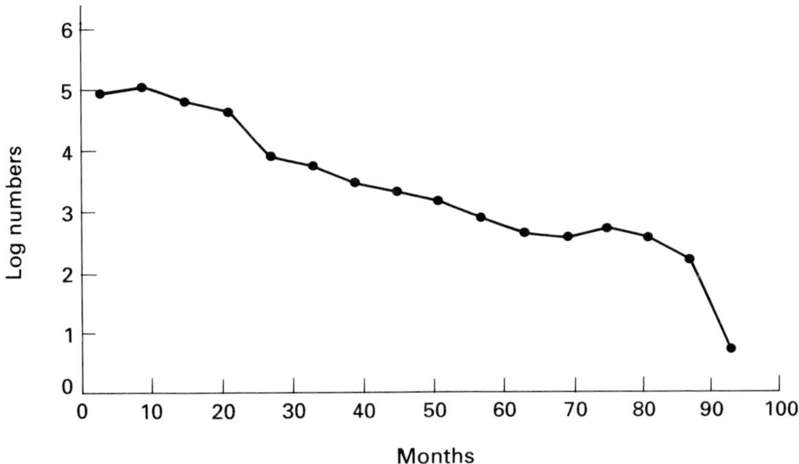

Fig. 11 Semilog plot of registrar numbers against duration in grade suggesting a fast and a slow decay.

parts of the country. There can be little doubt that prescriptive norms are in the air – the number of psychiatrists needed to change a light bulb (only one, but the bulb has really got to want to change) will be laid down. Demand and supply parameters will be better quantitated, and managerial decisions, based on financial power, will become paramount. If errors like the two tier system of GP referral, and the supremacy of waiting lists as an indication of need, are not to prevail then the profession must regain lost influence in policy making. Its arguments will need to be better informed and marshalled. Direction of labour – the apotheosis of manpower planning – is a real danger. The more discontented and disaffected the work force becomes, the more apathetic it will be. We must not train too many people for too few jobs, or allow gluts and dearths to develop in various specialties or in different parts of the country. A proper understanding of the principles and objectives of manpower planning – including its politics – behoves all who are engaged in medical administration, and that now means all of us.

I have touched on only two relatively trivial examples to illustrate possible modelling procedures. Similar analytical techniques can be applied to the outstanding issues troubling us at present. These include length of training, part-time training, contribution of foreign medical graduates from both the EC and elsewhere, the changing demands of an ageing population and manpower demands of applying new techniques, changes in disease incidence, and expected hours of work. Such a complex scenario will challenge would-be regulators to the uttermost. It may be impossible to devise administrative machinery which can cope with problems like these. Adam Smith's view would certainly be that only untrammelled enterprise and adaptation would work. Perhaps we need to consider that.

REFERENCE

1 Bartholomew DJ. Statistical approach to manpower planning. *Statistician* 1972;20:3.

PART 6
CARDIOLOGY

Hypertrophic cardiomyopathy: a new classification?

W. J. McKENNA, H. C. WATKINS & C. A. MacREA

Currently, cardiomyopathies are defined as idiopathic heart muscle disorders and are classified into two main types: hypertrophic and dilated [1]. This purely descriptive classification based on the structure and function of the heart has served clinicians well on purely clinical prognostic grounds over the past 30 years. The classification's descriptive nature does underscore our ignorance of aetiology and pathogenesis of these conditions. With the development of new molecular and immunological techniques there is clearly the potential to understand these conditions at more than a clinical level; but are we ready for a new classification? This paper examines this question in relation to hypertrophic cardiomyopathy in the light of recent developments in the understanding of the molecular genetics of this condition.

HISTORICAL PERSPECTIVE

Hypertrophic cardiomyopathy is defined as an idiopathic heart muscle disorder which is characterized by the presence of left and/or right ventricular hypertrophy in the absence of a systemic or cardiac cause. This definition of unexplained myocardial hypertrophy provides a diagnosis of exclusion. Problems arise when there are other potential causes of left ventricular hypertrophy, e.g. athletic training, obesity and systemic hypertension. The diagnostic criteria are also problematic in the young as the hypertrophy may not become apparent until after adolescent growth is completed. The diagnosis relies on a constellation of clinical features (rapid upstroke pulse, prominent left ventricular impulse, left ventricular outflow tract murmur) electrocardiographic abnormalities (left ventricular hypertrophy and repolarization changes, abnormal Q waves and intraventricular conduction defects) and echocardiographic abnormalities. Great reliance has come to be placed on the echocardiographic demonstration of left ventricular hypertrophy and this has provided the *sine qua non* of the condition [2].

Echocardiographic left ventricular hypertrophy is asymmetric septal in 50–60%, concentric or symmetrical in 20–30% and predominantly

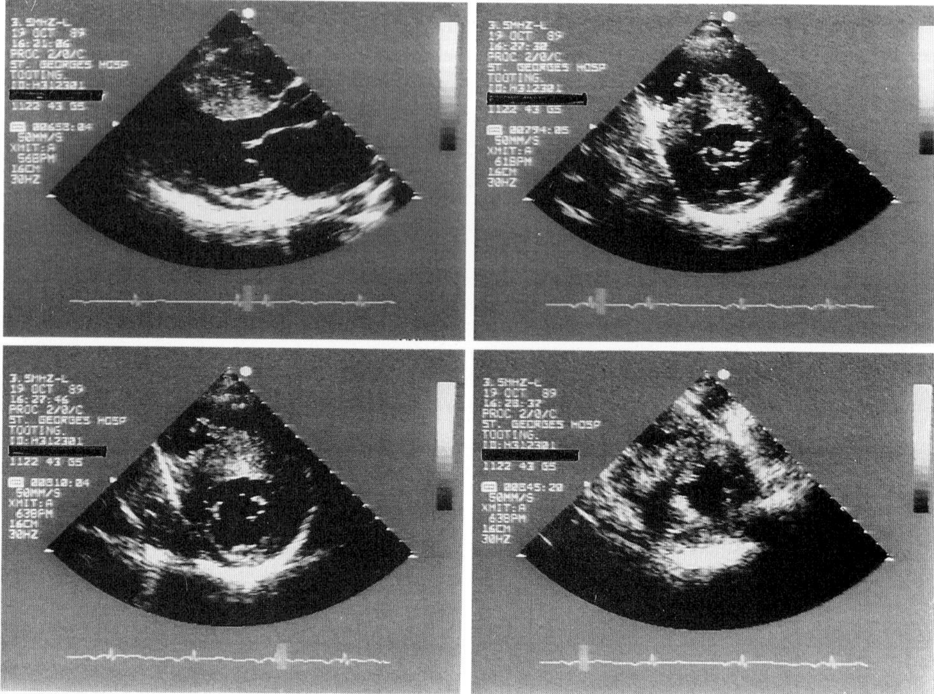

Fig. 1 Parasternal long-axis views (left) and short-axis at mitral valve level (right) showing asymmetric septal hypertrophy (top) and concentric hypertrophy (bottom) in two patients with hypertrophic cardiomyopathy.

distal ventricular in 10% of consecutive patients (Fig. 1) [3]. Though these are the commonest patterns, the hypertrophy may be confined to single segments of the left ventricle including the posterior wall, and the free wall at either mitral valve or papillary muscle level. In approximately a third of cases there is right ventricular hypertrophy; occasionally hypertrophy is confined to the right ventricle [4].

At postmortem examination the macroscopic correlates of the echocardiographic findings include increased heart weight, myocardial wall thickness and right ventricular involvement [5]. The characteristic histology shows myocyte disarray surrounding areas of increased loose connective tissue. This disorganization may involve up to 40% of myocardial sections, is not related to the severity of left ventricular hypertrophy and may indeed be present in myocardial areas that are not thickened. The major problem in the assessment of the condition is the inability to assess the extent and severity of myocyte disarray during life. The clinical correlates of the disarray are therefore largely speculative; the extent and severity of disarray is likely both to be a determinant of electrical instability and contribute to abnormalities of diastolic filling.

The spectrum of disease is wider than the phenotype which relies on the diagnostic presence of unexplained left ventricular hypertrophy. Families have been identified with many of the clinical features and characteristic histology, in the absence of increased left ventricular wall thickness during life or myocardial left ventricular hypertrophy at postmortem [6]. In one such family four members presented with sudden death. All had been previously asymptomatic. At postmortem all four had extensive myocyte disarray involving both the left and the right ventricle in the absence of increased wall thickness or heart weight. Similar families with autosomal dominant inheritance and myocyte disarray in the absence of hypertrophy, but in whom the predominant clinical presentation is with diastolic abnormalities, have been recognized. In one of these, clinical presentation was with atrial fibrillation associated with restrictive physiology. The proband died a disease-related death and was found at autopsy to have extensive disarray without hypertrophy. Screening of the family revealed electrocardiographic and echocardiographic evidence of marked diastolic abnormalities in the absence of left ventricular hypertrophy. Subsequently one of the younger members of this family has gone on to develop typical asymmetric septal hypertrophy.

One can view the diagnostic criteria for hypertrophic cardiomyopathy as a function of the limitation of the technology available. In the 1960s when stethoscopes and cardiac catheterization provided the main diagnostic tools the condition was considered to be a disease of left ventricular outflow tract obstruction, hence the terms 'hypertrophic obstructive cardiomyopathy', 'idiopathic hypertrophic subaortic stenosis' and 'muscular subaortic stenosis'. In the 1970s the development of M-mode echocardiography permitted visualization of what has turned out to be the thickest and thinnest myocardial segments, the upper anterior septum and the posterior wall respectively. The demonstration of asymmetric septal hypertrophy re-emphasized the asymmetric nature which had been first noticed by the pathologist Donald Teare and led to a decade where the condition was named asymmetric septal hypertrophy [5,7]. Indeed, some workers proposed that asymmetric septal hypertrophy was the genetically determined pathognomonic feature of the condition [8]. In the 1980s with the widespread availability of two-dimensional echocardiography and the capacity to image the entire heart it had become clear that many different patterns of hypertrophy can be present. When one considers that only 20% of patients with unexplained left ventricular hypertrophy actually have a left ventricular outflow tract gradient one can see the significant increase in the proportion of patients over the decades who fulfil the diagnostic criteria for hypertrophic cardiomyopathy. Recent pedigree analyses for molecular genetic work also suggest that clinicians may still be only appreciating the tip of the iceberg of this condition.

MOLECULAR GENETICS

During the past 5 years, one of the genes which causes hypertrophic cardiomyopathy has been discovered, several additional loci have been identified, disease-causing mutations are being introduced into transgenic animals and functional studies of diseased muscle have revealed abnormalities in the sarcomere function [9–14].

At the outset in the search for the gene, few would have claimed there was an obvious candidate gene. Many have considered left ventricular hypertrophy to be the *sine qua non* of the condition, and potential candidate genes included oncogenes and growth factors. At a histological level the phenotype, however, is myocyte disarray surrounding areas of increased loose connective tissue. One could reasonably ask which is the chicken and which is the egg? Are myocytes forced into disarray by the presence of increased loose connective tissue or is there something inherently wrong with the myocytes such that myofibrils and myocyte alignment becomes altered and the abnormal connective tissue is simply a secondary development. Was the likely gene a matrix protein or perhaps a contractile protein? The finding of point mutations in the DNA encoding β-cardiac myosin heavy chain in a large French Canadian family with hypertrophic cardiomyopathy surprised few, but had not been predicted [9,10]. In this family, all 21 affected individuals had an adenine for guanine substitution, which resulted in the change of a single amino acid from arginine to glutamine. The recognition that messenger RNA from the gene could be amplified from peripheral lymphocytes permits the screening of an individual patient for myosin mutations [15]. The use of RNase protection has proved to be an accurate if laborious method. To date, using this and other techniques, 17 missense mutations have been identified in hypertrophic cardiomyopathy patients. All of these mutations are single nucleotide substitutions, which result in the change of a single amino acid in the globular head or head-rod junction region of the myosin heavy chain. The evidence that these mutations are disease-causing is strong. They have only been found in individuals affected with hypertrophic cardiomyopathy and they have not been detected in unaffected relatives or in over 200 other unrelated individuals. The amino acid substitutions also affect residues which have been conserved throughout vertebrate evolution making them particularly likely to be of functional importance [10]. The ultimate proof, however, requires the introduction of the abnormal gene into a transgenic animal with the subsequent development of the phenotype. Such work is in progress. Nature, however, has already performed this experiment. We have screened the β-cardiac myosin heavy chain gene in individuals with sporadic hypertrophic cardiomyopathy who had typical clinical features, but unaffected parents. In two of seven such probands, missense mutations were identified (Arg723Cys and Glu924Lys); analyses demonstrated that neither proband had inherited the mutation from a parent (paternity proven) indicating that the mutations had arisen *de novo* [16] (Fig. 2). In one of the probands with the *de novo* mutation, the disease was passed on in the germline to her daughter [16]. *De novo* mutations, then, can cause both the familial and sporadic forms of hypertrophic cardiomyopathy. This indicates that sporadic and familial hypertrophic cardiomyopathy represent different parts of the spectrum of the same condition and this has important implications for management in relation to genetic counselling and risk factor stratification (see below).

PROGNOSIS

The natural history of hypertrophic cardiomyopathy is characterized by a slow progression of symptoms with a significant incidence of sudden death, which is highest in children (6% per year) and persists throughout adult life (2.5% per year) [1]. A clear profile of the high risk adult has emerged and non-invasive assessment identifies the vast majority of those at risk (negative predictive accuracy 95%) [17]. Risk factor stratification in the young is less accurate. The markers of high risk (syncope and family history of multiple sudden deaths) are highly specific but very insensitive and do not identify the majority of those younger individuals who go on to die suddenly. The finding of multiple mutations within the β-cardiac myosin heavy chain gene permits assessment of the influence of specific mutations on the course of the disease. The number of individuals from unrelated families that can be combined for analysis remains small and thus the conclusions are preliminary. Nevertheless, certain mutations are clearly associated with poor prognosis (e.g. Arg403Gln and Arg453Cys) whereas others (Val606Met) appear to be associated with particularly good prognosis [18] (Fig. 3). This latter mutation differs from the others in that it does not involve a charge change, and so would not be predicted to cause a severe disturbance in the structure and function of the myosin polypeptide. These data suggest that specific myosin mutations may be a determinant of survival and that knowledge of the precise defect may help management of patients, particularly in relation to risk factor stratification, which remains problematic in the young and those with sporadic disease.

PRECLINICAL DIAGNOSIS

The availability of techniques to screen for defects in the myosin gene in individual patients presents the possibility of preclinical diagnosis. This is especially relevant in teenagers who present diagnostic problems, par-

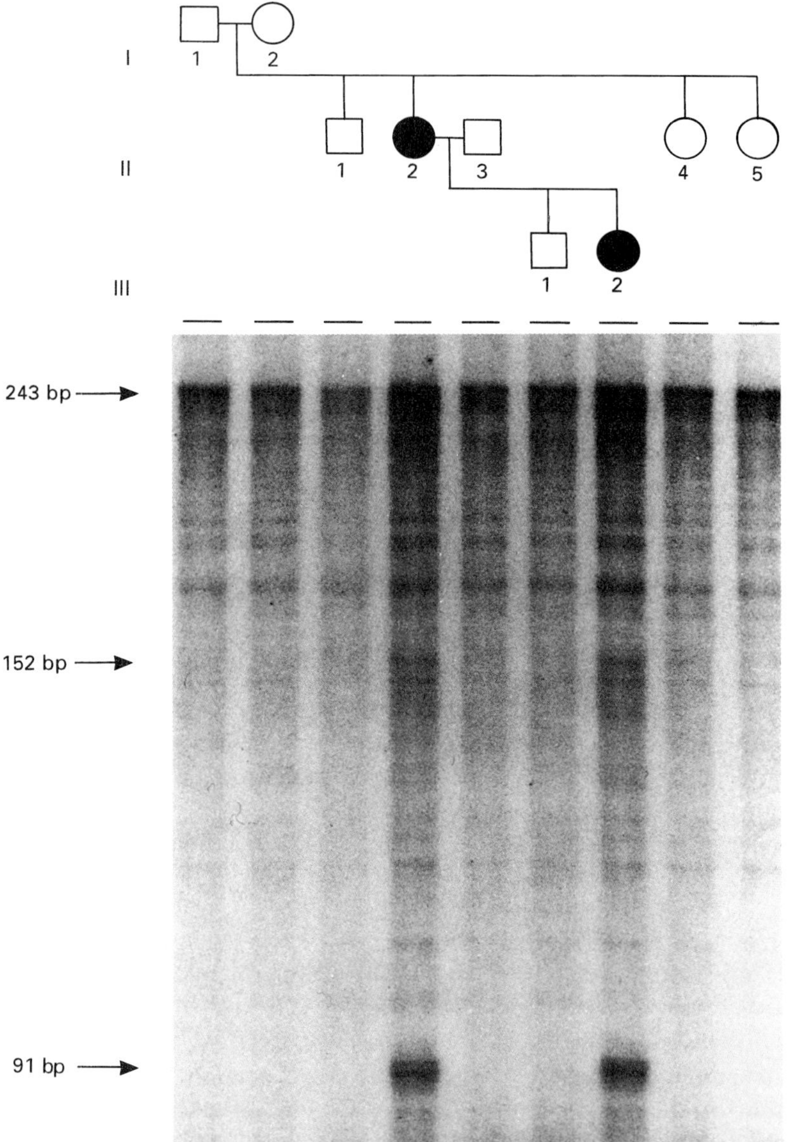

Fig. 2 Detection of the Glu924Lys mutation in exon 23 by RNase protection assay. The pedigree is shown above. *Squares* denote males and *circles* denote females; *solid symbols* denote those clinically affected and *open symbols* denote those unaffected. Below is an RNase protection assay of exon 23 DNA from each individual, in corresponding positions to those of the pedigree. Amplified DNA is hybridized to a ^{32}P-labelled RNA probe of normal β-cardiac myosin heavy chain sequence which is then digested with RNase A, resulting in cleavage at mismatched bases. The normal exon protects a 243 base fragment (arrow); the Glu924Lys mutation results in cleavage of this to fragments of 91 and 152 bases (arrows). Cleavage due to the nucleotide mismatch is present only in the clinically affected individuals II-2 and III-2. (Reproduced from the *Journal of Clinical Investigation* [16], by copyright permission of the American Society for Clinical Investigation.)

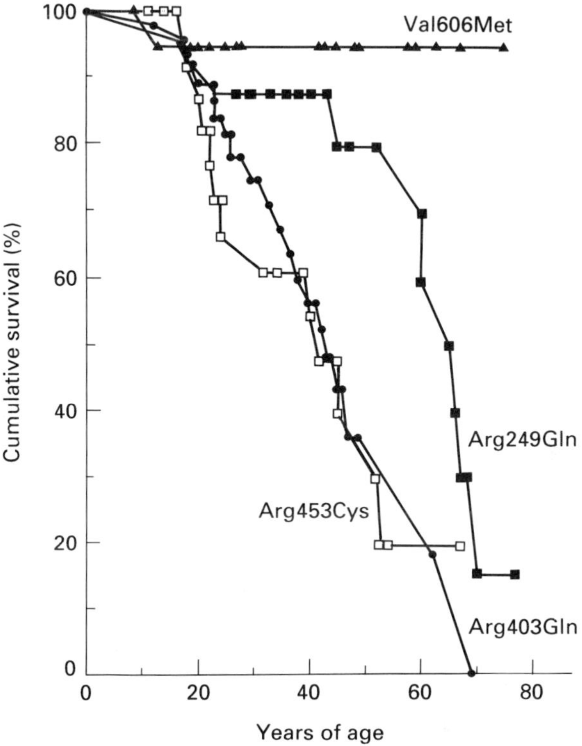

Fig. 3 Kaplan–Meier product-limit curves for the survival of family members, according to mutation. Curves are shown for families with each of four mutations. The curve for Arg453Cys refers to affected members in families with and without the hybrid gene. (Reprinted, by permission of the *New England Journal of Medicine* [18].)

ticularly when there has been a sudden death in a sibling. At present, DNA diagnosis remains a research tool, though it is probable that a clinical DNA test will ultimately be available. Important issues arise, including the need for concomitant genetic counselling, cost effectiveness and perhaps most important, a positive practical end-point for the patient. Can early diagnosis lead either to attenuation of the development of the disease at best, or if not, prevention of complications of the disease, particularly sudden death? No single specific therapy has been shown to improve prognosis in all patients with hypertrophic cardiomyopathy. Nevertheless, an approach to management which attempts to identify first high risk patients, and then the likely triggers of sudden death, can provide effective targeted therapy for approximately a third of high risk individuals. The most important triggers are amenable to specific therapy: paroxysmal atrial fibrillation – amiodarone; ischaemia – high dose verapamil; occult conduction disease – pacing; rapid atrioventricular conduction via an accessory pathway – ablation; and clinical ventricular tachycardia – amiodarone/implantable cardioverter defibrillator. In the remaining two-thirds of high risk patients, no predominant or likely trigger can be identified. Approximately half of these are adults with non-sustained ventricular tachycardia during electrocardiogram monitoring. In this subset, low dose amiodarone has been shown to be effective [19]. In the remaining third, efficacy of treatment is unproven and remains empiric in individual patients; available treatment modalities include amiodarone, myectomy and implantable cardioverter defibrillators for those who have experienced out of hospital ventricular fibrillation. Though management may require detailed characterization of patients in relation to likely risk, it is worth the effort because sudden death can be prevented.

A second important issue in relation to the use of a DNA diagnostic test for preclinical diagnosis is the degree to which the presence of a β-cardiac myosin heavy chain gene mutation predicts the outcome for any individual, particularly his/her risk of sudden death. This remains to be determined; as with any condition, preclinical screening programmes within families with hypertrophic cardiomyopathy will require careful evaluation of the clinical, psychosocial and financial implications.

GENETIC HETEROGENEITY

Myosin mutations cause disease in 30–50% of patients with sporadic and familial hypertrophic cardiomyopathy. There is, then, genetic heterogeneity. In addition to the hypertrophic cardiomyopathy locus on chromosome 14 (CMH1), there are three other loci identified [11–13]. These have been labelled by McCusick as the CMH2, 3 and 4 loci and are found on chromosome 1, 15 and 11 (Table 1). To date, disease genes at these loci have not been identified; candidate genes include a number of contractile proteins which are expressed in myocardium. Though the CMH1 (myosin) locus accounts for 30–50% of disease, the other three mapped loci each appear to account for a minority of the remaining disease. It is anticipated that there is at least one and perhaps several other genes, and thus the clinical entity of hypertrophic cardiomyopathy manifests considerable genetic heterogeneity.

Table 1 Disease loci for familial hypertrophic cardiomyopathy

Designation	Map position	Disease gene
CMH1	14q11–13	β-Cardiac myosin heavy chain
CMH2	1q3	Unknown
CMH3	15q2	Unknown
CMH4	11q1	Unknown

CONCLUSION

Is a new classification possible for hypertrophic cardiomyopathy? The molecular genetic advances of the past 5 years represent only the early 'shots' in understanding the molecular basis of hypertrophic cardiomyopathy. The identification of the other genes and an assessment of the genotype–phenotype relation will be necessary before the current descriptive diagnostic criteria can be supplanted. The way forward, however, is open and inviting.

REFERENCES

1 Goodwin JF. The frontiers of cardiomyopathy. *Br Heart J* 1982;48:1–18.
2 Maron BJ, Gottdiener JS, Epstein SE. Patterns and significance of distribution of left ventricular hypertrophy in hypertrophic cardiomyopathy. A wide angle, two dimensional echocardiographic study of 125 patients. *Am J Cardiol* 1981;48:418–428
3 Shapiro LM, McKenna WJ. Distribution of left ventricular hypertrophy in hypertrophic cardiomyopathy: a two-dimensional echocardiographic study. *J Am Coll Cardiol* 1983; 2:437–444.
4 McKenna WJ, Kleinebenne A, Nihoyannopoulos P, Foale R. Echocardiographic measurement of right ventricular wall thickness in hypertrophic cardiomyopathy: relation to clinical and prognostic features. *J Am Coll Cardiol* 1988;11:351–358.
5 Teare D. Asymmetrical hypertrophy of the heart in young adults. *Br Heart J* 1958; 20:1–8.
6 McKenna WJ, Stewart JT, Nihoyannopoulos P, *et al.* Hypertrophic cardiomyopathy without hypertrophy: two families with myocardial disarray in the absence of increased myocardial mass. *Br Heart J* 1990;63:287–290
7 Maron BJ, Epstein SE. Hypertrophic cardiomyopathy: a discussion of nomenclature. *Am J Cardiol* 1979;43:1242–1244.
8 Henry WL, Clark CE, Epstein SE. Asymmetric septal hypertrophy. Echocardiographic identification of the pathognomonic anatomic abnormality of IHSS. *Circulation* 1973; 47:225–233.
9 Jarcho JA, McKenna W, Pare JA, *et al.* Mapping a gene for familial hypertrophic cardiomyopathy to chromosome 14q1. *N Engl J Med* 1989;321:1372–1378.
10 Geisterfer Lowrance AA, Kass S, Tanigawa G, *et al.* A molecular basis for familial hypertrophic cardiomyopathy: a beta cardiac myosin heavy chain gene missense mutation. *Cell* 1990;62:999–1006.
11 Watkins H, MacRae C, Thierfelder L, *et al.* A disease locus for familial hypertrophic cardiomyopathy maps to chromosome 1q3. *Nature Genetics* 1993;3:333–337.
12 Thierfelder L, MacRae C, Watkins H, *et al.* A familial hypertrophic cardiomyopathy locus maps to chromosome 15q2. *Proc Natl Acad Sci USA* 1993;90:6270–6274.
13 Carrier L, Hengstenberg C, Beckmann JS, *et al.* Mapping of a novel gene for familial hypertrophic cardiomyopathy to chromosome 11. *Nature Genetics* 1993;4:311–313.
14 Cuda G, Fananapazir L, Zhu W-S, *et al.* Skeletal muscle expression and abnormal function of beta myosin in hypertrophic cardiomyopathy. *J Clin Invest* 1993;91: 2861–2865.
15 Rosenzweig A, Watkins H, Hwang DS, *et al.* Preclinical diagnosis of familial hypertrophic cardiomyopathy by genetic analysis of blood lymphocytes. *N Engl J Med* 1991;325:1753–1760.
16 Watkins H, Thierfelder L, Hwang DS, *et al.* Sporadic hypertrophic cardiomyopathy due to de novo myosin mutations. *J Clin Invest* 1992;90:1666–1671.
17 McKenna WJ, Camm AJ. Sudden death in hypertrophic cardiomyopathy. Assessment of patients at high risk. *Circulation* 1989;80:1489–1492.
18 Watkins H, Rosenzweig A, Hwang DS, *et al.* Characteristics and prognostic implica-

tions of myosin missense mutations in familial hypertrophic cardiomyopathy. *N Engl J Med* 1992;326:1108–1114.

19 McKenna WJ, Oakley CM, Krikler DM, Goodwin JF. Improved survival with amiodarone in patients with hypertrophic cardiomyopathy and ventricular tachycardia. *Br Heart J* 1985;53:412–416.

Viral myocarditis

L. K. BORYSIEWICZ

The infiltration of the myocardium with inflammatory cells is a common final end-point of a number of systemic diseases (Table 1), but is particularly identified in the context of acute virus infection. Historically, a clinical syndrome similar to viral myopericarditis was described in the middle of the nineteenth century, although obviously a viral aetiology was not proposed [1]. This association was first suggested in the context of both mumps and the flu epidemic of 1918 when cardiac pathology was identified in over 80% of fatal cases [2]. Enteroviruses were first causally implicated after sudden death with myocarditis in poliomyelitis [3]. As other viruses of this group were increasingly isolated from cases of myocarditis, an association with coxsackie virus group B (CVB) was established both in endemic and epidemic outbreaks [4]. Since that time the number of viruses associated with myocarditis has continued to increase with improved virological diagnosis (Table 2).

CLINICOPATHOLOGICAL DIAGNOSIS

Clinically myocarditis may vary from an inapparent to a fulminant illness, the diagnosis only being made at postmortem examination. The exact incidence and prevalence of this disorder is therefore difficult to establish. A number of reports have studied prevalence at postmortem but these must be interpreted with caution as population sampling error and diagnostic criteria vary between series. This has resulted in a proposed incidence at postmortem of 3.5–10% of cases of sudden death. Recently two large series have been published using the Dallas histological criteria [5] (Table 3): first, a 10-year autopsy series from Malmo, Sweden (1975–84) found myocarditis in 136:12747 (1.06%) [6]; second, 929 cases in 634440 postmortem cases in Japan from 1958–84 (0.15%) with fluctuations at 3–5 year intervals with a sustained rise after 1974 [7]. However, these series tend to identify rapidly fulminant cases and in view of the variable and often benign clinical course, they may significantly underestimate the clinical incidence of this disorder.

Diagnostically, the major advance has been the use of endomyocardial

Table 1 Causes of myocardial inflammation

Infection	
Viruses	
Parasites	
Trypanosoma cruzi	*Toxoplasma*
Filaria – Loa loa	*Schistosoma*
Trichinella	
Bacteria	
Staphylococcus	*Streptococcus*
Diphtheria	*Meningococcus*
Leptospira	*Legionella*
Lyme disease	
Fungi	
Aspergillus	*Crytococcus*
Candida	*Blastomyces*
Histoplasma	
Rickettsiae	
Chlamydia psittaci	*Coxiella*
Rocky Mountain spotted fever	Scrub typhus
Drugs	
Hypersensitivity reactions	
Specific drugs	
Paracetamol	Lithium
Doxorubicin	IL-2
Interferon α	
Toxins	
Lead	Arsenic
Animal bites	
Other systemic diseases	
Collagen vascular disease	
Sarcoidosis	
Hypothermia	
Hyperpyrexia	

Table 2 Viruses associated with myocarditis

RNA viruses	
Orthomyxoviruses	Influenza
Paramyxoviruses	Mumps
Rabies	
Arboviruses	Dengue
	Yellow fever
Retroviruses	HIV
Picornaviruses	Enteroviruses
	Polio
	CVA and CVB
	Echo
DNA viruses	
Herpesviruses	Herpes simplex virus (HSV)
	Varicella zoster virus (VZV)
	Epstein–Barr virus (EBV)
	Human cytomegalovirus (HCMV)

Table 3 Diagnostic categories for human myocarditis in endomyocardial biopsies – 'Dallas criteria'

Initial biopsy
No myocarditis
Borderline myocarditis
Active myocarditis
Follow-up biopsy
Ongoing (persistent) myocarditis
Resolving (healing) myocarditis
Resolved (healed) myocarditis
(All categories may or may not have associated fibrosis)

biopsy [8]. This has resulted in the establishment of accepted histopathological criteria – 'Dallas criteria' – to establish uniformity in reporting and investigating this disorder [5] (Table 3). However, the disease may be patchy. Thus, biopsy diagnosis is less sensitive than for detecting cardiac transplant rejection: on four to five samples examined at multiple levels sensitivity may be only 40–60% [9].

Although the histological picture provides a 'snapshot' of the disease process and may change rapidly [10], the availability of repeated biopsies has resulted in attempts to delineate a clinicopathological classification to help establish criteria to decide on therapy. This goal may be difficult to achieve because of the morphological similarity of the various pathogenic mechanisms (see below), but it may allow for a more accurate prognosis in the individual case. One classification [11] divides patients into:

1 'fulminant myocarditis' – with a fatal outcome or full recovery;

2 'acute myocarditis' – progressive dysfunction progressing to dilated cardiomyopathy;

3 'chronic myocarditis' – borderline histology tending to progress to dilated cardiomyopathy with ongoing inflammation. There appeared to be a variable response to immunosuppression in this group;

4 'persistent myocarditis' – chronic cardiac failure and no role for immunosuppression.

Whether this or other histologically-based classifications are of clinical value will depend on further studies. In addition, a number of clinical investigations have been used to predict severity of disease. Very few of these are of benefit in the acute case. Electrocardiogram abnormalities, especially those involving QRS abnormalities and left bundle branch block, have been identified as poor prognostic markers [12]. Rhythm disturbances in the context of myocarditis are well recognized and in experimental enterovirus infection, focal ultrastructural abnormalities have been identified in conducting tissue [13]. A number of imaging techniques have been used, including radionuclide scanning with gallium-67

[14] and technetium-99 pyrophosphate [15], to identify areas of inflammation. In addition, indium-111-labelled monoclonal antimyosin antibodies have been used to detect myocarditis, with a specificity of 58% and sensitivity of 100% [16]. However, these techniques have yet to be applied in larger patient studies.

Thus, a number of problems in the context of the individual case can be identified ranging from specific aetiology, assessment of severity and prognosis, pathogenesis, treatment and role of acute myocarditis in progression to dilated cardiomyopathy. It is difficult to address all these issues in man but animal models of viral myocarditis have been developed which may provide insights into the disorder.

VIRUSES ASSOCIATED WITH MYOCARDITIS

A number of viruses have been associated with myocarditis in humans (Table 2). It is difficult to isolate virus from affected myocardium in both postmortem specimens and biopsy material. Occasionally histological examination may detect characteristic viral inclusions such as those of human cytomegalovirus, and the clinical setting of the infection with absence of other aetiological agents may allow a putative diagnosis to be made, e.g. HIV myocarditis.

HIV myocarditis. The aetiology of HIV myocarditis is unknown, as many potential pathogens causing myocarditis occur more frequently in AIDS (Tables 1 and 2). The question remains as to whether HIV directly infects myocardial cells. Early studies failed to detect HIV by *in situ* hybridization (although HIV is present by polymerase chain reaction (PCR) of cardiac tissue, this could represent HIV in cells other than myocytes) but a number of reports claim direct localization. At postmortem, myocarditis is a common finding – 184:402 autopsies in 1991; yet an alternative causative agent is only identified in 15–20% of these [17]. As with viral myocarditis in HIV negative individuals the question of progression to dilated cardiomyopathy is of importance. Congestive cardiomyopathy is associated with a poor prognosis and often a terminal event. Although drugs may be associated with the development of this disorder it is important to note that the commonly used antiretroviral drugs – AZT, ddI and ddC – have not been implicated to date.

Enterovirus myocarditis. Historical, epidemic and serological information has provided a basis for implicating enteroviruses as a cause of myocarditis. However, it has proved difficult to establish Koch's postulates for these agents. It is unusual to isolate CVB by conventional culture techniques but enteroviruses have been detected in cardiac tissue by Northern blotting [18]. Unfortunately, this technique applied in inflammatory myositis has not been confirmed by subsequent PCR based studies [19]. However, in myocarditis *in situ* hybridization [20,21] and PCR [22], in patients with myocarditis and dilated cardiomyopathy, have detected enteroviral sequences. Interestingly, in patients where serology was compared with hybridization data, no correlation was observed between direct virus detection and presence of CVB immunoglobulin M (IgM) [23]. Cumulative studies found that 26% of 350 patients showed evidence of enterovirus on biopsy by *in situ* hybridization [9]. Furthermore, in 12 of 20 infants who died with acute CVB infection the myocardial cells expressed viral antigens, indicating that in the acute phase of the illness active replication and virus production occurs in these cells [24]. However, detection of virus genome or products neither establishes that it is necessarily pathogenic nor whether infection is persistent with limited gene expression.

Enteroviruses

The Picornaviridae are a large family of 27 nm non-enveloped, single-strand, 'positive-sense' RNA viruses, which include enteroviruses (polioviruses, CVA and CVB, echoviruses and numbered enteroviruses – 70+ serotypes), rhinoviruses (common cold viruses – 90+ serotypes), aphthoviruses (foot and mouth disease virus – 7 serotypes; no human pathogens) and cardioviruses (encephalomyocarditis virus (EMC), Mengo virus, uncommon human pathogens) [25]. The enterovirus genomic organization is that of a single strand 'positive-sense' RNA (equivalent to messenger RNA (mRNA)), encoding a single open reading frame translated into a virus polyprotein in the infected cell. This is processed by viral proteinase mediated cleavage.

The virus enters the cell by interaction with specific viral receptors, which for picornaviruses are of the immunoglobulin gene superfamily – poliovirus [26], rhinovirus – ICAM-1 [27] and echovirus VLA-2 [28] (Fig. 1). Virus entry is followed by uncoating and translation of the positive-strand RNA into the polyprotein. The RNA is bounded by a 5′ untranslated region which is a binding site for ribosomes without the need for a cap structure. This allows specific direction of virus protein synthesis in poliovirus as the viral proteinase cleaves cellular p220 inhibiting host cell protein synthesis. The polyprotein is cleaved into five structural proteins VP1–4 and VPg, two proteinases, a viral RNA polymerase and three other non-structural proteins. Meanwhile the viral genome is transcribed into a 'negative-sense' RNA strand which serves as a template for multiple daughter 'positive-sense' RNA strands to be incorporated into new virions. Encapsidation occurs in the cytoplasm by direct interaction of the structural proteins and infectious virus is released on cell lysis.

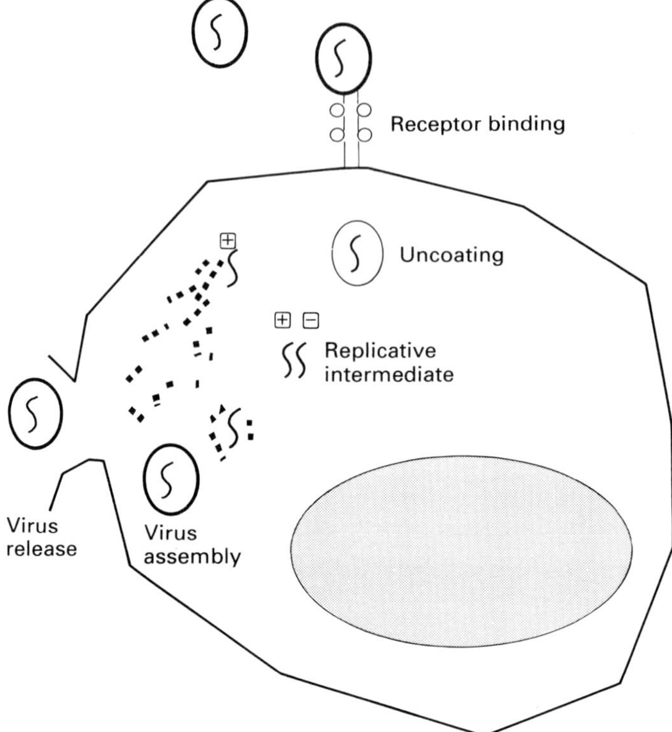

Fig. 1 Replicative virus cycle of enteroviruses.

Most *in vitro* infections with enteroviruses are rapidly lytic to the infected cell. However, it has been suggested that in a number of conditions persistence of enteroviruses in muscle may occur. In patients with chronic fatigue syndrome enteroviral RNA sequences were detected in 32:60 (53%) of patients, but also in 6:41 (15%) normal controls by PCR of reverse transcribed RNA [29]. Specific positive- and negative-strand probes have been used to determine the relative amounts of the two forms of the virus genome in skeletal muscle from these patients [30] and in cardiac muscle in patients with dilated cardiomyopathy [31]. In both instances a reduced ratio of positive:negative strand viral RNA was found. Such differences have also been detected by *in situ* hybridization in experimental murine enterovirus myocarditis [32]. Archard has proposed that persistence may be associated with a selection of virus variants defective in their control of viral RNA replication resulting in the accumulation of negative-strand RNA [31]. Although this may appear an attractive hypothesis such mutants have not been found.

In their replicative cycle, enteroviruses interfere with host cell metabolism in a number of ways which could impair myocardial cell function.

In vitro the beating of rat cardiac myofibres was inhibited by CVB-2 infection and directly associated with the development of viral cytopathic effect [33]. As yet it is unknown whether persistent viral infection is associated with functional impairment of cardiac muscle cells [34], but in other situations of virus persistence specialized cellular function can be impaired without direct cytopathology [35]. *In vivo* this direct virus mediated tissue injury may be augmented by the development of autoimmune and immunopathological responses.

PATHOGENESIS OF VIRAL MYOCARDITIS IN ANIMAL MODELS

Models of viral myocarditis have been established in mice with enteroviruses such as CVB-3 and -2, CVA-9, and EMC, as well as murine cytomegalovirus (MCMV) and reovirus (Table 4). Although similar agents have been used in other species, such as monkey, minipig, guinea pig, rabbit, rat and hamster, the availability of multiple inbred mouse strains allows the analysis of the genetic component of susceptibility to disease and various pathogenic mechanisms [36].

Do animal models of pathogenesis reflect human enteroviral myocarditis?

A number of murine models have been developed with a variety of myocarditic and non-myocarditic enteroviral strains, using animals with a different genetic background and of varying age [37]. It is clear that these factors play an important role in the nature of the disease process. Variation in the virus or the host will influence and ultimately explain the variation observed when different treatment protocols are used.

Role of virus factors in direct cardiac injury. There is ample evidence from *in vitro* studies that enteroviruses can infect isolated myocardial cells and induce direct cytopathic effect [33]. In the absence of an effective

Table 4 Examples of animal models of viral myocarditis

Virus	Species	Reference
CVB-2 and CVB-3	Mouse	Acute [37] Chronic [47]
CVB-1 and CVB-4		[37]
CVA-9	Mouse	[71]
EMC	Mouse	[74]
Reovirus	Mouse	[40]
MCMV	Mouse	[75]
Coronavirus	Rabbit	[76]

immune response as in SCID mice direct myocardial injury by enteroviruses is observed [38]. Mechanisms by which this may be mediated in the context of enterovirus infection have been discussed above, but to date although myocarditic variants of CVB-3, CVB-4 and EMC are well established, the molecular differences in myocarditic strains have not been identified.

Unlike picornaviruses, reovirus is a double-stranded, segmented RNA virus. The segmented nature of the virus genome has allowed the production of reassortant viruses which contain different combinations of gene segments from two parental viruses. Hence, when a phenotypic or disease variant is identified the reassortants can be used to define which segment co-segregates with the phenotypic marker of interest [39]. A myocarditic variant of this virus in neonatal mice (8B) was isolated after co-infection of mice with type 1 Lang and type 3 Dearing viruses. Using a panel of reassortants, a mutation in the M1 gene has been linked with the ability to induce myocarditis [40]. This gene encodes a viral core protein $\mu 1$ which is involved in virion structure but also viral RNA synthesis. In the case of enteroviruses, molecular differences in myocarditic variants may only be defined by direct sequencing of the virus genome, as has been performed to define neurotropic variants of poliovirus [41].

Other factors, including immunological damage (see below), are important but there may be a requirement for the continued presence of the virus even in chronic disease. In DBA/1J mice, no inflammatory lesions evolved in the absence of CSV replication, implying that suppression of virus replication is a valid therapeutic possibility to control myocarditis even late in the disease [42].

Induction of autoimmunity/immunopathology. In the intact animal, a high dose of virus will result in a significant mortality [37] but at sublethal doses the animal may initially recover only to succumb to later immune attack from virus induced autoantibodies [36] or a range of effector T cells [34]. In initial studies T-cell depletion protected mice against the development of myocarditis [43]. The nature of the T-cells mediating injury varies with the strain of mouse studied. CD8+ cytotoxic T-lymphocytes (CTL) have been defined which recognize and kill CVB infected cells by three distinct mechanisms:

1 the recognition of virus specific products in association with major histocompatibility complex (MHC) class I [44] (although in certain strains this killing may be mediated via CD4+ CTL and MHC class II);

2 the induction by the virus of CTL which kill normal cardiac muscle cells [45];

3 the induction of CTL which kill probably by recognition of host cell determinants expressed in CVB infected myocytes or if cardiac myocyte metabolism is perturbed [46].

Thus, there is a complex interaction which is in part determined by the host background and in turn is associated with the type of T-cell response that is generated and the nature/dose of the infecting virus. This strain susceptibility to the 'autoimmune' phase of myocarditis has been mapped to genes located on chromosome 17 linked to the MHC H-2 locus and on chromosome 14 in close proximity to a T-cell receptor locus [47].

As with the detection of virus, the presence of a specific immune response in an animal does not establish that this mediates injury *in vivo*. In addition to the abrogation of disease by removing or transferring disease by CTL, the mediators of cytotoxicity, pore-forming perforin molecules, have been found in infiltrating lymphocytes in experimental CVB-3 infection [48], and on the surface of damaged cardiac myocytes by electron microscopy in humans [49].

However, in other mice (DBA/2), CD4+, I-A^d restricted T cells mediate the acute inflammatory response to CVB-3 infection [50]. In other virus myocarditis such as MCMV, delayed-type hypersensitivity (DTH) mechanisms mediated by CD4+ cells may be important as determined by adoptive transfer and T-cell depletion studies [51]. Other mouse strains with CVB-3 myocarditis involve other effector cells: Balb/c – immature T cells [52]; natural killer cells [48]; $\gamma\delta$ T cells [53].

In addition to T-cell-mediated injury, CVB may induce autoantibodies that directly damage cardiac tissue. A CVB-4 neutralizing monoclonal antibody crossreacts with the amino terminal end of light meromyosin [54]. Furthermore, neutralizing antibodies induced by CVB-3 infection may mediate cardiac injury in adoptive transfer [55], and may be eluted from cardiac tissue [56]. It has also been shown that experimental myocarditis may be induced by isolated cardiac myosin with the induction of autoantibodies that are eluted from cardiac tissue [57]. However, other investigators have suggested that this may be a predominantly T-cell-mediated disease [58]. The importance of these observations in the context of human myocarditis is the frequent identification of autoantibodies directed against a number of cardiac myocyte components [59]. Some autoantibodies against the ADP/ATP carrier directly affect myocyte function [60], as may unfractionated serum from myocarditis patients.

Thus, autoantibodies are generated in both human and experimental infection which may impair contractility and induce inflammatory damage. What is less clear is whether in the context of viral myocarditis these antibodies are causal having been generated against virus but by molecular mimicry may crossreact with cardiac determinants [54,55], or are induced as a result of enterovirus damage exposing immunogenic determinants on cardiac muscle. The value of such responses in monitoring active myocardial damage is under investigation [59].

Whatever the mechanism inducing acute inflammatory damage in the myocardium, in experimental infection the process may result in chronic scarring and injury. With different variants of CVB-3, acute inflammation was observed in A/J mice, but only with myocarditic variants was chronic inflammation and deposition of disorganized collagen deposition observed at later stages [61]. The continued inflammatory damage is anatomically associated with areas of myocardium expressing virus antigens and by implication supporting active virus replication [42]. However, whether these observations represent the mechanism by which dilated cardiomyopathy may develop in humans (see below) is unknown.

TREATMENT OF MYOCARDITIS

A number of different therapies have been tried in murine enterovirus induced myocarditis, but no clear consensus or direction can be provided by the results (Table 5). In most studies exercise is detrimental in the acute phase of the disease [62]. Agents that may 'off-load' the myocardium – captopril [63,64], or reduce microvascular 'spasm' – verapamil [65], appear beneficial both in reducing the extent of inflammation and in improving outcome. Immunosuppression, whether with steroids, azathioprine, cyclophosphamide, cyclosporin or monoclonal antibodies, has had variable results especially in assessing survival. Although most of these agents suppress the inflammation they have no direct effect on outcome or paradoxically increase mortality. A further difficulty in interpretation of these results is the observation that 'immunomodulators', e.g. OK432 and lobenzarit, may be beneficial. These agents induce the release of a broad range of mediators. Therefore, the use of specific cytokines may be an attractive option. However, the

Table 5 Effect of treatment for murine enteroviral myocarditis

	Effect on myocardium		
Treatment	Necrosis	Infiltration	Mortality
Exercise	↑	↑	0
Captopril	↓	↓	0
Verapamil	↓	ND	ND
Immunosuppression			
Steroids	↓	↓	↑
Cyclophosphamide	↓	↓	↑
Anti-CD3	↓	↓	0
Cyclosporin/FK506	↓	ND	↓ ?
Immunostimulant	↓	ND	↓ ?
Antiviral therapy			
WIN 54954	↓	ND	0

selection of these will be difficult as certain cytokines, interleukin 1 (IL-1) and tumour necrosis factor (TNF), promote the development of myocarditis even in resistant strains of mice [66]. The variability of outcome in these experiments can only be fully explained by an underlying variability of myocarditis caused by age/host variation and the role of different pathogenic mechanisms that may operate.

Against this background the confusion that surrounds treatment in humans is understandable. The major unresolved issue is whether the use of immunosuppressive medication may be beneficial and this is currently being addressed in a prospective National Institutes of Health (NIH) Myocarditis study at the University of Utah. Until these results are available, it is possible that immunosuppression in recent onset dilated cardiomyopathy is only of marginal benefit [67] but may be of significant benefit to individual patients in the acute phase, especially those with histological 'borderline myocarditis' [68]. However, it remains to be established whether, as in the murine model, such treatment may be detrimental.

Although detailed analysis of the NIH trial at the University of Utah is still awaited a preliminary analysis has been reported [69]. The study involved patients with a less than 2 year history of congestive cardiac failure. In 2000 subjects only 200 were identified as having histological evidence of myocarditis and 111 entered into the study of additional cyclosporin and prednisone for 24 weeks with conventional heart failure therapy. There was no significant difference in outcome either functionally or in death rate. Furthermore, later review of histology only confirmed myocarditis in two-thirds of those entered, suggesting that this is overall a rare cause of heart failure in this group of subjects.

The role of antiviral agents has only been a theoretical option until the recent development of a number of specific agents. Ribavirin has been used in flu-associated myocarditis with no benefit [70]. WIN54954, a broad spectrum anti-picornavirus agent, has been studied in murine CVA9 myocarditis. Virus titres from the myocardium, and heart weight, were reduced at doses of 25–200 mg per kg even when the treatment was commenced 48–72 h post inoculation. However, the top dosage regimen induced neurotoxicity and any long-term benefit remains to be established [71]. This may be of particular importance if virus persistence is associated with later inflammation and disease progression, in which case this approach may be an important future therapy.

MYOCARDITIS: PROGNOSIS AND PROGRESSION TO DILATED CARDIOMYOPATHY

The natural history in most cases of myocarditis is towards natural resolution, although acute complications such as arrhythmias and a fulminant course are well recognized. However, it is unknown whether there is progression of acute myocarditis to chronic myocarditis and dilated cardiomyopathy. The incidence and prevalence of dilated cardiomyopathy is estimated at 7.5 per 100 000 per year and 8.3 per 100 000 respectively [72] with cases progressing to terminal cardiac failure and heart transplantation. If an association were established, then it is possible that treatment directed against initial injury could reduce this burden of morbidity. Direct studies suggest that enteroviruses may be associated with both diseases, yet from human studies only about 25% have evidence of enterovirus persistence. In CVB infection in the mouse, chronic progression of disease with fibrosis [61] is associated with virus persistence [42], although it is not clear to what extent such observations reflect dilated cardiomyopathy in man. This is further complicated in humans by the frequent observation of mononuclear infiltrates in biopsies from patients with clinical dilated cardiomyopathy [8]. Thus, there may be an inflammatory component to dilated cardiomyopathy but is clinical progression evident?

In 23 patients with biopsy proven clinical myocarditis followed prospectively, 12 (52%) developed dilated cardiomyopathy in a mean follow-up of 43 months [73]. Initial or follow-up histological features did not predict outcomes, whereas those who regained a normal ejection fraction by 6–8 months generally had a good prognosis. Alternatively, histological features of giant cells and chronic active myocarditis were found to progress to dilated cardiomyopathy in another study [11]. Thus, at present there is no definite predictive investigation in helping with establishing a prognosis in an individual case, other than clinical follow-up, measurement of left ventricular function and repeat biopsy where indicated. Further prospective studies are in progress in a number of centres and thus it is possible that this issue will be soon resolved.

SUMMARY

Viral myocarditis has been identified in humans and studied extensively in experimental animal models. In the latter, it is probable that a number of pathogenic mechanisms may operate including infection with variant viruses, host susceptibility, virus persistence and immunopathologically mediated tissue injury. These factors are not only determined by the nature of the infecting agent but also reflect the host genetic background. Such observations may explain the variability of this disorder in humans with regard to prognosis, response to treatment and disease progression to dilated cardiomyopathy. Unfortunately, the mechanisms involved in these processes in humans remain poorly understood therefore making a rational approach to management difficult, and underlining the need for further studies of myocarditis in humans.

REFERENCES

1 Woodruff JF. Viral myocarditis: a review. *Am J Pathol* 1980;101:426–479.
2 Lucke B, Wight T, Kime E. Pathologic anatomy and bacteriology of influenza: epidemic of autumn, 1918. *Arch Intern Med* 1919;24:154–237.
3 Saphir O, Wile SA. Myocarditis in poliomyelitis. *Am J Med Sci* 1942;203:781–788.
4 Helin M, Savola J, Lapinleimu K. Cardiac manifestations during a coxsackie B5 epidemic. *Br Med J* 1968;3:97–99.
5 Artez HT. Myocarditis. The Dallas Criteria. *Human Pathol* 1987;18:3–14.
6 Gravanis MB, Sternby NH. Incidence of myocarditis. A 10-year autopsy study from Malmo, Sweden. *Arch Pathol Lab Med* 1991;115:390–392.
7 Okada R, Kawai S, Kasyuya H. Nonspecific myocarditis: a statistical and clinicopathological study of autopsy cases. *Jap Circulation J* 1989;53:40–48.
8 Olsen EGJ. The value of endomyocardial biopsies in myocarditis and dilated cardiomyopathy. *Eur Heart J* 1991;12(Suppl D):10–12.
9 McManus M, Chow LH, Radio SJ, *et al.* Progress and challenges in the pathological diagnosis of myocarditis. *Eur Heart J* 1991;12(Suppl D):18–21.
10 Keogh AM, Billingham ME, Schroeder JS. Rapid histological changes in endomyocardial biopsy specimens after myocarditis. *Br Heart J* 1990;64:406–408.
11 Lieberman EB, Hutchins GM, Herskowitz A, *et al.* Clinicopathological description of myocarditis. *J Am Coll Cardiol* 1991;18:1617–1626.
12 Morgera T, Lenarda AD, Dreas L, *et al.* Electrocardiography of myocarditis revisited: clinical and prognostic significance of electrocardiographic changes. *Am Heart J* 1992; 124:455–467.
13 Terasaki F, James TN, Nakayama Y, *et al.* Ultrastructural alterations of the conduction system in mice exhibiting sinus arrest or heart block during coxsackievirus B3 acute myocarditis. *Am Heart J* 1992;123:439–452.
14 Veluvolu P, Kamrani F, Horton DP, *et al.* Acute transient myocarditis. Evaluation by gallium scanning. *Clin Nucl Med* 1992;17:411–413.
15 Kao CH, Wang SJ, Yeh SH. Detection of coxsackie B virus myocarditis on Tc-99m PYP myocardial imaging. *Clin Nucl Med* 1992;17:48–51.
16 Peters NS, Poole-Wilson PA. Myocarditis – continuing clinical and pathologic confusion. *Am Heart J* 1991;121:942–947.
17 Kaul S, Fishbein M, Siegel RJ. Cardiac manifestations of acquired immune deficiency syndrome: a 1991 update. *Am Heart J* 1991;122:535–544.
18 Bowles NE, Richardson PJ, Olsen EGJ, Archard LC. Detection of Coxsackie B virus myocardial biopsy samples from patients with myocarditis and dilated cardiomyopathy. *Lancet* 1986;i:1120–1123.
19 Leff RL, Love LA, Miller FW, *et al.* Viruses in idiopathic inflammatory myopathies: absence of candidate viral genomes in muscle. *Lancet* 1992;339:1192–1195.
20 Kandolf R, Amies D, Kirschner P, *et al.* *In situ* detection of enteroviral genomes in myocardial cells by nucleic acid hybridisation: an approach to the diagnosis of viral heart disease. *Proc Natl Acad Sci USA* 1987;84:6272–6276.
21 Kandolf R, Klingel K, Mertsching H, *et al.* Molecular studies on enteroviral heart disease: patterns of acute and persistent infections. *Eur Heart J* 1991;12(Suppl D): 49–55.
22 Jin O, Sole MJ, Butany JW, *et al.* Detection of enterovirus RNA in myocardial biopsies from patients with myocarditis and cardiomyopathy using gene amplification by polymerase chain reaction. *Circulation* 1990;82:8–16.
23 Tracy S, Chapman NM, McManus BM, *et al.* A molecular and serologic evaluation of enteroviral involvement in human myocarditis. *J Mol Cell Cardiol* 1990;22:403–414.
24 Foulis AK, Farquharson MA, Cameron SO, *et al.* A search for the presence of the enteroviral capsid protein VP1 in pancreases of patients with type 1 (insulin-dependent) diabetes and pancreases and hearts of infants who died of coxsackie viral myocarditis. *Diabetologia* 1990;33:290–298.
25 Palmenberg AC. Genome organisation, translation and processing in picornaviruses. In: Rowlands DJ, Mayo MA, Mahy BWJ, eds. *The Molecular Biology of the Positive Strand*

RNA Viruses; FEMS Symposium 32. 1st edn. London: Academic Press, 1987:1–16.
26 Koike S, Taya C, Kurata T, *et al.* Transgenic mice susceptible to poliovirus. *Proc Natl Acad Sci USA* 1991;88:951–955.
27 Greve JM, Davis G, Meyer AM, *et al.* The major human rhinovirus receptor is ICAM-1. *Cell* 1989;56:839–847.
28 Bergelson JM, Shepley MP, Chan BMC, *et al.* Identification of the integrin VLA-2 as a receptor for Echovirus I. *Science* 1992;255:1718–1720.
29 Gow JW, Behan WMH, Clements GB, *et al.* Enteroviral RNA sequences detected by polymerase chain reaction in muscle of patients with postviral fatigue syndrome. *Br Med J* 1991;302:692–696.
30 Cunningham L, Bowles NE, Lane RJM, *et al.* Persistence of enterovirus RNA in chronic fatigue syndrome is associated with the abnormal production of equal amounts of positive and negative strands of enteroviral RNA. *J Gen Virol* 1990;71:1399–1402.
31 Archard LC, Bowles NE, Cunningham L, *et al.* Molecular probes for detection of persisting enterovirus infection of human heart and their prognostic value. *Eur Heart J* 1991;12(Suppl D):56–59.
32 Hohenadl C, Klingel K, Mertsching J, *et al.* Strand-specific detection of enteroviral RNA in myocardial tissue by an in situ hybridisation. *Mol Cell Probes* 1991;5:11–20.
33 Yang YZ, Yuan WL, Guo Q, *et al.* Effect of dexamethasone on coxsackie virus B2-infected rat beating heart cells in culture. *Eur Heart J* 1991;12(Suppl D):39–43.
34 Huber SA. Viral myocarditis – a tale of two diseases. *Lab Invest* 1992;66:1–3.
35 Oldstone MBA, Rodriguez M, Daughaday WH, Lampert PW. Viral perturbation of endocrine function: disordered cell function leads to disturbed homeostasis and disease. *Nature* 1984;307:278–281.
36 Rose NR, Neumann DA, Herskowitz A. Coxsackie virus myocarditis. *Adv Intern Med* 1992;37:411–429.
37 Reyes MP, Lerner AM. Animal models of coxsackie virus myocarditis. In: Kawai C, Abelmann WH, ed. *Pathogenesis of Myocarditis and Cardiomyopathy: Recent Experimental and Clinical Studies.* 1st edn. Tokyo: University of Tokyo Press, 1987:37–48.
38 Chow LH, Beisel KW, McManus BM. Enteroviral infection of mice with severe combined immunodeficiency: evidence for direct viral pathogenesis of myocardial injury. *Lab Invest* 1992;66:24–31.
39 Tyler KL, Fields BN. Reoviridae. In: Fields BN, Knipe DM, eds. *Virology*, Vol. 2. 2nd edn. New York: Raven Press, 1990:1271–1328.
40 Sherry B, Fields BN. The reovirus M1 gene, encoding a viral core protein, is associated with the myocarditic phenotype of a reovirus variant. *J Virol* 1989;63:4850–4856.
41 Evans DMA, Dunn G, Minor PD, *et al.* Increased neurovirulence associated with a single nucleotide change in a non-coding region of the Sabin type 3 poliovaccine genome. *Nature* 1985;314:548–550.
42 Kingel K, Hohenadl C, Canu A, *et al.* Ongoing enterovirus-induced myocarditis is associated with persistent heart muscle infection: quantitative analysis of virus replication, tissue damage and inflammation. *Proc Natl Acad Sci USA* 1992;89:314–318.
43 Woodruff JF, Woodruff JJ. Involvement of T lymphocytes in the pathogenesis of coxsackie virus B3 heart disease. *J Immunol* 1974;113:1726–1734.
44 Huber SA, Lodge PA. Coxsackievirus B3 myocarditis. Identification of different pathogenic mechanisms in DBA/2 and Balb/c mice. *Am J Pathol* 1986;122:284–291.
45 Huber SA, Job LP, Auld KR. Sex-related differences in the rapid production of cytotoxic spleen cells active against uninfected myofibers during coxsackie virus B3 infection. *J Immunol* 1981;126:1336–1340.
46 Huber SA, Heintz N, Tracy R. Coxsackievirus B3-induced myocarditis. Virus and actinomycin D treatment of myocytes induces novel antigens recognised by cytolytic T lymphocytes. *J Immunol* 1988;141:3214–3219.
47 Traystman MD, Chow LH, McManus BM, *et al.* Susceptibility to Coxsackie virus B3-induced chronic myocarditis maps near the murine TCRα and Myhcα loci on chromosome 14. *Am J Pathol* 1991;138:721–726.
48 Seko Y, Shinikai Y, Kawasaki A, *et al.* Expression of perforin in infiltrating cells in murine hearts with acute myocarditis caused by coxsackie virus B3. *Circulation* 1991; 84:788–795.

49 Young LH, Joag SV, Zheng LM, *et al*. Perforin-mediated myocardial damage in acute myocarditis. *Lancet* 1990;336:1019–1021.

50 Blay R, Simpson K, Leslie K, Huber SA. Coxsackie virus-induced disease: $CD4^+$ cells initiate both myocarditis and pancreatitis in DBA/2 mice. *Am J Pathol* 1989;135: 899–907.

51 Craighead JE, Martin WB, Huber SA. Role of $CD4^+$ (Helper) T cells in the pathogenesis of murine cytomegalovirus myocarditis. *Lab Invest* 1992;66:755–761.

52 Kishimoto C, Abelmann WH. *In vivo* significance of T cells in the development of coxsackie virus B3 myocarditis in mice: immature but antigen-specific T cells aggravate cardiac injury. *Circulation Res* 1990;67:589–598.

53 Huber SA, Moraska A, Choate M. T cells expressing the $\gamma\delta$ T cell receptor potentiate coxsackie virus B3-induced myocarditis. *J Virol* 1992;66:6541–6546.

54 Beisel KW, Srinivasappa J, Prabhakar BS. Molecular cloning of a heart antigen that cross-reacts with a neutralising antibody to coxsackie virus B4. *Eur Heart J* 1991; 12(Suppl D):60–64.

55 Gauntt CJ, Arizpe HM, Higdon AL, *et al*. Anti-coxsackie virus B3 neutralising antibodies with pathological potential. *Eur Heart J* 1991;12(Suppl D):124–129.

56 Neumann DA, Lane JR, LaFond-Walker A, *et al*. Elution of autoantibodies from the hearts of coxsackie virus-infected mice. *Eur Heart J* 1991;12(Suppl D):113–116.

57 Neumann DA, Lane JR, Wulff SM, *et al*. *In vivo* deposition of myosin specific autoantibodies in the hearts of mice with experimental autoimmune myocarditis. *J Immunol* 1992;148:3806–3813.

58 Smith SC, Allen PM. Myosin-induced acute myocarditis is a T cell-mediated disease. *J Immunol* 1991;147:2141–2147.

59 Maisch B, Outzen H, Roth D, *et al*. Prognostic determinants in conventionally treated myocarditis – focus on antimyolemmal antibodies. *Eur Heart J* 1991;12(Suppl D):81–87.

60 Schulze K, Becker BF, Scultheiss HP. Antibodies to the ADP/ATP carrier, an autoantigen in myocarditis and dilated cardiomyopathy, penetrate into myocardial cells and disturb energy metabolism *in vivo*. *Circulation Res* 1989;64:179–192.

61 Leslie KO, Schwartz J, Simpson K, Huber SA. Progressive interstitial collagen deposition in coxsackie virus B3-induced murine myocarditis. *Am J Pathol* 1990;136:683–693.

62 Ilback N-G, Fohlman J, Friman G. Exercise in coxsackie B3 myocarditis: effects on heart lymphocyte subpopulations and the inflammatory reaction. *Am Heart J* 1989; 117:1298–1302.

63 Rezkalla S, Kloner RA, Khatib G, Khatib R. Beneficial effects of captopril in acute coxsackie virus B3 murine myocarditis. *Circulation* 1990;81:1039–1046.

64 Rezkalla S, Kloner RA, Khatib G, Khatib R. Effect of delayed captopril therapy on left ventricular mass and myonecrosis during acute coxsackie virus murine myocarditis. *Am Heart J* 1990;120:1377–1381.

65 Dong R, Liu P, Wee L, *et al*. Verapamil ameliorates the clinical and pathological course of murine myocarditis. *J Clin Invest* 1992;90:2022–2030.

66 Lane JR, Neumann DA, Lafond-Walker A, *et al*. Interleukin 1 or tumor necrosis factor can promote coxsackie B3-induced myocarditis in resistant B10.A mice. *J Exp Med* 1992,175:1123–1129.

67 Latham RD, Mulrow JP, Virmani R, *et al*. Recently diagnosed idiopathic dilated cardiomyopathy: incidence of myocarditis and efficacy of prednisolone therapy. *Am Heart J* 1989;117:876–882.

68 Jones SR, Herskowitz A, Hutchins GM, Baughman KL. Effects of immunosuppressive therapy in biopsy-proved myocarditis and borderline myocarditis on left ventricular function. *Am J Cardiol* 1991;68:370–376.

69 Davies MJ, Ward DE. How can myocarditis be diagnosed and should it be treated? *Br Heart J* 1992;68:346–347.

70 Ray CG, Icenogle TB, Minnich LL, *et al*. The use of intravenous ribavirin to treat influenza virus-associated acute myocarditis. *J Infect Dis* 1989;159:829–836.

71 See DM, Tilles JG. Treatment of coxsackie virus A9 myocarditis in mice with WIN 54954. *Antimicrob Ag Chemotherapy* 1992;36:425–428.

72 Williams DG, Olsen EGJ. Prevalence of overt dilated cardiomyopathy in two regions of England. *Br Heart J* 1985;54:153–155.

73 Quigley PJ, Richardson PJ, Meany BT, *et al.* Long-term follow-up of acute myocarditis. Correlation of ventricular function and outcome. *Eur Heart J* 1987;8(Suppl J):39–42.
74 Matsumori A. Lessons from animal experiments in myocarditis. *Herz* 1992;17:107–111.
75 Lawson CM, O'Donoghue H, Bartholomaeus WN, Reed WD. Genetic control of mouse-cytomegalovirus induced myocarditis. *Immunology* 1989;69:20–26.
76 Edwards S, Small JD, Geratz JD, *et al.* An experimental model for myocarditis and congestive cardiac failure after rabbit coronavirus infection. *J Infect Dis* 1992;165: 134–140.

Chronic heart failure: recent developments

G. JACKSON

INTRODUCTION

Chronic cardiac failure has a poor prognosis with over 50% of people dying in 5 years and only 1 in 4 of those referred to hospital living longer than 3 years. However, these figures apply to the era before angiotensin converting enzyme (ACE) inhibitors and with the development of these agents a new and important means of treatment has emerged. We now have the ability not only to influence the quality of life but also to lengthen life. The main focus of this presentation will relate to the recent trials and their practical implications.

The incidence of heart failure rises steeply above age 75 years (Fig. 1) [1] and it is often this age group who are omitted from studies. Furthermore, any thoughts on the treatment or prevention of asymptomatic left ventricular dysfunction in the presence or absence of previous infarction might therefore be reasonably focused on those between 65 and 75 years and yet this has not so far been the case.

THE TRIALS

It is essential to remember that in all the studies correctable mechanical causes (e.g. aortic stenosis) have been excluded and systolic pump failure rather than diastolic failure is the pathophysiology.

The VeHeFT-1 [2] study compared placebo, prazosin and a high dose combination of hydralazine and isosorbide dinitrate (ISDN) in moderate heart failure and showed that the combination of hydralazine and ISDN improved survival (Fig. 2). At about the same time CONSENSUS 1 [3] reported on a comparison of enalapril and placebo in severe heart failure revealing a 31% reduction in mortality from active therapy. The SOLVD treatment trial [4] then compared enalapril with placebo in mild to moderate heart failure demonstrating a 23% reduction in mortality and significantly reduced hospitalization for heart failure (Fig. 3). Set in the clinical context, the implications from SOLVD were that if an ACE inhibitor was given to 1000 patients with chronic heart

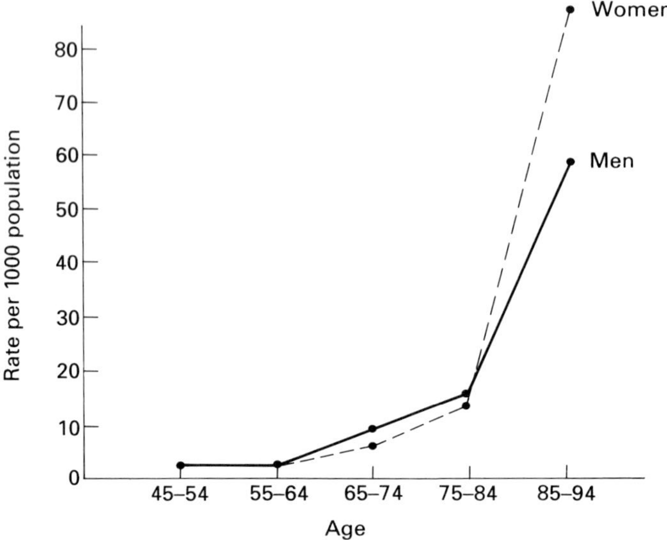

Fig. 1 Incidence of heart failure. (By permission from Kannel and Belanger [1].) By the year 2001 there will be 22% of people aged over 75 years, and a massive 69% increase in those aged over 85 years. The potential benefits of successful therapy for this condition can be easily seen.

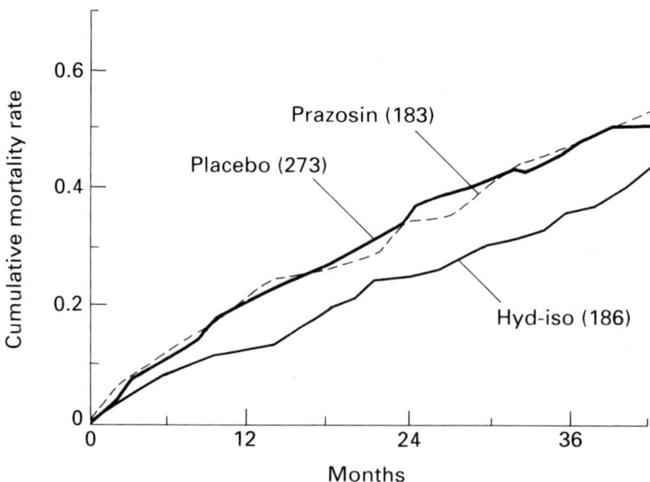

Fig. 2 V-HeFT-1: Mortality–risk reduction in patients treated with isosorbide dinitrate and hydralazine for mild to moderate heart failure. (By permission from Cohn *et al.* [2].)

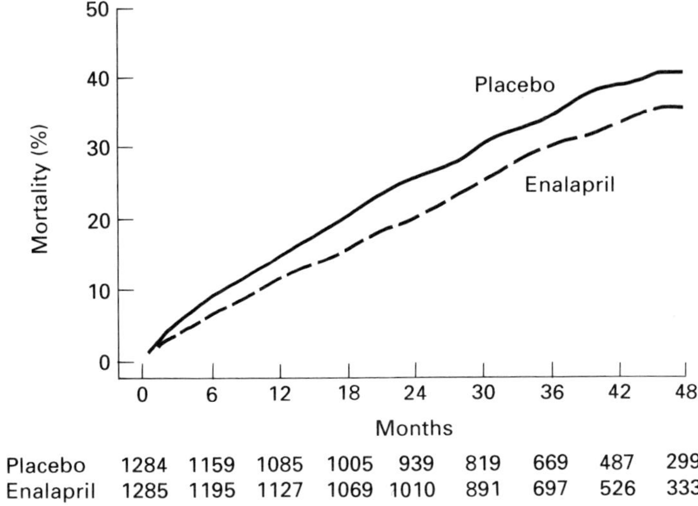

Fig. 3 Mortality curves for placebo and enalapril in SOLVD ($P = 0.0036$). The numbers of patients alive in each group at the end of each period are shown at the bottom of the figure. (By permission from SOLVD [4].)

failure for one year, 17 deaths and 67 hospitalizations for chronic heart failure would be avoided. VeHeFT-2 [5] compared the hydralazine/ISDN combination with enalapril in mild to moderate heart failure and showed superior survival figures with enalapril and only a low incidence of adverse effects with enalapril. However, a 21% incidence of headache causing cessation of therapy occurred with hydralazine/ISDN compared to only 7% on enalapril. Adverse effects from enalapril were similarly low in SOLVD treatment and CONSENSUS 1 even though the latter involved severe cases. The smaller Munich Heart Failure Trial [6] compared captopril with placebo looking principally at progression of mild to moderate heart failure and demonstrated a reduction from 26.4 to 10.8% from active therapy. A very interesting study – the HY-C trial [7] – compared hydralazine and nitrates to captopril and nitrates where the nitrates were used in titration to achieve a wedge pressure of 15 mmHg. Eighty-four per cent of captopril patients needed nitrates to achieve the target wedge pressure suggesting a possible combination therapy strategy particularly as the actuarial one year survival rate was 81% on captopril compared with 51% on hydralazine (Fig. 4).

Turning now to asymptomatic left ventricular dysfunction, the rationale for trying to delay progression not only relates to symptoms – the prognosis worsens as the left ventricle dilates and this particularly applies post infarction where remodelling can begin in the first few days. In SOLVD [8] prevention with enalapril significantly reduced the amount of chronic heart failure, myocardial infarction and the need for hospital

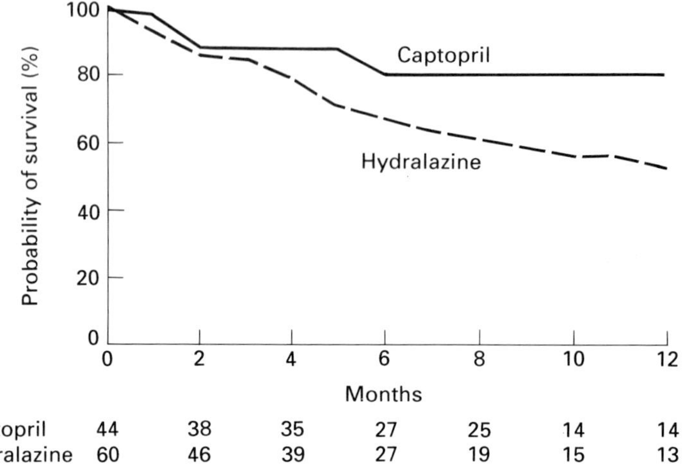

Fig. 4 Kaplan–Meier survival curves for the 104 patients discharged on the oral vasodilator regime of captopril or hydralazine plus ISDN (HY-C Trial). (By permission from Fonarow *et al.* [7].)

admission but not overall mortality though the trend was positive at 8%. Eighty per cent of these cases were post infarction and the criteria for entry was an ejection fraction (EF) of 35% or less.

SAVE [9] compared captopril with placebo in the presence of asymptomatic left ventricular dysfunction (EF less than 40%) post infarction commencing therapy at 3–14 (median 11) days. Captopril caused a 19% reduction in mortality and a 37% fall in the development of severe heart failure (Fig. 5). Side-effects were minimal with only 32 out of 1115 patients being unable to sustain therapy.

IMPLICATIONS FROM THE TRIALS

1 In symptomatic heart failure ACE inhibitors should be used as soon as possible whether symptoms are controlled on diuretics or not.

2 If they are not tolerated hydralazine/ISDN should be considered as an alternative.

3 Isosorbide mononitrate (ISMN) added to ACE inhibition may improve matters further.

4 In asymptomatic left ventricular dysfunction post infarct ACE inhibitors should be initiated. In other patients we need further information.

5 Dosages were in general higher than currently used in clinical practice with a target of captopril 50 mg three times a day in SAVE (79% achieved this) and enalapril 20 mg daily in SOLVD and VeHeFT-2. We almost

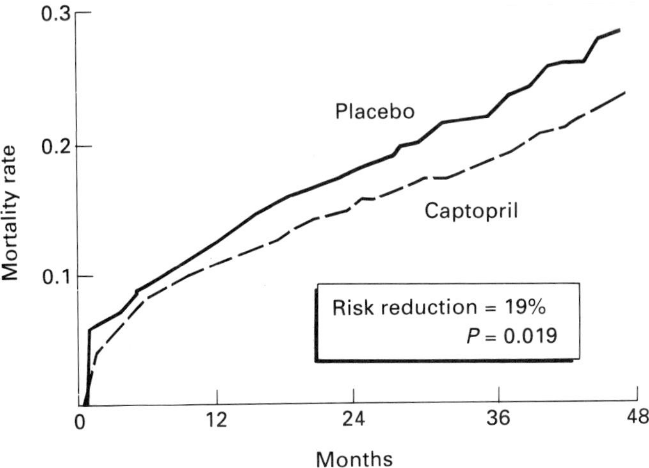

Fig. 5 SAVE: Cumulative mortality from all causes in the study groups. (By permission from Pfeffer *et al.* [9].)

certainly underdose these agents in general but in the elderly we do need to be cautious. The objective is to achieve a level of captopril 50 mg two or three times a day, invariably with isosorbide mononitrate (20 mg twice a day).

6 These trials do not include the elderly and contain highly selected and observed patients. As the ACE inhibitors become more widely used adverse effects may increase so the encouraging figures should not encourage complacent monitoring.

MAKING THE DIAGNOSIS

After establishing the benefits of ACE inhibitors in particular but vasodilators in general, it follows that the diagnosis of heart failure must be precise. We are all aware of the typical symptoms and signs but sometimes the pain of angina is perceived as breathlessness due to the tight restrictive feeling often felt. It is important therefore to probe what is meant by breathlessness. We should consider echocardiography in all cases, not only to establish systolic dysfunction but to rule out a mechanical cause, in particular aortic and mitral valve disease whose murmurs may be difficult to hear in the presence of a low output, and diastolic failure when the ventricle is stiff and relaxes poorly but systolic function is preserved. Diastolic dysfunction is treated differently usually with agents to prolong filling time by slowing heart rate (e.g. β-blockers) and calcium antagonists to relax the ventricle.

INITIATING THERAPY

In general we need to advise on weight loss, cessation of smoking, moderation of alcohol and a reduction in salt intake. Exercise will need to be limited in severe cases but should be encouraged as progress is made. Agents which may exacerbate or cause the chronic heart failure must be discontinued if at all possible (e.g. β-blockers, calcium antagonists, non-steroidal anti-inflammatory agents and salt-containing antacids). For more severe cases a home visit will be needed to see if any adjustments are necessary to facilitate activity, e.g. bed downstairs, ground level toilet or even rehousing if in a hilly district with a lot of steps or stairs.

DIURETICS

Symptomatic heart failure needs diuretic therapy as ACE inhibition alone is not as effective. Caution is needed with potassium sparing agents if ACE inhibitors are coprescribed but the combination may be necessary if ACE inhibition alone does not sustain potassium levels. As diuretics are prescribed ACE inhibitors should be initiated. Excessive diuresis causing dehydration may lead to hypotension; the introduction of ACE inhibitors and their earlier use can reduce the need for diuretics, which is more socially acceptable. Frusemide or bumetanide are the agents of choice and must be given intravenously in more severe cases to guarantee bioavailability. Increasingly, low dose loop diuretics and low dose thiazides are being used in combination as the additive effects are less likely to interfere with daily life due to the more gradual action of the thiazides. Regular monitoring of urea and electrolytes and creatinine will ensure safe initiation and continuation of therapy.

DIGOXIN

Several trials have now established that this is effective in sinus rhythm both acutely and long term, particularly when there is cardiomegaly and a gallop rhythm [10]. It may be used with all other agents and the average dose in 0.25 mg daily. Less will be needed with impaired renal function and in the elderly and as toxicity relates in part to potassium levels, these should be monitored at the commencement of therapy and regularly if other agents are being adjusted.

Digoxin does reduce symptoms, reduces hospital admissions and improves exercise ability, and when carefully used, side-effects are not as frequent as believed – in several trials hardly more than placebo. Digoxin has not so far been shown to lengthen life; trials are now in progress. Where heart failure and atrial fibrillation (AF) coexist, digoxin is essential therapy, as is warfarin. Digoxin carries no risk of hypotension or dehydration. Thus, it has a place as an alternative to ACE inhibitors if hypotension is a problem and has a place in combination. It should be used more frequently.

ANTICOAGULANTS

These are essential when AF is present but must also be considered in the presence of severe left ventricular dysfunction because of an increased risk of deep venous thrombosis, and pulmonary and systemic embolism, which may in part explain the sudden death rate which ends life in 40% of chronic heart failure patients. Where warfarin is contraindicated aspirin forms a less satisfactory alternative. There is a pressing need for trials of anticoagulants in chronic heart failure as it is my impression that they are being underemployed.

FLOSEQUINAN

This is a new balanced venous and arterial vasodilator which is symptomatically effective when added in to ACE inhibitors, or when these are contraindicated, in a dosage of up to 150 mg daily [11]. Unfortunately, a mortality trial (not yet published) comparing flosequinan 50, 75 and 100 mg once daily with placebo added to ACE inhibitor in severe failure demonstrated an increased death rate on flosequinan 100 mg daily. Whilst initial results looking at symptoms and haemodynamics remain encouraging with no evidence of tolerance and a low incidence of side-effects, mainly headache, there remains a doubtful role for flosequinan even at 50 mg daily unless clearcut symptomatic benefit can be established at this lower dosage.

CALCIUM ANTAGONISTS

No beneficial data exist other than in mild failure when angina coexists where one can argue that a nitrate would be safer [12]. Several studies have shown adverse effects from nifedipine demonstrating that the gamble of offsetting negative inotropic effects with peripheral vasodilators cannot be sanctioned. With far safer options (ACE inhibitors, nitrates) it is difficult to accept the need for more studies of calcium antagonists even if they are more vascular specific such as amlodipine or felodipine. Let us hope no patient will be deprived benefits already achieved from ACE inhibitors when entering upcoming calcium antagonist studies.

AMIODARONE

This is the least negatively inotropic antiarrhythmic agent and recent studies suggest it improves prognosis when complex ventricular arrhythmias and left ventricular dysfunction coexist post infarction [13]. Its extension into other areas is likely and there is an increasing role for ACE/amiodarone/anticoagulants in carefully selected areas. Screening at-risk patients with 24–48 hour ambulatory monitoring may therefore become as routine as screening with echocardiography.

PHOSPHODIESTERASE INHIBITORS

In chronic heart failure oral milrinone reduces life expectancy [14]. These agents have a short-term intravenous role but in chronic failure they are contraindicated orally.

β-BLOCKADE

Used more in Scandinavia than elsewhere [15] β-blockers may well have a role when angina and mild (controlled) failure coexist. Though xamoterol, the agent with the most partial agonist activity (43%), worsened survival in severe chronic heart failure it may be effective here also. It remains, however, a potentially dangerous avenue to pursue and requires hospital supervision for initiation. There is still a place for the use of conventional β-blockers or xamoterol but one should be mindful that the arguments in favour of ACE inhibitors and digoxin tend to overwhelm those in favour of β-blockers. Several trials are due to report which may help clarify their usage.

SURGERY

Occasionally reversible ischaemia contributes to left ventricular dysfunction and coronary artery bypass grafting may be helpful, especially if angina coexists. *Cardiomyoplasty*, which involves wrapping the latissimus dorsi round the heart and using pacing stimulation to boost systole, is now under evaluation. *Heart transplantation* offers an 80% 5-year survival for the lucky few who acquire a donor heart. Late coronary disease is an increasing problem now that rejection is treatable.

CONCLUSION

In chronic heart failure due to systolic heart failure an accurate diagnosis needs to be made as early as possible for symptomatic and prognostic reasons. All patients must be considered for an ACE inhibitor whether symptomatic or with asymptomatic left ventricular dysfunction. There is no doubt that the basis of therapy is a diuretic and ACE inhibitor in combination. Early use of nitrates should also be considered. There are arguments in favour of digoxin, anticoagulants and amiodarone in selected cases and more patients should be anticoagulated and digoxin should be considered earlier. There is no good reason for increasing the use of calcium antagonists and one should be cautious with regard to β-blockade with or without partial agonist activity.

In the future a combination of diuretic, ACE inhibitor and nitrate and digoxin and warfarin will be in standard use. Routine 24-hour electrocardiograms will be needed if the amiodarone studies continue to be positive. This may seem a large number of drugs for a patient to take but when only 25% of chronic heart failure patients reach 3 years, and quality and quantity of life can be improved, it is an acceptable price to pay.

REFERENCES

1 Kannel WB, Belanger AJ. Epidemiology of heart failure. *Am Heart J* 1991;121: 951–957.

2 Cohn JN, Archibald DG, Ziesche S, *et al.* Effects of vasodilator therapy on mortality in chronic congestive heart failure. *N Engl J Med* 1986;314:1547–1552.

3 CONSENSUS Trial Study Group. Effects of enalapril on mortality in severe congestive heart failure. Results of the Co-operative North Scandinavian Enalapril Survival Study (CONSENSUS). *N Engl J Med* 1987;316:1429–1435.

4 SOLVD Investigators. Effects of enalapril on survival of patients with reduced left ventricular ejection fractions and congestive heart failure. *N Engl J Med* 1991;325: 293–302.

5 Cohn JN, Johnson G, Ziesche S, *et al.* A comparison of enalapril with hydralazine–isosorbide dinitrate in the treatment of chronic congestive heart failure. *N Engl J Med* 1991;325:303–310.

6 Kleber FX, Niemoller L, Doering W. Impact of converting enzyme inhibition on progression of chronic heart failure. Results of the Munich Mild Heart Failure Trial. *Br Heart J* 1992;67:289–296.

7 Fonarow GC, Chelimsky-Fallick C, Stevenson LW, *et al.* Effect of direct vaso-dilation with hydralazine versus angiotensin-converting enzyme inhibition with captopril on mortality in advanced heart failure: The Hy-C Trial. *J Am Coll Cardiol* 1992;19: 842–850.

8 SOLVD Investigators. Effect of enalapril on mortality and the development of heart failure in asymptomatic patients with reduced left ventricular ejection fractions. *N Engl J Med* 1992;327:685–691.

9 Pfeffer MA, Braunwald E, Moye LA, *et al.* Effect of captopril on mortality and morbidity in patients with left ventricular dysfunction after myocardial infarction. Results of the Survival and Left Ventricular Enlargement Trial (SAVE). *N Engl J Med* 1992;327(10):669–677.

10 Kulick DL, Rahimtoola SH. Current role of digitalis therapy in patients with congestive heart failure. *JAMA* 1991;265:2995–2997.

11 Cowley AJ, Wynne RD, Stainer K, *et al.* Flosequinan in heart failure: acute haemodynamics and longer term symptomatic effects. *Br Med J* 1988;297:169–172.

12 Editorial. Calcium antagonist caution. *Lancet* 1991;i:885–886.

13 Burkhart F, Pfisterer M, Kiowski W, *et al.* Effect of anti-arrhythmic therapy on mortality in survivors of myocardial infarction with asymptomatic complex ventricular

arrhythmias: Basel Anti-arrhythmic Study of Infarct Survival. *J Am Coll Cardiol* 1990; 16(7):1711–1718.

14 Packer M, Carver JR, Rodeheffer RJ, *et al.* Effect of oral milrinone on mortality in severe chronic heart failure. *N Engl J Med* 1991;325:1468–1475.

15 Waagstein F, Caidahl K, Wallentin I, Bergh C-H, Hjalmarson A. Long-term β-blockade in dilated cardiomyopathy. Effects of short- and long-term metoprolol treatment followed by withdrawal and readministration of metoprolol. *Circulation* 1989;80: 551–563.

Coagulability, thrombosis and vascular disease

T. W. MEADE

There have been three main stimuli to the reawakening of interest in thrombosis as a major determinant of ischaemic heart disease (IHD). One was the promising early results of randomized controlled trials of aspirin in the secondary prevention of myocardial infarction (MI) [1]. The second was resolution of the debate between pathologists as to whether thrombosis causes or is the consequence of MI, when the advent of thrombolytic therapy and the growing use of angiography showed the high frequency of total coronary occlusion during MI [2]. Even then, however, the place of thrombosis in sudden coronary death still remained controversial and it was not until the particularly careful autopsy studies of Davies and Thomas [3] that the almost universal occurrence of at least a degree of thrombosis in sudden coronary death was acknowledged. The third is the growing recognition of strong associations between haemostatic variables and the onset of IHD [4].

There had, however, been much earlier epidemiological recognition of a thrombotic component in IHD. Thus, Morris [5] showed a high prevalence of advanced atheroma – about 30% – in the first decade of the century, i.e. before the start of the great rise in IHD mortality in the 1920s. Morris also showed that there was no increase in advanced atheroma (if anything, prevalence fell) to accompany the rise in IHD mortality. These observations clearly indicated an increase in some process other than atherogenesis. Morris [5] suggested that the increase in smoking in men during the First World War might have contributed to the rise in clinically manifest IHD and there is indeed evidence that smoking may lead to IHD predominantly through its thrombogenic effects, although it almost certainly promotes atherogenesis as well [4]. In further epidemiological studies of the pathology of IHD, Morris and Crawford [6] showed that there was no relationship between the degree of physical activity at work and the extent of atheroma at autopsy but that there was an inverse relationship in the case of lumen occlusion – the heavier the work the lower the prevalence of occlusion. The relationship was strongest for myocardial infarction, those in heavy occupations during life showing a very substantial degree of protection compared with those in light occupations. The protective effect against IHD of vigorous exercise during leisure has now also been demonstrated [7]. There is no reasonable doubt that the association is one of cause and effect and that exercise (like smoking) influences the onset of IHD largely through short-term effects on thrombotic potential (see for example, reference [8]).

Coronary artery thrombi are due to platelet aggregates and to the deposition of fibrin in varying proportions. The very rapid adhesion of platelets to damaged endothelium and then to each other is central to arterial thrombosis. It is, however, fibrin which gives many developing thrombi their ultimate stability and volume. A recent biochemical (as distinct from morphological) study showed that fibrin formation and platelet activation are probably equally important in the early hours of MI [9] emphasizing that the mechanical obstruction of the coronary artery is due to two main processes, with the implication that the most effective approach to antithrombotic therapy may involve the simultaneous use of platelet active agents and anticoagulants.

Given that there is a major thrombotic contribution to IHD in particular, but also to stroke, an obvious question is the extent to which those at risk can be characterized on account of a thrombotic tendency and how far any such tendency can, in turn, be defined in terms of measures of haemostatic function. So far, coagulation factor assays have proved more useful than platelet function tests though this reflects the unsatisfactory nature of the latter and not the importance of platelets in arterial thrombosis. Of possible platelet function tests, spontaneous aggregation [10] and platelet size [11] are related to the risk of recurrent MI but there is so far no satisfactory way of relating platelet function to the risk of a first episode. However, one feature of the coagulation system – summarized in Fig. 1 – is that both thrombin and fibrinogen have substantial effects on platelet aggregability as well as their better known clotting functions and it may indeed be [12] that platelet behaviour is determined at least as much by plasma influences as by any intrinsic properties of the platelets themselves. Figure 1 also shows that the traditional distinction between the extrinsic and intrinsic coagulation pathways is an oversimplification. Thus, dietary fat probably influences coagulability through the activation of factor VII (extrinsic system) by factor XII (intrinsic system). The factor VII activation of factor IX is another example. Nonetheless, there is increasing evidence [13] that it is the extrinsic system, initiated by the complexing of factor VII with tissue factor, that mainly determines the degree of coagulability.

Current interest chiefly centres on two clotting factors, factor VII and fibrinogen.

Factor VII mainly circulates in a single chain form. On complexing with tissue factor (e.g. from an atheromatous plaque) single-chain VII is

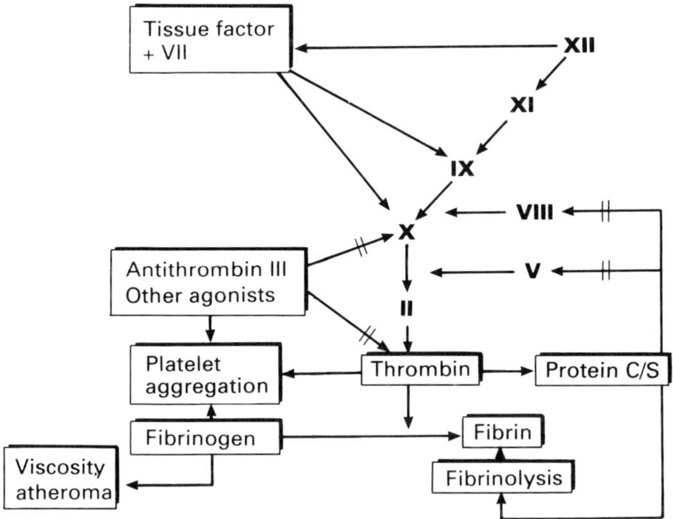

Fig. 1 Summary of coagulation system showing inter-relationships with platelets and the fibrinolytic system. Unbarred lines indicate activation, barred lines indicate inhibition. The scheme indicates the position of different factors, without distinguishing between inactive (zymogen) and active forms, e.g. conversion of factor X to activated X, Xa by IXa, itself derived from factor IX. Non-coagulation cofactors, e.g. calcium ions, also not shown.

converted to the two-chain form, which is up to 100 times more active than the former. Based on a biological activity assay system that is sensitive to the two-chain form, high factor VII levels were strongly associated with the subsequent incidence of IHD in the Northwick Park Heart Study (NPHS) [14], particularly in the case of fatal events. Several cross-sectional and prevalence studies also show higher factor VII levels in cases than controls [4]. There is a direct relationship between the levels of factor VII and markers of thrombin generation, suggesting that factor VII activity is at least a valid index of the degree of coagulability. Whether the degree of factor VII activity itself contributes to the latter (as distinct from simply reflecting it) is unresolved, although there is some evidence that it does directly influence coagulability [4]. The general epidemiological features of factor VII are consistent with its involvement in IHD. For example, increasing age, oral contraceptive use, the menopause, diabetes, obesity and in particular high dietary fat consumption are all associated with raised factor VII levels. Thus, in both observational and experimental studies, there is a direct relationship between fat intake and factor VII activity [15]. One possibility is that large negatively charged and triglyceride-rich lipoproteins (e.g. chylomicrons and very low density lipoproteins) activate the intrinsic pathway which, in turn, activates factor VII. Figure 2 illustrates the long-term atherogenic effect of diet in IHD and its much shorter-term

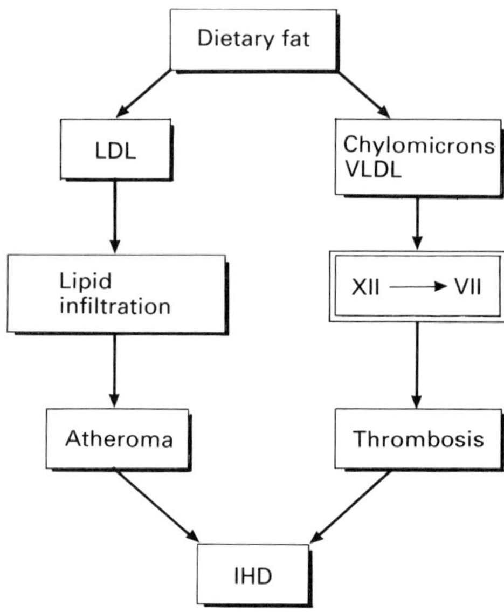

Fig. 2 Diet and IHD: atherogenic and thrombogenic pathways. LDL, Low-density lipoprotein; VLDL, very low-density lipoprotein.

thrombogenic effect. It is still often claimed that dietary intervention is unlikely to be effective in adults in whom significant atheroma has often already developed and that it is, therefore, only children and young adults who stand to benefit. If, however, dietary fat intake does have short-term thrombogenic effects, this conclusion is largely misplaced and adults already affected by a significant degree of atheroma probably stand to benefit considerably.

Several prospective studies show an independent relationship between fibrinogen and the incidence of IHD [4] which, at face value, is of the same magnitude as for cholesterol and IHD. However, because of the greater within-person variability in fibrinogen, the true relationship is probably rather stronger than for cholesterol. In the prospective studies with adequate numbers of older participants, there is also an association between high fibrinogen levels and the incidence of stroke in men that is of the same order as for IHD [16,17]. Since the association between cholesterol and stroke is probably not as clear as for IHD, the fibrinogen level may be a particularly useful index of the risk of major cardiovascular disease, defined as the sum of IHD and stroke. High fibrinogen levels also appear to predict the recurrence of IHD in those surviving a first episode [18]. Only one of the prospective studies has included sufficiently large numbers of women, in whom high levels are also associated with IHD incidence though not very clearly with stroke (probably because of small numbers of events) [17]. High fibrinogen levels are undoubtedly associated with the progression of peripheral vascular disease in terms of worsening symptoms [19], loss of patency after vein grafting [20] and of mortality from cardiovascular disease [21]. It is also likely that fibrinogen levels influence the initial onset of peripheral vascular disease [22]. Some of the prospective studies suggest there may be synergy between high fibrinogen levels and hypertension in the onset of IHD and stroke.

Fibrinogen is an acute phase protein. High levels might, therefore, simply reflect the underlying degree of arterial wall damage, bearing in mind that atheroma has many of the characteristics of an inflammatory response. Even if this were the full explanation for the association between fibrinogen and clinically manifest arterial disease, the strong and independent nature of the association still provides an opportunity for improved precision in identifying those at risk. The balance of evidence suggests, however, that – whatever their determinants – high fibrinogen levels are of direct, pathogenetic significance. This important point can usefully be considered in two stages. First, regardless of their origins, are high fibrinogen levels likely to predispose to thrombosis? Second, what are the origins of high levels? Figure 3 summarizes the pathways through which high fibrinogen levels may predispose to thrombosis and clinical events and (considered in more detail later) the characteristics associated with high or low levels. The influence of fibrinogen on viscosity and the relationship, in turn, of viscosity to IHD is the pathway for which there is probably the strongest evidence at present, one of the prospective studies showing a strong association between plasma viscosity (as well as fibrinogen) and the incidence of IHD [23]. Until recently, perhaps the

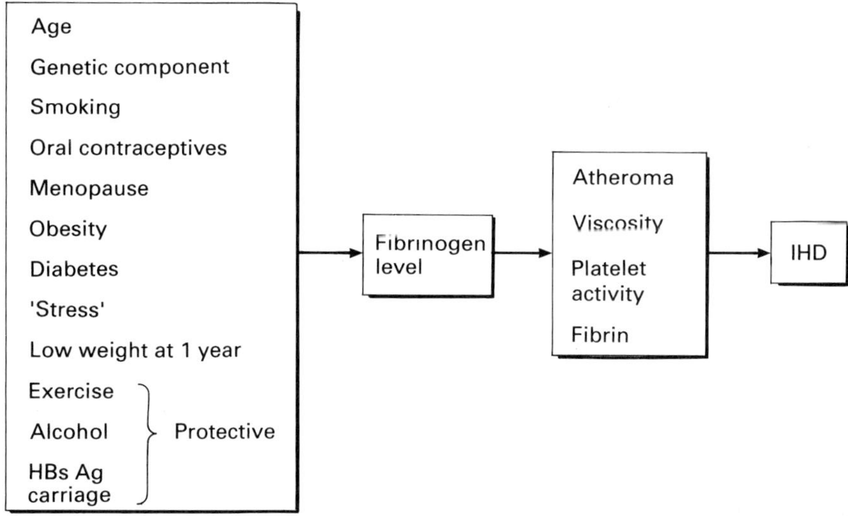

Fig. 3 Summary of determinants and thrombogenic pathways of fibrinogen in pathogenesis of IHD.

most controversial explanation for a causal role for fibrinogen in IHD was the postulated effects of high levels on fibrin deposition. It was argued that circulating levels of fibrinogen exceed those required for haemostasis, although this observation does not preclude the possibility that high levels may nevertheless predispose to the somewhat different process of thrombogenesis. However, these theoretical considerations have now been replaced by experimental results in animals and in studies using human plasma which leave little doubt that when coagulation is initiated, the starting fibrinogen level directly influences the amount of fibrin deposited [24–26]. There is consistent evidence that fibrinogen levels within the physiological range influence platelet aggregability [27,28]. Finally, there is growing evidence for the involvement of fibrinogen in the onset and development of the atheromatous lesion itself [29]. In summary, therefore, there are several pathways through which high fibrinogen levels are likely to increase the risk of thrombosis, whatever their origins. Even if these include an acute or chronic phase contribution, this contribution is likely to be functionally significant. Figure 3 also shows the personal characteristics apparently influencing fibrinogen levels. One of the strongest is smoking, though it is important to recognize that fibrinogen is also strongly associated with IHD in non-smokers. The full return to non-smoking fibrinogen levels in those who discontinue smoking may take several years, paralleling the time course in the decline in the risk of IHD itself in ex-smokers. The extent to which fibrinogen levels are genetically determined, which may be substantial, represents a component of high levels that cannot be explained as a response to atheroma. In fact, fibrinogen levels are probably influenced by nearly all the major IHD risk factors – either adversely as with smoking, obesity and diabetes, or beneficially in the case of moderate alcohol consumption and strenuous physical activity. The one obvious exception is the absence of any apparent influence of diet, particularly dietary fat intake. (It is possible that fish oil lowers fibrinogen, though the evidence on this point is equivocal.) In summary, high fibrinogen levels appear to be a major channel through which likely determinants of IHD are translated into a number of pathways influencing thrombogenesis and clinically manifest disease.

OTHER HAEMOSTATIC VARIABLES

Evidence from prospective and cross-sectional studies and in haemophiliacs suggests that factor VIII may also be involved in IHD [14,30,31]. Recent findings from the Northwick Park Hospital Study, summarized in Table 1, show that poor fibrinolytic activity is strongly associated with subsequent IHD in younger men. High plasminogen activator inhibitor (PAI) levels may also influence the recurrence of myocardial infarction in

Table 1 Median values of fibrinolytic activity (100 per dilute blood clot lysis time in hours) at entry to the NPHS according to IHD incidence subsequently

Age (years)	IHD	No IHD
40–49	15.6	26.7
(*N*)	(32)	(511)
50–59	25.1	25.1
(*N*)	(94)	(537)
60–64	27.3	25.1
(*N*)	(52)	(156)

younger individuals [32]. The potential importance of fibrinolytic activity in IHD has of course been highlighted by the success of thrombolytic therapy in early MI.

PRACTICAL IMPLICATIONS

If prospective screening for IHD is considered justifiable (which is controversial), it is clearly valuable to include newer measures that make a substantial, independent contribution to predictive ability. Fibrinogen meets these criteria. Less controversial is opportunistic screening, involving only those who themselves decide to consult their physicians who may then, in turn, select only some for further investigation. Here, there is a growing case for the measurement of fibrinogen as part of the routine investigation of those considered for other reasons to be at risk of thrombotic events, whether these are first events or recurrences. Two practical considerations arise. One is the within-person variability of fibrinogen. More than one and ideally three or four estimations should be carried out to establish an individual's habitual level. The second is differences between laboratories in methods for measuring fibrinogen and in the absolute levels of their reference ranges. In general, different methods for determining fibrinogen (clot weight, clotting time or immunological) give results that are highly correlated. Furthermore, associations with fibrinogen, e.g. according to current, previous or never smoking status, are remarkably consistent from one study to another. But absolute values may vary considerably. To move towards the kind of standardization of cholesterol measurements that is now widely practised, an international standard for fibrinogen has recently been established and is likely to facilitate the comparison of results from different laboratories. For some time to come, however, clinical decisions will in many cases still have to be based on the values and reference ranges in separate laboratories.

As already indicated, the practical value of factor VII activity measurements is currently limited by the rather different performance of the available assays and the probable need to consider assay systems sensitive to two-chain VII. In the general investigation of 'hypercoagulability', the measurement of activation peptides such as fragment 1.2 or fibrinopeptide A, indicating the production and the action of thrombin respectively, is likely to be increasingly useful in establishing risk and in deciding about management.

The value of platelet-active agents in the secondary prevention of IHD (including unstable angina) and stroke is beyond dispute, the reduction in risk of further major cardiovascular events being about 25%. Currently, aspirin and streptokinase are mandatory (unless contraindicated) in the early stages of suspected myocardial infarction, and in the longer term aspirin is increasingly routine in the secondary prevention of further major episodes in those who have recovered from MI or stroke and in unstable angina. Although not formally tested in all these circumstances, there is increasing reason to believe that a dose of no more than 75 mg aspirin daily is effective [33,34] and lower doses are of course accompanied by less bleeding. The value of aspirin in the primary prevention of IHD (i.e. the prevention of a first episode) is much less clear. Furthermore, it is possible though not certain that aspirin in this context may somewhat increase the risk of stroke, possibly because of an increase in cerebral haemorrhage.

The demonstration of a habitually raised fibrinogen level is already being used in different ways. Of lifestyle modifications, much the most important is the avoidance or discontinuation of smoking although, once again, it is important to remember that levels in ex-smokers remain above non-smoking levels for several years, as does the risk of IHD itself, even though both start to fall fairly quickly. Encouraging smoking cessation is not of course dependent on knowing the fibrinogen level (and has other objectives besides preventing IHD) but it is probably justifiable to give special attention to those with raised levels, particularly younger subjects. The beneficial effect of strenuous exercise on fibrinogen now provides both doctors and patients with a further incentive towards prevention. Another approach is to use a high fibrinogen level as a marker of risk in helping to decide, e.g. whether to prescribe aspirin even though this has no effect on the fibrinogen level itself. Undoubtedly, definitive randomized controlled trials to establish how far IHD incidence can be reduced by fibrinogen lowering agents are now needed.

A second generation of oral anticoagulant trials, from The Netherlands and Norway [35,36], which have taken advantage of requirements for satisfactory trials not fully appreciated earlier on, have reinforced the value of oral anticoagulants. The implications of these trials are by no means academic, even allowing the value and easier administration of aspirin in this context. First, the indications are that oral anticoagulation may be slightly more effective than aspirin, although the extent to which the two regimens have been directly compared is at present limited. Even a small advantage in a condition as common as IHD may have substantial implications. Second, however, there is increasing and so far very consistent evidence from trials concerned with the management and prevention of venous thrombosis, the prevention of thromboembolism in atrial fibrillation and in the management of patients undergoing heart valve surgery, that much lower than conventional intensity oral anticoagulation may be equally effective while carrying a lower risk of bleeding and also reducing the requirement for frequent blood testing and dose monitoring [37]. Third, recent trials also suggest that the simultaneous modification of platelet function and fibrin formation is substantially more effective than modifying either process on its own [38,39]. Contrary to general expectation, the concurrent use of aspirin and warfarin, particularly at low International Normalized Ratio values in carefully selected individuals, does not lead to an unacceptable increase in serious bleeding, though minor episodes (e.g. bruising and nose-bleeds) certainly do increase [40].

If, as seems likely, thrombogenesis is the structural event immediately preceding and leading to major IHD, it may be the optimal point for intervention, whether by lifestyle or pharmacological methods. This approach is of course entirely compatible with also trying to modify the risk factors and other pathways leading up to thrombosis.

REFERENCES

1 Elwood PC, Cochrane AL, Burr ML, *et al.* A randomized controlled trial of acetylsalicylic acid in the secondary prevention of mortality from myocardial infarction. *Br Med J* 1974;i:436–440.

2 DeWood MA, Spores J, Notske R, *et al.* Prevalence of total coronary occlusion during the early hours of transmural myocardial infarction. *N Engl J Med* 1980;303:897–901.

3 Davies MJ, Thomas A. Thrombosis and acute coronary-artery lesions in sudden cardiac ischemic death. *N Engl J Med* 1984;310:1137–1140.

4 Meade TW. The epidemiology of atheroma, thrombosis and ischaemic heart disease. In: Bloom AL, Forbes CD, Thomas DP, Tuddenham EDG, eds. *Haemostasis and Thrombosis.* 3rd edn. Edinburgh: Churchill Livingstone 1994 (in press).

5 Morris JN. Recent history of coronary disease. *Lancet* 1951;ii:1053–1057, 1111–1120.

6 Morris JN, Crawford MD. Coronary heart disease and physical activity of work. Evidence of a national necropsy survey. *Br Med J* 1958;ii:1486–1496.

7 Morris JN, Clayton DG, Everitt MG, *et al.* Exercise in leisure time: coronary attack and death rates. *Br Heart J* 1990;63:325–334.

8 Connelly JB, Cooper JA, Meade TW. Strenuous exercise and plasma fibrinogen. *Br Heart J* 1992;67:351–354.

9 Rapold HJ, Haeberli A, Kuemmerli H, *et al.* Fibrin formation and platelet activation in patients with myocardial infarction and normal coronary arteries. *Eur Heart J* 1989;10: 323–333.

10 Trip MD, Cats VM, van Capelle FJL, Vreeken J. Platelet hyperreactivity and prognosis in survivors of myocardial infarction. *N Engl J Med* 1990;332:1549–1554.

11 Martin JF, Bath PM, Burr ML. Influence of platelet size on outcome after myocardial

infarction. *Lancet* 1991;330:1409–1411.
12 Lowe GDO, Forbes CD. Platelet aggregation, haematocrit and fibrinogen. *Lancet* 1985;i:395–396.
13 Meade TW, Miller GJ, Rosenberg RD. Characteristics associated with the risk of arterial thrombosis and the prethrombotic state. In: Fuster V, Verstraete M, eds. *Thrombosis in Cardiovascular Disorders*. WB Saunders Co, 1992:79–98.
14 Meade TW, Mellows S, Brozovic M, *et al.* Haemostatic function and ischaemic heart disease: principal results of the Northwick Park Heart Study. *Lancet* 1986;ii:533–537.
15 Miller GJ. Fibrinogen, factor VII and other haemostatic variables; roles in primary and secondary prevention of coronary heart disease. *Cardiovascular Risk Factors* 1992;2: 361–367.
16 Wilhelmsen L, Svardsudd K, Korsan-Bengtsen K, *et al.* Fibrinogen as a risk factor for stroke and myocardial infarction. *N Engl J Med* 1984;311:501–505.
17 Kannel WB, Wolf PA, Castelli WP, D'Agostino RB. Fibrinogen and risk of cardiovascular disease. *JAMA* 1987;258:1183–1186.
18 Haines AP, Howard D, North WRS, *et al.* Haemostatic variables and the outcome of myocardial infarction. *Thrombos Haemostas* 1983;50:800–803.
19 Dormandy JA, Hoare E, Khattab AH, *et al.* Prognostic significance of rheological and biochemical findings in patients with intermittent claudication. *Br Med J* 1973;iv: 581–583.
20 Wiseman S, Kenchington G, Dain R, *et al.* Influence of smoking and plasma factors on patency of femoropopliteal vein grafts. *Br Med J* 1989;299:643–646.
21 Banerjee AK, Pearson J, Gilliland EL, *et al.* A six year prospective study of fibrinogen and other risk factors associated with mortality in stable claudicants. *Thrombos Haemostas* 1992;68:261–263.
22 Kannel WB, D'Agostino RB. Update of fibrinogen as a major cardiovascular risk factor. The Framingham Study. *J Am Coll Cardiol* 1990;15:156a.
23 Yarnell JWG, Baker IA, Sweetnam PM, *et al.* Fibrinogen, viscosity, and white blood cell count are major risk factors for ischemic heart disease. The Caerphilly and Speedwell Collaborative Heart Disease Studies. *Circulation* 1991;83:836–844.
24 Gurewich V, Lipinski B, Hyde E, *et al.* The effect of the fibrinogen concentration and the leukocyte count on intravascular fibrin deposition from soluble fibrin monomer complexes. *Thrombos Haemostas* 1976;36:605–614.
25 Chooi CC, Gallus AS. Acute phase reaction, fibrinogen level and thrombus size. *Thrombos Res* 1989;53:493–501.
26 Naski MC, Shafer JA. A kinetic model for the a-thrombin-catalyzed conversion of plasma levels of fibrinogen to fibrin in the presence of antithrombin III. *J Biol Chem* 1991;266:13003–13010.
27 Meade TW, Vickers MV, Thompson SG, Stirling Y, *et al.* Epidemiological characteristics of platelet aggregability. *Br Med J* 1985;290:428–432.
28 Meade TW, Vickers MV, Thompson SG, Seghatchian MJ. The effect of physiological levels of fibrinogen on platelet aggregation. *Thrombos Res* 1985;38:527–534.
29 Smith EB, Keen GA, Grant A, Stirk C. Fate of fibrinogen in human intima. *Arteriosclerosis* 1990;10:263–275.
30 Egeberg O. Clotting factor levels in patients with coronary atherosclerosis. *Scand J Clin Lab Invest* 1962;14:253–258.
31 Rosendaal FR, Varekamp I, Smit C, *et al.* Mortality and causes of death in Dutch haemophiliacs 1973–86. *Br J Haematol* 1989;71:71–76.
32 Hamsten A, de Faire U, Wallius G, *et al.* Plasminogen activator inhibitor in plasma: risk factor for recurrent myocardial infarction. *Lancet* 1987;ii:988–990.
33 RISC group. Risk of myocardial infarction and death during treatment with low dose aspirin and intravenous heparin in men with unstable coronary artery disease. *Lancet* 1990;336:827–830.
34 SALT Collaborative Group. Swedish aspirin low-dose trial (SALT) of 75 mg aspirin as secondary prophylaxis after cerebrovascular ischaemic events. *Lancet* 1991;338:1345–1349.
35 Sixty-Plus Reinfarction Study Research Group. A double-blind trial to assess long-term

oral anticoagulant therapy in elderly patients after myocardial infarction. *Lancet* 1980;ii: 989–994.
36 Smith P, Arnesen H, Holme I. The effect of warfarin on mortality and reinfarction after myocardial infarction. *N Engl J Med* 1990;323:147–152.
37 Meade TW. Low intensity oral anticoagulation. In: Poller L, Thompson JM, eds. *Thrombosis and its Management*. Churchill Livingstone, 1992:84–97.
38 ISIS-2 Collaborative Group. Randomised trial of intravenous streptokinase, oral aspirin, both or neither among 17187 cases of suspected acute myocardial infarction. *Lancet* 1988;ii:349–360.
39 Turpie AGG, Gent M, Laupacis A, *et al.* A comparison of aspirin with placebo in patients treated with warfarin after heart valve replacement. *N Engl J Med* 1993;329: 524–529.
40 Meade TW, Roderick PJ, Brennan PJ, *et al.* Extra-cranial bleeding and other symptoms due to low dose aspirin and low intensity oral anticoagulation. *Thrombos Haemostas* 1992;68:1–6.

PART 7
ENDOCRINOLOGY

Endocrine hypertension: liquorice and allsorts of steroids

P. M. STEWART

INTRODUCTION

Endocrine hypertension is by and large synonymous with adrenal hypertension. Whilst hypertension occurs in primary hyperparathyroidism, acromegaly and in some patients taking oestrogens, the mechanism of the hypertension remains obscure and they will not be discussed further [1]. Endocrine hypertension is rare, accounting for approximately 1% of all subjects with hypertension, and the causes are listed in Table 1. This article cannot be comprehensive, but shall focus attention primarily on a common cause (primary aldosteronism) and a rare cause (11β-hydroxysteroid dehydrogenase deficiency) of mineralocorticoid hypertension and will combine clinical and laboratory-based research to highlight recent advances in this field. Finally the presentation, diagnosis and treatment of the patient presenting with a phaeochromocytoma will be discussed.

MINERALOCORTICOID HYPERTENSION

The adrenal cortex produces two classes of corticosteroid hormone, glucocorticoids (cortisol) produced predominantly from the zona fasciculata and reticularis and mineralocorticoid (aldosterone) produced exclusively by the zona glomerulosa. The distal nephron, the distal colon and salivary glands are important targets for mineralocorticoid action in humans. In the distal nephron, aldosterone causes sodium retention and potassium excretion, with concomitant loss of hydrogen ions resulting in a metabolic alkalosis. Mineralocorticoid hypertension is therefore mediated initially by volume expansion. There is associated suppression of the renin–angiotensin system and hypokalaemia. Cardiac output rises initially but is replaced within weeks of the onset of hypertension with an increase in peripheral vascular resistance. Although rare, mineralocorticoid hypertension is an important diagnosis to make as it may be secondary to a resectable adrenal tumour or signify other endocrine pathology. It should be excluded in any patients with hypertension and hypokalaemia. A

Table 1 Causes of endocrine hypertension

Mineralocorticoid excess
Primary aldosteronism
Aldosterone secreting adenoma
Unilateral/bilateral idiopathic adrenal hyperplasia
Dexamethasone-suppressible hyperplasia
Hyperdeoxycorticosteronism
Deoxycorticosterone-secreting adrenal adenoma
Congenital adrenal hyperplasia
11β-hydroxylase deficiency
17α-hydroxylase deficiency
11β-hydroxysteroid dehydrogenase deficiency
The syndrome of apparent mineralocorticoid excess
Liquorice, carbenoxolone ingestion
Secondary aldosteronism
Renovascular hypertension
Malignant hypertension
Diuretic therapy
Primary hyperreninism
Miscellaneous
Cushing's syndrome
Liddle's syndrome
Exogenous steroids (cortisol, fludrocortisone)
Glucocorticoid resistance
Phaeochromocytoma
Miscellaneous
Acromegaly
Hyperparathyroidism
Hyper- and hypothyroidism
Glucocorticoid excess
Oestrogen and androgen-related hypertension

proposed scheme for evaluating a patient with hypertension and hypokalaemia is shown in Fig. 1.

Primary aldosteronism

This is the commonest cause of mineralocorticoid hypertension [2]. Approximately 70% of such patients will have an autonomous, aldosterone producing adrenal adenoma (APA). Increasingly recognized (25–30% of patients), however, is a condition called bilateral idiopathic adrenal hyperplasia (IHA). A very small subgroup of patients will have either adrenal carcinomas or dexamethasone-suppressible hyperplasia (DSH). In normal subjects, aldosterone secretion from the adrenal zona glomerulosa is under the control of angiotensin II (AII), potassium and adrenocorticotrophic hormone (ACTH). In contrast to patients with APA, aldosterone secretion in patients with IHA is almost exclusively under the control of AII, and as such has been regarded as a continuum

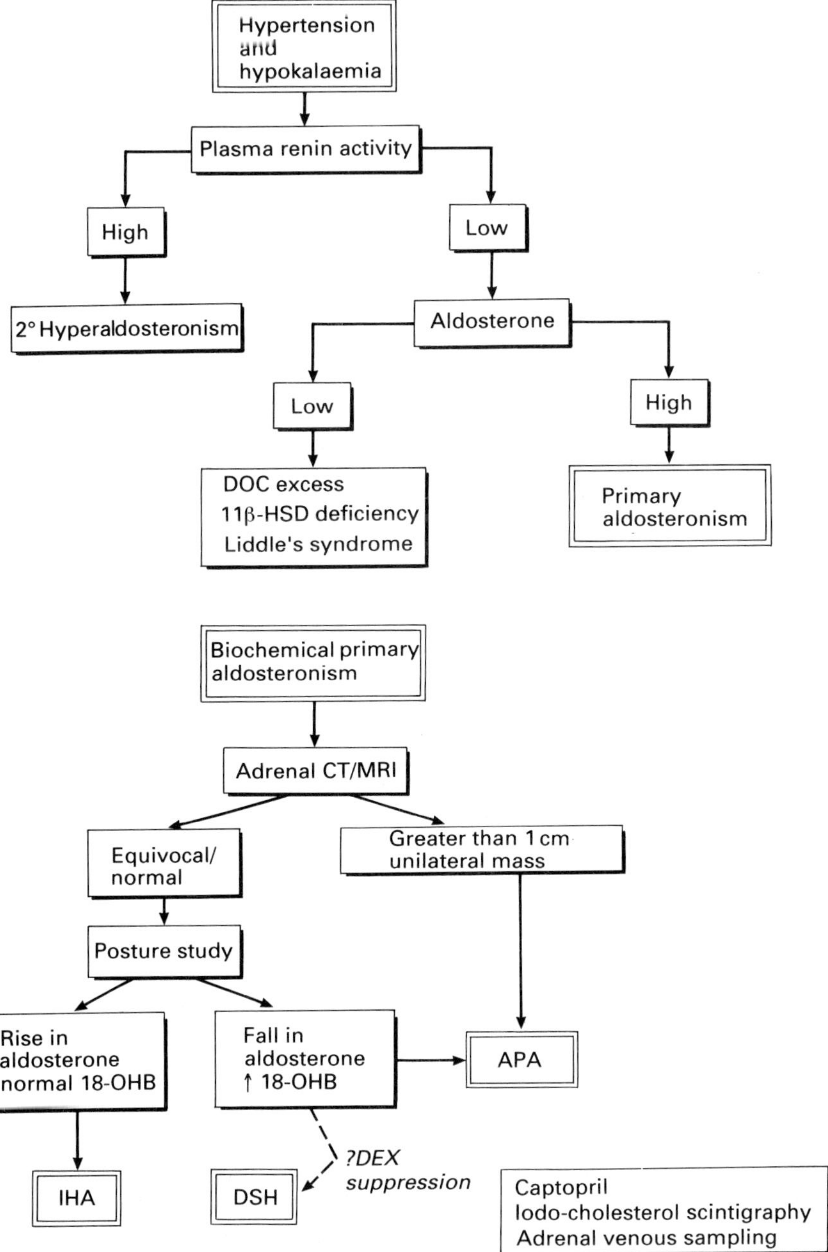

Fig. 1 Proposed scheme for the investigation of a patient with hypokalaemia and hypertension, and for the differential diagnosis of primary hyperaldosteronism. APA, Aldosterone producing adenoma; IHA, idiopathic adrenal hyperplasia; DSH, dexamethasone-suppressible hyperplasia.

of the spectrum of low-renin essential hypertension. DSH is a rare condition inherited as an autosomal dominant trait and characterized by inappropriate aldosterone secretion under the control of ACTH [3]. In contrast to APA and IHA, plasma aldosterone rises within 30–60 minutes following the administration of ACTH and both the hypertension and hypokalaemia respond to suppressive therapy with dexamethasone. The secretion of intermediate steroids in the synthesis of aldosterone (18-hydroxycorticosterone, 18-hydroxycortisol) may also be used to diagnose the condition, these metabolites being grossly elevated in DSH, less so in APA, and normal in IHA [4].

The differential diagnosis of APA, IHA and DSH is of some importance. Whilst surgery restores normokalaemia in APA and lowers blood pressure in over 50% of cases, it is an ineffective treatment for IHA and DSH. Various diagnostic tests have therefore been employed to differentiate these conditions [5,6]. Posture studies have an overall sensitivity of 75%. Plasma renin, aldosterone, cortisol and 18OH-corticosterone (or 18OH-cortisol) are measured at 08.00 hours in the supine position and then again at 12.00 hours, the subject having been erect for at least 60 minutes. Because of the AII control of aldosterone secretion in IHA, aldosterone levels rise when erect, but are unaltered or show a slight fall in APA. A marked fall in aldosterone levels between 08.00 and 12.00 hours as ACTH levels fall (hence the cortisol measurement) would be suggestive of DSH. The captopril test, by blocking endogenous AII levels, may be a more sensitive modification of the posture study, aldosterone levels falling after a bolus dose of captopril in IHA, but remaining unchanged in APA.

Computerized tomography (CT) or magnetic resonance imaging (MRI) of the adrenals will usually detect adenomas greater than 1 cm in size, and adrenal scintigraphy using iodo-cholesterol scanning (following dexamethasone suppression) has a sensitivity of approximately 70%. However, adrenal incidentalomas do occur, and biochemical testing must be performed together with radiological studies. The most sensitive localizing investigation is adrenal venous sampling and although the right adrenal vein can be difficult to cannulate, this study may be required to differentiate confidently between APA and IHA.

The treatment of primary aldosteronism depends on the cause. Patients with APA should be considered for surgery but treated medically for at least 1 month beforehand with a mineralocorticoid antagonist (spironolactone or amiloride). Because of its long half-life, spironolactone should be discontinued 2–3 days prior to surgery to prevent postoperative hyperkalaemia. Medical treatment, again with either spironolactone or amiloride, is indicated for patients with IHA. Patients with DSH respond well to a suppressive dose of dexamethasone.

Recently the molecular basis for DSH has been characterized. Two related cytochrome P450 genes, 11β-hydroxylase 1 and 2, located on chromosome 8q, are required for the synthesis of aldosterone and have been cloned and characterized [7]. The product of the P450 11β1 gene converts deoxycorticosterone (DOC) to corticosterone in the zona glomerulosa and 11-deoxycortisol to cortisol in the zona fasciculata. Its action is regulated by ACTH (Fig. 2). P450 11β2 converts corticosterone to aldosterone via 18-hydroxycorticosterone in the zona glomerulosa and is regulated by AII. Recent studies have shown that DSH results from unequal crossover between the 11β1 and 11β2 genes, resulting in a chimaeric gene comprising 5′ sequences of 11β1 and 3′ sequences of 11β2. The product of this gene is expressed in the zona fasciculata, resulting in an enzyme which can convert DOC to aldosterone but which is now regulated by ACTH [8]. This has been confirmed in several large kindreds of patients with DSH.

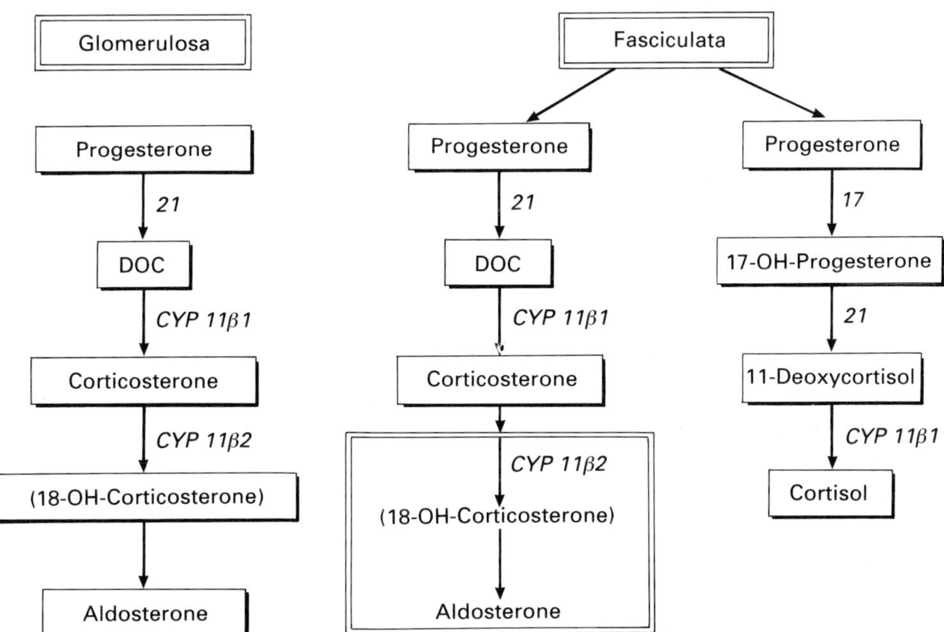

Fig. 2 Adrenal steroidogenesis in the zona fasciculata and glomerulosa to produce cortisol and aldosterone respectively. In dexamethasone-suppressible hyperplasia, aldosterone is secreted from the zona fasciculata (boxed area) from the product of a chimaeric gene containing CYP P450 11β1 and 11β2 sequences. DOC, Deoxycorticosterone.

11β-hydroxysteroid dehydrogenase deficiency (11β-HSD)

Congenital 11β-HSD deficiency: the syndrome of apparent mineralocorticoid excess

11β-HSD is responsible for the interconversion of the active glucocorticoid cortisol to its inactive metabolite cortisone. Congenital deficiency of 11β-HSD was first described in 1974 but characterized further by Ulick *et al.* in 1979 [9]. Since then only around 50 patients have been described. Typically the patient is a child who presents with severe (and often fatal) mineralocorticoid hypertension and hypokalaemia. Failure to thrive, weight loss, short stature and symptoms from hypokalaemic nephropathy (polyuria, thirst, nocturia) are the usual features [10]. Patients have suppressed plasma renin activity but also very low aldosterone levels. Until recently the mineralocorticoid responsible was unknown, hence the label 'syndrome of apparent mineralocorticoid excess' (AME).

The condition can be diagnosed from a characteristic urinary steroid metabolite profile, with an increase in the ratio of cortisol metabolites (tetrahydrocortisols, tetrahydro F (THF), allo-THF) to cortisone metabolites (tetrahydrocortisone, tetrahydrone E (THE)). In normals the THF+allo-THF/THE ratio is approximately 1; in AME values of 7–70 are found (Fig. 3). Although the plasma cortisol half-life is high, circulating cortisol levels remain normal because of the negative ACTH feedback mechanism. We have had the opportunity to study the first adult case of AME. Our detailed metabolic balance studies indicated that cortisol was acting as a potent mineralocorticoid in this condition. Thus cortisol administration resulted in profound sodium retention, kaliuresis with suppression of the renin–angiotensin system, weight gain and hypertension. Dexamethasone (which is not metabolized by 11β-HSD) suppressed endogenous cortisol secretion, restored normokalaemia and lowered blood pressure [11].

More recently a variant of AME has been described in three patients, again with hypertension and hypokalaemia, the so-called type II AME. Whilst the plasma cortisol half-life is prolonged and cortisol secretion rate reduced, the THF+allo-THF/THE ratio is entirely normal. The full enzyme defect in these patients has not been characterized, but the electrolyte abnormality and hypertension again respond to dexamethasone [12].

Acquired 11β-HSD deficiency: liquorice ingestion

Liquorice has been used for centuries in the Far East as a component of traditional Chinese herbal medicine. However, its mineralocorticoid side-

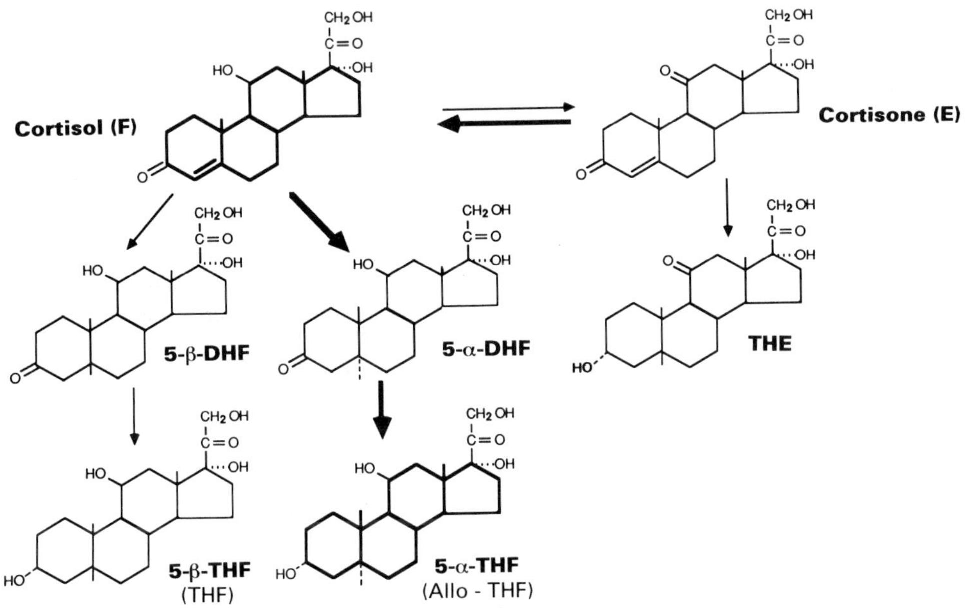

Fig. 3 The interconversion of cortisol to cortisone by 11β-HSD is shown. Bold arrows reflect the principal routes of metabolism in apparent mineralocorticoid excess and liquorice ingestion.

effects were first appreciated in Holland in the late 1940s. There Reevers first prescribed a liquorice extract (*succus liquiritiae*) for the treatment of dyspepsia. It was certainly effective but 20% of his patients returned with ankle swelling, heart failure and mineralocorticoid hypertension [13]. The active mineralocorticoids in liquorice are glycyrrhizic acid (GI) and its hydrolytic product glycyrrhetinic acid (GE), and since the original observations of Reevers, many patients with liquorice-induced mineralocorticoid excess have been reported.

Hypokalaemia can be a major problem, resulting in rhabdomyolysis and cardiac arrhythmias [14,15]. These mineralocorticoid side-effects had been widely attributed to a direct action of GI and GE on the mineralocorticoid receptor. However, studies performed in patients with Addison's disease, and also in animals following bilateral adrenalectomy, revealed that liquorice was without biological activity unless also administered with a small dose of glucocorticoid. We therefore studied the effect of liquorice in normal volunteers on metabolic balance. The sodium retention and hypokalaemia induced by liquorice was associated with inhibition of 11β-HSD activity, as shown by an increase in the plasma cortisol half-life and an increase in the THF+allo-THF/THE ratio [16]. Subsequent studies in both animals [17] and humans [18] support our observation that liquorice acts as a mineralocorticoid indirectly through inhibition of 11β-HSD.

Carbenoxolone, the anti-ulcer drug, is the synthetic derivative of GE which also results in mineralocorticoid side-effects. Whilst there are subtle differences on 11β-HSD activity between liquorice and carbenoxolone, the same mechanism predominates, i.e. indirect mineralocorticoid effect through inhibition of cortisol metabolism [19].

The biological significance of 11β-HSD

It was clear from studying patients with AME and liquorice ingestion that cortisol and not aldosterone was the preferred mineralocorticoid. Studies on the expressed mineralocorticoid receptor (MR) indicated, rather surprisingly, that the cortisol and aldosterone had an equal affinity for this receptor [20]. How then, in the face of cortisol concentrations 100–1000 times greater than aldosterone, did aldosterone occupy the MR *in vivo*? From our clinical observations, we [21] and others [22] went on to show that renal 11β-HSD permits a much lower concentration of aldosterone to occupy the MR by shuttling cortisol to inactive cortisone. When 11β-HSD activity is impaired, i.e. in AME or following liquorice ingestion, cortisol becomes a highly potent mineralocorticoid. This has led to a significant amount of research as to the role and nature of 11β-HSD within animal and human tissues. The enzyme is widely expressed and recent evidence now also indicates that 11β-HSD, by converting cortisol to cortisone at the tissue level, also regulates ligand exposure to the glucocorticoid receptor. Debate continues as to the nature of 11β-HSD within mineralocorticoid target tissues and it is possible that there are multiple isoforms of the enzyme, one perhaps involved in glucocorticoid hormone action, another in protecting the MR [23].

Clinically, the tissue control of corticosteroid hormone action by 11β-HSD has unlimited applications. Defective 11β-HSD activity has been documented in patients with essential hypertension, renal failure, alcohol-induced pseudo-Cushing's syndrome and ectopic ACTH syndrome. Alterations in tissue levels of hormone, largely independent of circulating levels, have many ramifications for endocrinology as a whole, not just 11β-HSD and gluco-/mineralocorticoid hormone action [24].

In summary, mineralocorticoid hypertension is rare but should be excluded in any patients with hypertension and hypokalaemia. Our further understanding of its mechanisms has revealed novel insights into the control of salt and water balance, steroid hormone action within the kidney and adrenal steroidogenesis.

PHAEOCHROMOCYTOMA

This condition refers to tumours of sympathogonial cells which secrete adrenaline, noradrenaline and dopamine. Technically phaeochromocytoma refers to a tumour arising in the adrenal medulla and paraganglioma outside the adrenal, but the term phaeochromocytoma has been adopted as a generic one to encompass both of these sites. The clinical features are extremely variable and often quite bizarre. The classical symptoms are headache (80% of cases), sweating (70%), palpitations (60%) and pallor (42%). Nausea, tremor, anxiety, epigastric pain, chest pain, weakness and dyspnoea are also experienced in up to 20% of cases. Hypertension is almost invariable but is sustained in only 50% of cases, occurring in the remainder only during an attack. Paradoxically, postural hypotension may be a feature, secondary to a reduction in plasma volume [25,26].

As with other secondary forms of hypertension, the diagnosis is made by a combination of biochemical and radiological studies. A timed analysis of the urinary excretion of free catecholamines, metanephrines or vanillylmandelic acid is required, during which period the patient should not take interfering substances, such as nuts, bananas and drugs, such as methyldopa, theophyllines, and sympathomimetics, which may produce a false positive result. Plasma catecholamines may be a more sensitive assay in some laboratories. The tumour can usually be localized by CT scanning. However, 10% of tumours are extra-adrenal and 2% extra-abdominal. In these cases, CT scanning may be combined with isotope scanning with ^{131}I-labelled meta-iodobenzylguanidine (MIBG) [27].

Surgery is the optimum therapy for patients with phaeochromocytomas. However, surgery is associated with considerable morbidity and mortality unless the patient is adequately prepared. α-Blockers such as phenoxybenzamine, phentolamine and prazosin are required to reduce peripheral vascular resistance but have to be given for some weeks prior to surgery to restore plasma volume. All too often surgery is performed on a patient treated with α-blockers for too short a duration; hypertension may not be a problem at surgery, but the vasodilation that occurs following removal of the source of catecholamines, on top of the reduced plasma volume, can result in profound postoperative shock. Indeed we frequently use intravenous saline in addition to α-blockade preoperatively to ensure an adequate plasma volume. β-Blockers are usually also required to counteract the tachycardia secondary to α-blockade. However, they should never be prescribed without concomitant α-blockade, as the unopposed α-adrenergic stimulation results in worsening hypertension. Ten per cent of phaeochromocytomas are malignant. In such cases, high doses of ^{131}I-MIBG have been used with some success.

Endocrine hypertension is a rare condition. Symptoms in such patients are few, and a high index of suspicion is required if a secondary cause of hypertension is to be uncovered. When we are privileged to see such cases it gives us a great opportunity to understand better the mechanisms of hypertension, many of which are no doubt of relevance to patients with essential hypertension.

REFERENCES

1 Fraser R, Davies DL, Connell JMC. Hormones and hypertension. *Clin Endocrinol* 1989;31:701–746.

2 Conn JW, Knopf RF, Nesbit RM. Clinical characteristics of primary aldosteronism from an analysis of 145 cases. *Am J Surg* 1964;107:159–172.

3 Ganguly A, Melada GA, Leutscher JA, Dowdy AJ. Control of plasma aldosterone in primary aldosteronism. *J Clin Endocrinol Metab* 1973;37:765–775.

4 Gomez-Sanchez CE, Montgomery M, Ganguly A, *et al.* Elevated urinary excretion of 18-oxocortisol in glucocorticoid-suppressible hyperaldosteronism. *J Clin Endocrinol Metab* 1984;59:1022–1024.

5 Mantero F, Rocco S, Carpene G, *et al.* Diagnostic and therapeutic procedures in primary aldosteronism. In: Mantero F, Vescei P, eds. *Corticosteroids and Peptide Hormones in Hypertension*. New York: Raven Press, 1987:231–241.

6 Young WF, Glee GG. Primary aldosteronism: Diagnostic evaluation. *Endocrinol Metab Clin North Am* 1988;17:367–395.

7 Curnow KM, Tusie-Luna MT, Pascoe L, *et al.* The product of the CYP11β2 gene is required for aldosterone biosynthesis in the human adrenal cortex. *Mol Endocrinol* 1991;5:1513–1522.

8 Lifton RP, Dluhy RG, Powers M, *et al.* A chimaeric 11β-hydroxylase/aldosterone synthase gene causes glucocorticoid-remediable aldosteronism and human hypertension. *Nature* 1992;355:262–265.

9 Ulick S, Levine LS, Gunczler P, *et al.* A syndrome of apparent mineralocorticoid excess associated with defects in the peripheral metabolism of cortisol. *J Clin Endocrinol Metab* 1979;49:757–764.

10 Shackleton CHL, Stewart PM. The hypertension of apparent mineralocorticoid excess syndrome. In: Biglieri EG, Melby JC, eds. *Endocrine Hypertension*. New York: Raven Press, 1990:155–173.

11 Stewart PM, Corrie JET, Shackleton CHL, Edwards CRW. Syndrome of apparent mineralocorticoid excess: A defect in the cortisol-cortisone shuttle. *J Clin Invest* 1988;82:340–349.

12 Ulick S, Tedde R, Mantero F. Pathogenesis of the type 2 variant of the syndrome of apparent mineralocorticoid excess. *J Clin Endocrinol Metab* 1990;70:200–206.

13 Reevers F. Behandling van uleus ventriculi in uleus duodeni met succus liquiritiae. *Nederl T Geneesk* 1948;92:2968–2971.

14 Blachley JD, Knochel JP. Tobacco chewer's hypokalaemia: liquorice revisited. *N Engl J Med* 1980;302:784–785.

15 Neilson I, Pedersen RN. Life-threatening hypokalaemia caused by liquorice. *Lancet* 1984;i:1305.

16 Stewart PM, Wallace AM, Valentino R, *et al.* Mineralocorticoid activity of liquorice: 11β-hydroxysteroid dehydrogenase comes of age. *Lancet* 1987;ii:821–824.

17 Monder C, Stewart PM, Lakshmi V, *et al.* Licorice inhibits corticosteroid 11β-dehydrogenase of rat kidney and liver: *in vivo* and *in vitro* studies. *Endocrinology* 1989;125:1046–1053.

18 Farese RV, Biglieri EG, Shackleton CHL, *et al.* Licorice-induced hypermineralocorticoidism. *N Engl J Med* 1991;325:1225–1227.

19 Stewart PM, Wallace AM, Atherden SM, *et al.* Mineralocorticoid activity of car-

benoxolone: contrasting effects of carbenoxolone and liquorice on 11β-hydroxysteroid dehydrogenase activity in man. *Clin Sci* 1990;78:49–52.
20 Arriza JL, Weinberger C, Cerelli G, *et al.* Cloning of human mineralocorticoid receptor complementary DNA: Structural and functional kinship with the glucocorticoid receptor. *Science* 1987;237:268–275.
21 Edwards CRW, Stewart PM, Burt D, *et al.* Localisation of 11β-hydroxysteroid dehydrogenase: Tissue-specific protector of the mineralocorticoid receptor. *Lancet* 1988; ii:986–989.
22 Funder JW, Pearce PT, Smith R, Smith AI. Mineralocorticoid action: target tissue specificity is enzyme, not receptor, mediated. *Science* 1988;242:583–585.
23 Walker BR, Moisan MP. Multiple isoforms of the cortisol-cortisone shuttle. *J Endocrinol* 1992;133:1–3.
24 Stewart PM, Sheppard MC. Novel aspects of hormone action: intracellular ligand supply and its control by a series of tissue specific enzymes. *Mol Cell Endocrinol* 1992;83:C13–C18.
25 Engelman K. Phaeochromocytoma. *Clin Endocrinol Metab* 1977;6:769–797.
26 Ball SG. Phaeochromocytoma. In: Robertson JIS, ed. *Handbook of Hypertension.* Amsterdam: Elsevier, 1983;2:238–275.
27 Francis IR, Glazer GM, Shapiro B, *et al.* Complementary roles of CT scanning and ^{131}I-MIBG scintigraphy in the diagnosis of phaeochromocytoma. *Am J Radiol* 1983; 141:719–725.

Growth hormone treatment

C. G. D. BROOK

The height which an individual attains is determined by the base from which he or she starts (birth length), the rate of growth and its duration. Growth *in utero* and during most of the first year of life is determined predominantly by nutritional influences. Thus, the first 70 cm of a child's growth is largely (not exclusively) hormone independent.

In the latter half of the first year of life, the childhood phase of growth takes over and, other things being equal, the rate of growth at this age is determined by the amplitude of pulsatile growth hormone secretion [1]. Childhood growth continues until the pubertal contribution of sex steroids is entrained, in girls at approximately 11 years, when about 140 cm of height has been attained, and at 13 years and 150 cm in boys. During this phase of growth, growth hormone and sex steroids are synergistic in developing the adolescent growth spurt.

From this tripartite model of growth, it will be understood that the time to use growth hormone therapeutically is during the childhood years. Patients with panhypopituitarism may be assisted to avoid hypoglycaemia in the early months of life by the use of growth hormone; it is certainly also indicated for a failing endogenous secretion at puberty but the main time for its use is in childhood.

GROWTH HORMONE AND GROWTH

As already indicated, the amplitude of pulsatile growth hormone secretion determines the rate at which children grow. The nature of the asymptotic relationship (Fig. 1) is extremely important: it indicates that the children growing most slowly and having least growth hormone secretion will respond best to an increment of growth hormone. Children with a lesser degree of growth hormone insufficiency and a greater pretreatment height velocity need a much greater increment of growth hormone (on the x axis in the figure) to produce a similar increment of height velocity (on the y axis). Thus, the relationship between the response to treatment and pretreatment growth hormone status is also asymptotic, the curve being the inverse of the one shown in Fig. 1. With

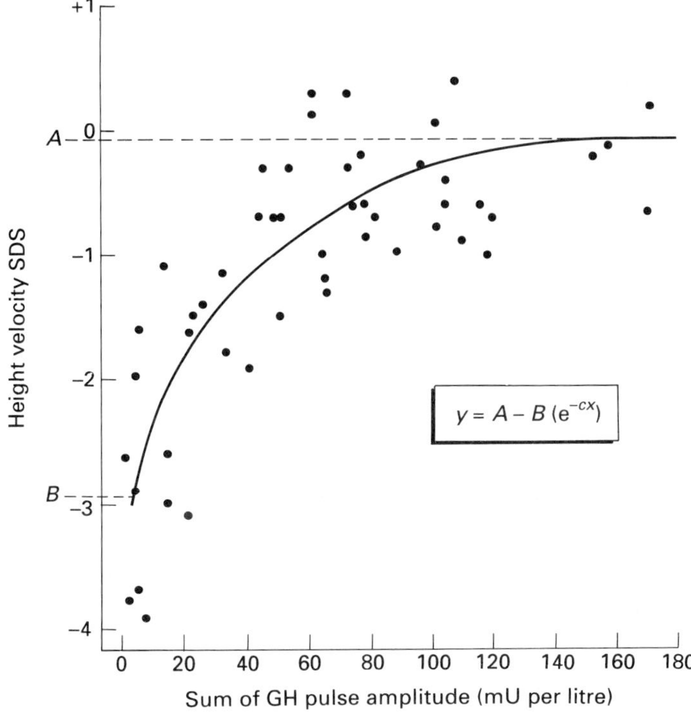

Fig. 1 Relation between the amplitude of pulsatile growth hormone secretion and height velocity standard deviation score (SDS) in 50 short prepubertal children. Note the asymptotic nature of the relationship. The calculated asymptote B coincides with the rate at which children with the deletion of the growth hormone gene grow. The asymptote A in this population approaches zero but must enter the positive range because otherwise tall children in general and pituitary giants in particular would not exist. The nature of the asymptotic relationship determines that children growing most slowly with least growth hormone secretion respond best to treatment. (By permission from Hindmarsh *et al.* [1].)

these two asymptotic curves in opposite directions, it will be appreciated that the relationship between pretreatment height velocity and response is linear with a negative slope [2].

Within a group of children with a similar pretreatment height velocity, a classical pharmacological dose–response curve exists between the dose of growth hormone administered and the response achieved. This means that it is possible to draw a family of curves for the response expected in any group of children depending on the dose of growth hormone administered (Fig. 2). The slopes of the curves in Fig. 2 are identical (only the intercepts differ) but where the skeleton is abnormal, the same slope cannot be assumed and, generally speaking, slopes for children who are not normal (including Turner syndrome) are lower and flatter than those in Fig. 2 [3].

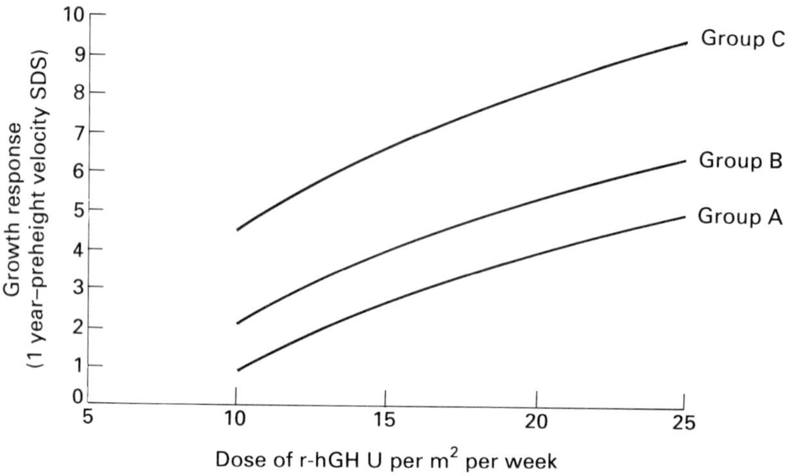

Fig. 2 Dose–response curves for human growth hormone (difference between first treatment year and pretreatment height velocity). Group C are children with idiopathic isolated growth hormone insufficiency growing with a pretreatment height velocity standard deviation score (SDS) less than −2 SD below the mean for age and sex. Group A are a group of normal children: a low dose of growth hormone will have a negligible effect on increasing growth velocity. To achieve a level similar to the response in group C, a doubling of growth hormone dosage is required. Group B, defined by a pretreatment height velocity SDS between −0.8 and −2.0, have partial growth hormone insufficiency: the importance of their curve is that it has a shape identical to that of groups A and C; only the intercepts differ.

INDICATIONS FOR GROWTH HORMONE TREATMENT

In the absence of the other disease processes causing a low growth velocity, abnormality of growth hormone secretion is the most probable explanation of low growth velocity during childhood. This can be demonstrated through measurements of growth hormone secretion, either occurring naturally or provoked by various stimuli [4], but since any child given growth hormone will grow more quickly, the place of such tests requires thought by the clinician.

On the assumption that a child growing slowly has an insufficiency of growth hormone secretion, the administration of growth hormone in a dose 15 U per m^2 per week (0.5 U per kg per week) will produce a predictable response according to the pretreatment growth velocity [2]. If the child fails to respond as expected, the diagnosis is wrong, there are problems with compliance with the therapeutic regimen or, exceptionally rarely, there is a reason for the growth hormone message not being received, which equates to a wrong diagnosis. Antibody production to the highly purified synthetic growth hormone preparations currently available is a problem only for patients with deletion of the growth hormone gene, an extremely rare condition which should have been diagnosed by the failure ever to register a measurable quantity of growth hormone in blood.

Low growth velocity due to growth hormone insufficiency is the only absolute indication for the use of growth hormone. Growth hormone has been used for this indication for more than 3 decades. Although growth hormone treatment alters body composition and causes transient carbohydrate intolerance and lipid abnormalities, it has been a treatment remarkably free of side-effects. Nevertheless, the initial preparations were derived from pituitary glands taken from postmortem examination and, very unfortunately, it has now become clear that some of the patients from whom the pituitary glands were taken had died of Creutzfeldt–Jacob disease.

The infective agent of this condition, a prion, is extremely difficult to destroy without destroying the delicate structure of a peptide hormone and consequently a number of patients worldwide have become infected with Creutzfeldt–Jacob disease and have died as a result of using pituitary extracted growth hormone. When this problem was realized in 1985, pituitary growth hormone was withdrawn from the vast majority of countries. Growth hormone manufactured by the techniques of molecular biology was introduced in 1986 and has been used exclusively ever since in most countries. In the author's opinion, it would be unethical to use pituitary extracted growth hormone in 1993.

Concern has recently been expressed about a connection between growth hormone and leukaemia. Twenty-nine cases of leukaemia have been reported in children treated with growth hormone, 11 in the USA, 10 in Japan and eight in Europe. Of the 11 in the USA, eight had previous neoplastic disease, which is known to be associated with other second malignancies including leukaemia, and three had idiopathic growth hormone insufficiency. In Japan, two had neoplastic disease, seven idiopathic growth hormone insufficiency and one had a syndrome predisposing to leukaemia. In Europe, three had predisposing conditions and five had growth hormone insufficiency. These figures work out to a count of one case per 350 000 person years, an observed/expected risk ratio of 3.3. Omitting children with previous malignant diseases and predisposing causes, there are 15 patients with idiopathic growth hormone insufficiency, giving an observed/expected ratio of 1.7.

In the biggest post marketing surveillance series in the USA and Canada, 29 000 children have been treated with growth hormone over 120 000 patient years. Approximately 2800 of these patients start and stop growth hormone each year and taking all cases of leukaemia in North America the risk ratio of developing leukaemia is 3.0, but in children without a predisposing cause to leukaemia the risk ratio has been calculated to fall to 1.0, which is no different from the normal risk in childhood. There is no evidence that growth hormone causes a recurrence of brain tumours. No other side-effects have been reported.

POSSIBLE USES OF GROWTH HORMONE

When the supply by synthetic growth hormone became unlimited except by cost in 1986, numerous trials of its use were set in train [5]. In nearly all of them (Turner syndrome, skeletal dysplasia, renal failure, etc.) initial responses were favourable, even though the dose that had to be used to obtain such responses was considerably greater than those for use in children with growth hormone insufficiency [6]. It soon became clear, therefore, that any child given growth hormone would grow more quickly, assuming an adequate dose was used.

There are two components of response to such treatment, one in the short term and the other whether final height can be influenced. In order to achieve the latter, two ingredients are required: first the continuation of an increase in growth velocity year after year and, second, the continuation of growth for an adequate length of time.

As time has gone by, it has become clear that the maintenance of an increased growth velocity year after year in patients on treatment with growth hormone is difficult to achieve. The explanation is not clear and it must in theory be possible to maintain such a growth rate because if it were not, tall people in general and pituitary giants in particular would not exist. In therapeutic practice, it has been extremely difficult to maintain a greater than average growth velocity in any groups of children: those who are growth hormone insufficient experience catch-up and then maintain an average growth velocity, realizing the growth potential available to them at the time of diagnosis [7]. They do not become excessively tall because a sufficiently fast velocity is not maintained indefinitely.

Growth hormone has profound effects on the gonadal response to gonadotrophin secretion and shortens the duration of puberty [8]. This means that it is possible to lose what has been gained initially in the short term, not only by the waning effect of treatment but also by shortening the period of availability for response. For this reason, although results are available showing the short-term advantage of growth hormone therapy, which is not to be ignored, the long-term responses will not become available until final heights have been reported in children who entered the trials of growth hormone for what have come to be called wider indications.

Turner syndrome

Nowhere is this problem better exemplified than in the Turner syndrome. Growth hormone given in a dose of 30 U per m^2 per week increases the rate of growth of patients with the Turner syndrome. Doses smaller than this are not more effective than low-dose sex steroids in the short term [3]. It seems probable that growth hormone will achieve a final increment of height of 8–10 cm in girls with the Turner syndrome [9], but as 75% of this gain is probably attainable by the long-term and judicious use of low-dose sex steroids at a fraction of the cost and without daily injections [3], Turner syndrome cannot be regarded as an absolute indication for the use of growth hormone.

Skeletal dysplasias

One of the reasons for what some would regard as the disappointing response of the Turner syndrome to treatment with growth hormone is the abnormal skeleton characteristic of the mesenchymal defect in that condition. In other skeletal dysplasias, such as achondroplasia, hypochondroplasia and multiple epiphyseal dysplasia, similar constraints apply [10]. The particular hallmark of skeletal dysplasias is the failure of realization of the pubertal growth spurt. In view of the waning response of all conditions to growth hormone, it seems likely that if only one course of growth hormone therapy is to be made available to a patient with a skeletal dysplasia, that course perhaps should be aimed at maximizing pubertal growth rather than being exhibited earlier in childhood. These therapies are still under investigation and the general prescription of growth hormone for patients with skeletal dysplasias is certainly not recommended at the time of writing.

Renal disease

In chronic renal failure and after transplants, there are nearly always complicating variables, such as the use of steroids or other immunosuppressive agents, and dietary or metabolic problems. For this reason, although growth hormone has been effective in a majority of children with such problems when the other variables have been corrected, the general prescription of growth hormone for this indication cannot yet be recommended.

Corticosteroids

For many diseases in paediatric practice, steroid medication is life saving (e.g. asthma, collagen vascular diseases, rheumatoid arthritis, nephrotic syndrome) but the major side-effect is a diminution of growth velocity. The exact mechanism by which steroids reduce growth velocity is not known, but it is not due to the generation of insulin-like growth factor 1 (IGF-1) in response to what is clearly normal growth hormone secretion. It is probably downstream of IGF-1 at cartilage level. Thus, the use of growth hormone to spare the growth-retarding side-effects of steroids has been very disappointing. The anabolic effects of growth hormone in terms of protein turnover and muscle strength have not been adequately addressed.

Use in adult patients

Adult patients with hypopituitarism have disappointing lifestyles in terms of achievement of academic, social and personal goals and it has been clearly demonstrated that such patients do better with growth hormone [11]. It seems likely that this will move from a relative indication to a more general prescription. The use of growth hormone to reverse severe catabolic states secondary to surgery, trauma or burns has not been adequately studied but there may be a marginal acceleration in wound healing and beneficial effects on nerve growth which have yet to be realized. Whether the effect will be of sufficient magnitude to justify the use of growth hormone in these situations remains to be determined.

CONTRAINDICATIONS

Growth hormone is expensive. It has to be given by daily subcutaneous injections, which is a considerable burden for some patients. Although growth hormone usage is remarkably free of side-effects, there are well-established consequences of administering growth hormone which could have deleterious long-term consequences: it is a powerful lipolytic agent so that free fatty acids rise on treatment; it has an anti-insulin activity, so that there is relative carbohydrate intolerance in treated patients; it causes water retention, so there is a marginal rise in blood pressure which is particularly troublesome in older patients. The combination of glucose intolerance, mobilization of free fatty acids and hypertension should be enough to deter physicians from employing growth hormone when the effects are doubtful and the disease is not particularly serious, because the risk–benefit equation tips unfavourably.

In view of the physiology of growth and growth hormone secretion [1], it was not surprising that normal children responded to growth hormone therapy with an increase in growth rate [12] as time has gone by. It has become clear that normal children may gain only a few centimetres after many years of growth hormone treatment, because there is no abnormality to correct [13], and our recent unpublished data using growth hormone for 7 years confirms that the maximum increment in final height is not likely to exceed 0.5 SD over that predicted at the start of treatment. This is confirmed elsewhere (Albertsson-Wikland, personal communication). In my opinion the use of growth hormone in normal children is contraindicated.

Children who have not entered puberty in their early teens continue to grow along the childhood growth curve at an increasingly slow rate. Such patients have a relative insufficiency of growth hormone by any of the usual tests [4], but they should not be given growth hormone. What they need is sex steroids [14]. If they are given growth hormone, their rate of progress through puberty will be accelerated and they may become shorter than they would otherwise have become (own unpublished data). For patients who are showing pubertal signs and yet growing inadequately, it may be possible to demonstrate an insufficiency of growth hormone and such patients should, of course, be treated in the usual manner as above for the absolute indication of growth hormone insufficiency.

The use of growth hormone as an anabolic agent by athletes is contraindicated for the reasons outlined above. Accelerated atherosclerosis must be a serious risk in such situations. For any of the wider indications, growth hormone should not be used in one-off cases until the long-term effects of the trials of growth hormone in such conditions have been reported. There is no place for the one-off prescription at the time of writing.

SUMMARY

Growth hormone treatment is safe and the effects are predictable. The only absolute indication for the use of growth hormone is for patients with congenital or acquired insufficiency of growth hormone secretion. For such patients, the sooner the insufficiency of their hormone secretion is corrected, the better will be the long-term result. Thus, patients after radiotherapy should be treated earlier and on the basis of a low growth velocity and not be expected to become short before treatment is employed.

Data about the wider indications for growth hormone are rapidly becoming available in terms of final heights achieved. Until these have been reported and assessed, growth hormone should not be used on a one-off basis. Growth hormone should not be given to normal people or to patients suffering the side-effects of steroids.

REFERENCES

1 Hindmarsh P, Smith PJ, Brook CGD, Matthews DR. The relationship between height velocity and growth hormone secretion in short prepubertal children. *Clin Endocrinol* 1987;27:581–591.
2 Darendeliler F, Hindmarsh PC, Brook CGD. Dose–response curves for treatment with biosynthetic human growth hormone. *J Endocrinol* 1990;125:311–316.
3 Bainbridge JWB, Spoudeas HA, Massarano AA, *et al.* The application of the infancy–childhood–puberty model of growth to the management of the Turner syndrome. In: Rouke MB, Rosenfeld RG, eds. *Turner syndrome: Growth Promoting Therapies.* Amsterdam: Excerpta Medica, 1991:159–167.
4 Brook CGD, Hindmarsh PC. Tests for growth hormone secretion. *Arch Dis Child* 1991;66:85–87.
5 Hindmarsh PC, Bridges N, Brook CGD. Wider indications for treatment with biosynthetic human growth hormone in children. *Clin Endocrinol* 1991;34:417–427.
6 Darendeliler F, Hindmarsh PC, Brook CGD. Non-conventional use of growth hormone. *Horm Res* 1990;33:128–136.
7 Bundak R, Hindmarsh PC, Smith PJ, Brook CGD. Long-term auxologic effects of human growth hormone. *J Pediatr* 1988;112:875–879.
8 Darendeliler F, Hindmarsh PC, Preece MA, Cox L, Brook CGD. Growth hormone increases rate of pubertal maturation. *Acta Endocrinol* 1990;122(3):414–416.
9 Rosenfield RG, Long term effects of growth hormone and oxandrolone on height in Turner syndrome: five year result. In: Rouke MB, Rosenfeld RG, eds. *Turner Syndrome: Growth Promoting Therapies.* Amsterdam: Excerpta Medica, 1991:159–167.
10 Appan A, Laurent S, Chapman M, *et al.* Growth and growth hormone therapy in hypochondroplasia. *Acta Paediatr Scand* 1990;79:796–803.
11 Salomon F, Cuneo RC, Hesp R, Sönksen MD. The effects of treatment with recombinant human growth hormone on body composition and metabolism in adults with growth hormone deficiency. *N Engl J Med* 1989;321:1797–1803.
12 Hindmarsh PC, Brook CGD. Effect of growth hormone on short normal children. *Br Med J* 1987;295:573–577.
13 Hindmarsh PC, Pringle PJ, Di Silvio L, Brook CGD. Effects of 3 years of growth hormone therapy in short normal children. *Acta Paediatr Scand* 1990;366:6–12.
14 Buyukgebiz A, Hindmarsh PC, Brook CGD. Treatment of constitutional delay of growth and puberty with oxandrolone compared with growth hormone. *Arch Dis Child* 1990;65:448–452.

Polycystic ovary syndrome: reproductive and metabolic implications

S. FRANKS, S. ROBINSON & D. JOHNSTON

PREVALENCE AND SIGNIFICANCE OF POLYCYSTIC OVARIES IN REPRODUCTIVE DISORDERS

The classic features of polycystic ovary syndrome (PCOS) are anovulation, hyperandrogenism and obesity but the ability, in recent years, to identify polycystic ovaries by pelvic ultrasonography has led to a reappraisal of the presentation and aetiology of PCOS [1]. It is now evident that the spectrum of clinical features of women with polycystic ovaries ranges from menstrual disturbance without hirsutism – but with biochemical evidence of hyperandrogenism – to hirsutism in women with regular, ovulatory cycles. According to two large, ultrasound-based studies, obesity (body mass index (BMI) in excess of 25 kg per m^2) occurs in only 35% of subjects with polycystic ovaries but has a significant influence on clinical and biochemical phenotype [2,3].

On analysis of results from ultrasound examination of women attending a single gynaecological endocrine clinic, polycystic ovaries were found in 87% of women with oligomenorrhoea, and 32% of those with amenorrhoea [1,4]. These data are consistent with the reported 73% prevalence of PCOS – as diagnosed on clinical and biochemical criteria – in women with anovulatory infertility [5]. More surprisingly perhaps, polycystic ovaries were present in 87% of women with hirsutism and regular menses. In a further study, polycystic ovaries were detected in over 80% of women with spontaneous ovulatory cycles who had a history of early pregnancy loss [6]. The high frequency of polycystic ovaries in women with reproductive disorders prompted us to investigate the prevalence of this ovarian appearance in the normal population. Twenty-two per cent of a series of 257 women were found to have polycystic ovaries [7]. All considered themselves to be normal and had not had occasion to consult a doctor about menstrual disturbances or hirsutism. Nevertheless, the majority of women with a polycystic ovary appearance on ultrasound had a clinical 'marker' of this, i.e. irregular menses or objective evidence of mild hirsutism.

Despite the heterogeneity of clinical presentation, there are biochemical features which are common to all groups of women with polycystic ovaries, notably hyperandrogenaemia and hypersecretion of luteinizing hormone (LH) [1,8]. A very recent study suggests that, regardless of the presenting features in the probands, the presence of polycystic ovaries is inherited as an autosomal dominant trait and is associated with premature, male-pattern balding in female relatives [9]. This suggests that an 'abnormality' of androgen metabolism may be central to the aetiology of PCOS whether the proband presents with anovulation or hirsutism (or both). The heterogeneity of clinical features is likely to be due to the interaction of this central genetic abnormality with environmental and/or other genetic factors.

It is now becoming clear that one of the most important factors which determine the clinical features in a woman with polycystic ovaries and hyperandrogenism is the presence or absence of hyperinsulinaemia and insulin resistance.

HYPERINSULINAEMIA, INSULIN RESISTANCE AND OVULATION

Hyperinsulinaemia is now recognized to be a feature of PCOS. Women with PCOS are relatively hyperinsulinaemic and insulin resistant when compared with weight-matched controls [10–12]. Interestingly, however, hyperinsulinaemia and insulin resistance appear to be confined to women with *anovulation*; these features are not found in equally hyperandrogenaemic women with polycystic ovaries who have regular menstrual cycles [13,14] (Fig. 1). This raises the possibility that hyper-

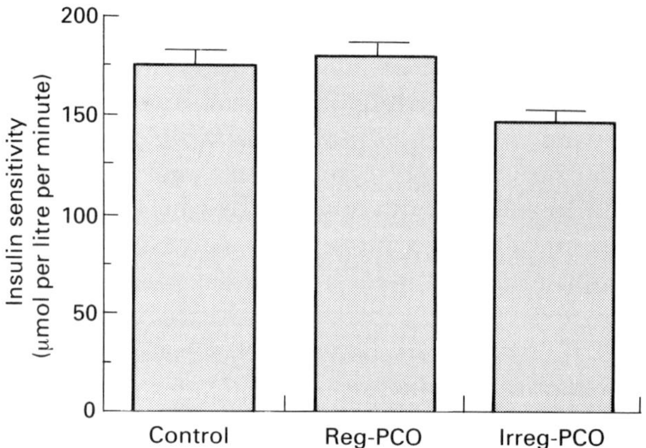

Fig. 1 Insulin sensitivity (mean (SE)) in women with PCOS who had regular (reg-PCO) or irregular (irreg-PCO) periods and in weight-matched (paired) controls. Insulin sensitivity was significantly reduced in both lean and obese women with PCOS and anovulation. (Data from Robinson *et al.* [14].)

insulinaemia and/or insulin resistance may be involved in the mechanism of anovulation in women with ovarian hyperandrogenism. In other words, the presence or absence of hyperinsulinaemia/insulin resistance affects the clinical phenotype. In this context it is noteworthy that weight reduction in obese anovulatory women with polycystic ovaries is accompanied by a reduction in fasting and glucose-stimulated plasma insulin concentrations and associated with regulation of menstrual cycles [15]. The mechanism by which disturbances of insulin secretion or action affect ovarian function remains unclear but recent data suggest that the granulosa cells of ovaries from women with anovulation and polycystic ovaries are not resistant to the action of insulin; i.e. hyperinsulinaemia rather than insulin resistance may be the aetiological factor (Mason, Willis, Gilling-Smith and Franks, unpublished data).

METABOLIC CONSEQUENCES OF PCOS: GLUCOSE HOMEOSTASIS AND LIPOPROTEIN/LIPID METABOLISM

Dunaif *et al.*, in a large study of anovulatory women with PCOS, found that 20% of obese PCOS subjects had impaired glucose tolerance or frank diabetes [11]. These disturbances of glucose/insulin homeostasis are associated with abnormalities of energy expenditure and of lipid metabolism. In a recent study, we demonstrated that whereas resting energy expenditure was similar in PCOS and control subjects, postprandial thermogenesis (PPT) was significantly reduced in women with PCOS [16]. Lower PPT was associated with impaired insulin sensitivity. These findings suggest a possible mechanism for a predisposition to weight gain in women with PCOS.

Abnormalities of lipoprotein/lipid metabolism have also been noted in women with PCOS [17,18]. Our own studies have confirmed this, and shown that obese women with PCOS have higher plasma concentrations of triglycerides than obese controls, and that both obese and lean women with PCOS have reduced high-density lipoprotein 2 (HDL_2) cholesterol compared with weight-matched control groups [19] (Fig. 2). Insulin sensitivity was also positively correlated with serum concentrations of HDL_2 cholesterol ($r_s = 0.48$, $P < 0.01$); i.e. the greater the insulin resistance, the lower the level of HDL_2 cholesterol. Such results are consistent with the observation that women with PCOS may be at increased risk of cardiovascular disease [17,18,20].

SUMMARY

PCOS is the most common cause of hirsutism and of anovulatory infertility; it may also have a role in recurrent miscarriage. Hyperinsulinaemia

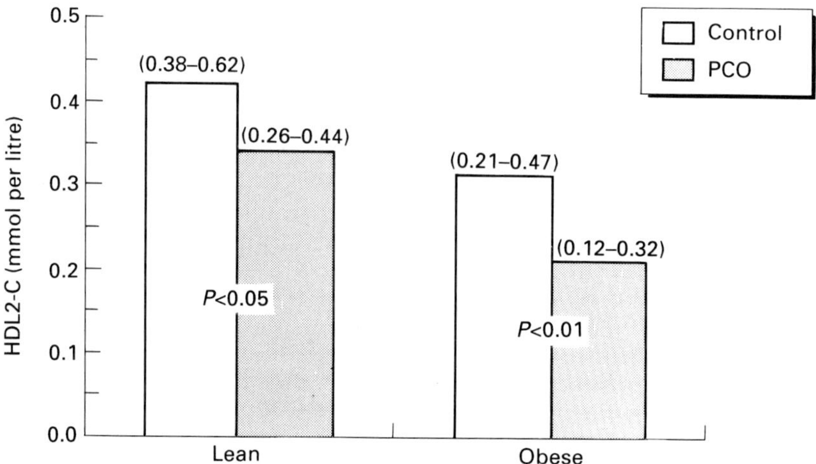

Fig. 2 Plasma concentrations of HDL_2 cholesterol (HDL2-C) in lean and obese women with PCOS compared with weight-matched controls. Results are the median and range.

and insulin resistance in PCOS are features of anovulatory subjects but not of those with regular cycles, suggesting that disturbances of insulin secretion may be involved in the mechanism of anovulation in PCOS.

The metabolic implications of hyperinsulinaemia/insulin resistance in PCOS include apparently increased risks of non-insulin-dependent diabetes mellitus and cardiovascular disease. PCOS is associated with subnormal plasma concentrations of HDL_2 cholesterol, and the latter is inversely correlated with plasma insulin concentrations and insulin sensitivity.

REFERENCES

1 Franks S. Polycystic ovary syndrome: a changing perspective. *Clin Endocrinol* 1989;51: 87–120.

2 Conway GS, Honour JW, Jacobs HS. Heterogeneity of the polycystic ovary syndrome: clinical, endocrine and ultrasound features in 556 patients. *Clin Endocrinol* 1989;30: 459–470.

3 Kiddy DS, Sharp PS, White DM, *et al.* Differences in clinical and endocrine features between obese and non-obese subjects with polycystic ovary syndrome: an analysis of 263 consecutive cases. *Clin Endocrinol* 1990;2:213–220.

4 Adams J, Polson DW, Franks S. Prevalence of polycystic ovaries in women with anovulation and idiopathic hirsutism. *Br Med J* 1986;293:355–359.

5 Hull MG. Epidemiology of infertility and polycystic ovarian disease: endocrinological and demographic studies. *Gynecol Endocrinol* 1987;1:235–245.

6 Sagle M, Bishop K, Ridley N, *et al.* Recurrent early miscarriage and polycystic ovaries. *Br Med J* 1988;297:1027–1028.

7 Polson DW, Adams J, Wadsworth J, Franks S. Polycystic ovaries – a common finding in normal women. *Lancet* 1988;i:870–872.

8 Franks S. The ubiquitous polycystic ovary. *J Endocrinol* 1991;129:317–319.

9 Carey AH, Chan K, White DM, *et al.* Evidence for a single gene effect in polycystic ovaries and male pattern baldness. *Clin Endocrinol* 1993;38:653–658.

10 Chang RJ, Nakamura RM, Judd HL, Kaplan SA. Insulin resistance in nonobese patients with polycystic ovarian disease. *J Clin Endocrinol Metab* 1983;57:356–359.
11 Dunaif A, Graf M, Mandeli J, *et al.* Characterization of groups of hyperandrogenic women with acanthosis nigricans, impaired glucose tolerance, and/or hyperinsulinemia. *J Clin Endocrinol Metab* 1987;65:499–507.
12 Dunaif A, Segal KR, Futterweit W, Dobrjansky A. Profound peripheral insulin resistance, independent of obesity, in polycystic ovary syndrome. *Diabetes* 1989;38: 1165–1174.
13 Sharp PS, Kiddy DS, Reed MJ, *et al.* Correlation of plasma insulin and insulin-like growth factor-1 with indices of androgen transport and metabolism in women with polycystic ovary syndrome. *Clin Endocrinol* 1991;35:253–257.
14 Robinson S, Kiddy DS, Gelding S, *et al.* The relationship of insulin sensitivity to menstrual pattern in women with hyperandrogenism and polycystic ovaries. *Clin Endocrinol* 1993;39:351–355.
15 Kiddy DS, Hamilton-Fairley D, Bush A, *et al.* Improvement in endocrine and ovarian function during dietary treatment of obese women with polycystic ovary syndrome. *Clin Endocrinol* 1992;36:105–111.
16 Robinson S, Chan S-P, Spacey S, *et al.* Post prandial thermogenesis is reduced in polycystic ovary syndrome and is associated with increased insulin resistance. *Clin Endocrinol* 1992;36:537–543.
17 Wild RA, Painter PC, Coulson PB, *et al.* Lipoprotein lipid concentrations and cardiovascular risk in women with polycystic ovary syndrome. *J Clin Endocrinol Metab* 1985;61:946–951.
18 Conway GS, Agrawal R, Betteridge DJ, Jacobs HS. Risk factors for cardiovascular disease in lean and obese women with polycystic ovary syndrome. *Clin Endocrinol* 1992;37:119–125.
19 Robinson S, Kiddy D, Henderson AD, *et al.* Insulin resistance is increased and HDL_2 cholesterol decreased in polycystic ovary syndrome. *J Endocrinol* 1991;66:(Abstract)66.
20 Dahlgren E, Janson PO, Johansson S, *et al.* Polycystic ovary syndrome and risk for myocardial infarction – evaluated from a risk factor model based on a prospective population study of women. *Acta Obstet Gynecol Scand* 1992;71:599–604.

Controversies in the management of hyperthyroidism and hypothyroidism

A. D. TOFT

It is remarkable that there should still be debate about the management of the hyperthyroidism of Graves' disease as there have been three choices of treatment for over 40 years. Standard teaching has been that the initial treatment in patients under 40–45 years of age is with an antithyroid drug for about 18 months with a recommendation for surgery should relapse occur. Older patients are treated with iodine-131. Of course management varies from centre to centre and between countries and these differences have been highlighted in recent surveys of practice in Europe and in the USA. For example, the preferred treatment of a 43-year-old female presenting with hyperthyroidism of moderate severity due to Graves' disease who did not plan further pregnancies was anti-thyroid drugs (77%) by European physicians but iodine-131 (69%) by their North American counterparts. There was an even greater contrast in choice of therapy when the index case was changed to that of a 19-year-old female. One-third of physicians in the USA regarded iodine-131 as most appropriate, whereas the corresponding figure in Europe was only 4%. The more liberal use of iodine-131 is finding favour with an increasing number of physicians in the UK [1], but is permanent hypo-thyroidism the only significant adverse effect? At the same time, there are reports that high remission rates can be achieved by the use of an unusual combination of antithyroid drugs and thyroxine [2]. Surgery would seem to be the loser in the face of these two developments.

It is even more surprising that any problems with thyroxine replacement therapy are perceived as primary hypothyroidism has been a very satisfying disorder to treat for over a century, most patients being restored to normal health and activities within a few months of presentation. Controversy, however, has arisen following the development of sensitive assays for thyrotrophin (TSH) which have raised the question of whether an undetectable serum TSH concentration is an indication of overtreatment when recorded in asymptomatic patients receiving thyroxine as replacement, rather than suppressive, therapy. And, once started, is the usual exhortation that thyroxine treatment is lifelong necessarily correct?

The use of TSH measurements as a first-line test of thyroid function identifies patients with subclinical hypothyroidism – the unsatisfactory term used to describe clinically euthyroid and asymptomatic patients in whom the only biochemical abnormality is a raised serum TSH concentration. Should such individuals be treated with thyroxine or simply observed?

MANAGEMENT OF THE HYPERTHYROIDISM OF GRAVES' DISEASE

Iodine-131 therapy

Iodine uptake

There is a tendency to dismiss the value of routine thyroid gland uptake measurements using technetium-99m, iodine-123 or iodine-131 in the management of hyperthyroidism. Certainly they have little role in confirming a clinical diagnosis of hyperthyroidism, given the greater sensitivity and specificity of assays for serum TSH and free and total thyroxine (T_4) and triiodothyronine (T_3), but are invaluable in determining the cause of thyrotoxicosis. In particular, a negligible uptake will identify those patients with postpartum or silent thyroiditis, subacute (de Quervain's) thyroiditis, thyrotoxicosis factitia, or exposure to iodine in whom treatment with iodine-131 is contraindicated. Indeed the iodine-containing antidysrhythmic agent, amiodarone, is an increasing cause of hyperthyroidism which may present many months after drug withdrawal due to a long half-life of elimination. Uptake measurements should be performed in all patients who are candidates for treatment with iodine-131 if unnecessary or ineffective therapy is to be avoided.

A more liberal policy?

Those in favour of the more widespread use of iodine-131 therapy for hyperthyroidism would argue that it is cheap, easy to administer and effective as a single dose in the majority of cases. By giving a relatively large dose of 555 MBq most patients will be hypothyroid within a year and subsequent care can pass to the general practitioner. The initial anxieties about an increase in incidence of post-treatment thyroid carcinoma and leukaemia have evaporated. Furthermore, the gonadal irradiation averages 0.8–1.4 rem, similar to that for a barium enema or intravenous pyelogram and it has not been possible to show an association between incidental or therapeutic irradiation with iodine-131, even in children and adolescents, and congenital abnormalities in subsequent offspring – although the series are small.

So why not advocate a policy of iodine-131 therapy for all non-pregnant patients with Graves' disease? First, the public has a heightened awareness of the dangers of radioactivity as a result of widely reported accidents at nuclear power stations. A significant minority, even among those over the age of 40–45 years for whom this treatment modality has always been the first choice, may refuse such an option, particularly when therapy is dependent upon adhering to the UK Ionising Radiation Regulations of 1985 with the resultant disruption, albeit temporary, socially, domestically and at the workplace. Second, there are adverse effects of iodine-131 therapy which have only recently been described and cannot be dismissed lightly. These are damage to the parafollicular C-cells, an increased incidence of gastric carcinoma, and development or worsening of ophthalmopathy.

Calcitonin deficiency. Although intrathyroidal C-cells do not concentrate iodine-131, they could be damaged indirectly due to their contiguity to follicular cells. There are recent reports of a reduction in both basal and intravenous calcium-stimulated calcitonin concentrations in patients who have been treated with iodine-131 for hyperthyroidism, more marked in those with Graves' disease than toxic multinodular goitre [3]. The consequences of long-term calcitonin deficiency are not known but may include osteoporosis. This is particularly relevant as most patients treated with iodine-131 will develop hypothyroidism, and thyroxine in a dose sufficient to suppress serum TSH concentrations may reduce bone density.

Gastric carcinoma. Mortality studies of hyperthyroid patients are scarce. However, a recent Swedish report analyzed cancer mortality in more than 10 000 patients (with an average age of 56 years at the time of treatment with iodine-131) and found that there was a significantly increased risk of death from cancer of the stomach more than 10 years after exposure [4]. The probability of a radiation-induced cancer is proportional to the radiation dose received by the organ in question. It is perhaps not surprising, therefore, that an excess mortality from gastric carcinoma has been demonstrated as, after the thyroid, the stomach receives the greatest amount of radiation following a therapeutic dose of iodine-131 for hyperthyroidism. (Thyroid cancer does not develop because the relatively large radiation dose either kills or sterilizes the follicular cells.)

The latest methods for predicting excess cancer risks following radiation exposure indicate that, for most radiosensitive organs, there will be an increasing risk of attributable cancer with time. This is because, after a latent period of a few years, the pattern of appearance of radiation-induced cancer is thought to follow a constant multiple of the 'natural' baseline rates, which themselves invariably increase with age. If people are young at the time of exposure they simply have more life ahead of them in which radiation-induced cancers can be expressed, so that their cumulative lifetime risk is higher than for someone exposed at an older age. Although there are large uncertainties in the models used to predict the pattern of appearance of individual types of radiogenic cancer, it would appear that there might be a 1% chance of stomach cancer in a 15-year-old treated with 400 MBq iodine-131 for Graves' disease. This, taken together with the Swedish study, is a cogent argument against reducing the long-established age threshold for radioiodine treatment of hyperthyroidism in the UK.

Ophthalmopathy. Although a large retrospective study has shown no influence of the type of treatment of the hyperthyroidism of Graves' disease on the clinical course of the ophthalmopathy [5], there is accumulating anecdotal evidence that the eye disease may worsen most often after iodine-131 therapy. The anecdotes are now supported by a prospective study in which ophthalmopathy developed or was exacerbated in one-third of patients treated with iodine-131 and was twice as frequent, and of more severity, than in those treated with antithyroid drugs or surgery (Fig. 1) [6]. In this study younger patients did not receive iodine-131. Furthermore, serum TSH concentrations were raised in some patients following radioiodine but the other two groups were given thyroxine either in combination with antithyroid drugs or soon after surgery to prevent any degree of thyroid failure.

There are, therefore, still more questions than answers. Does the deleterious effect of iodine-131 on ophthalmopathy hold true for all age

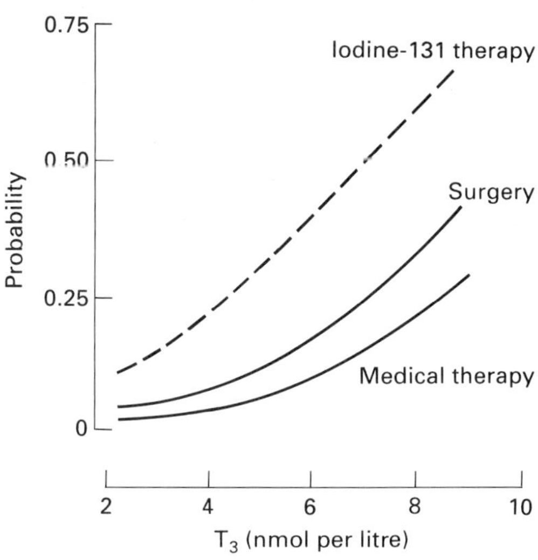

Fig. 1 The influence of pretreatment serum total T_3 concentrations and the type of therapy on the risk of the development or worsening of ophthalmopathy in patients with hyperthyroidism due to Graves' disease. (Reprinted, by permission of the *New England Journal of Medicine* [6].)

groups? Corticosteroids, presumably by their immunosuppressive effect, given at the time of iodine-131 therapy and for 3–4 months thereafter, prevent the progression of mild ophthalmopathy [7]. Would antithyroid drugs prescribed before and for 6–8 weeks after radioiodine administration exert the same beneficial effect? Clinical experience suggests that any tendency to hypothyroidism makes ophthalmopathy worse. Is there a role, therefore, for early treatment with thyroxine, thereby preventing a rise in serum TSH concentrations which is likely to occur 2–3 months after treatment in those patients developing hypothyroidism within the first 6 months? What is the significance of the increased concentration of TSH-receptor antibodies, which follows iodine-131 therapy but neither of the other two treatment modalities?

Until these various issues are resolved, it would seem sensible to avoid the use of iodine-131 in patients with moderate or severe ophthalmopathy. An alternative is the combination of carbimazole 40 mg daily and thyroxine 150–200 μg daily. This regimen is based on two principles: first, the hope that the well-established immunosuppressive action of carbimazole will inhibit the retrobulbar immune response and, second, to ensure an undetectable serum TSH concentration and thereby minimize thyroid antigen expression.

Antithyroid drugs: a renaissance?

The natural history of the hyperthyroidism of Graves' disease in most patients is alternating episodes of relapse and remission each lasting many months. Despite their immunosuppressive action, the antithyroid drugs do not seem to modify this pattern and it is not surprising, therefore, that even after prolonged treatment the relapse rate is approximately 50%, the majority of recurrences developing during the first 2 years. This state of affairs has been viewed by patients and physicians alike as unsatisfactory and was the reason for the popularity of thyroid surgery as a primary treatment of hyperthyroidism in the 1970s and for the increasing enthusiasm for iodine-131 therapy during the last few years. However, medical treatment of Graves' disease may soon enjoy a renaissance based on a remarkable study in which patients were treated with an antithyroid drug and thyroxine for 18 months and then thyroxine alone for a further 3 years. The relapse rate during that period was less than 2% compared with 35% for patients treated with methimazole alone [2]. Similarly, the administration of thyroxine during the second half of pregnancy and for 12 months after delivery in patients with Graves' disease is effective not only in decreasing the levels of antibodies to the TSH receptor but also in preventing the postpartum recurrence of hyperthyroidism [8]. If these results, reported from Japan, are confirmed, the management of Graves' disease will be revolutionized.

MANAGEMENT OF PRIMARY HYPOTHYROIDISM

Overt hypothyroidism

As a result of the ready availability of assays for TSH and better supervision through computerized follow-up of patients taking thyroxine replacement therapy, undertreatment is becoming unusual. In a recent study only 3.5% of patients had raised serum TSH concentrations but TSH was undetectable in 60% [9]. Does it matter if serum TSH is suppressed to less than 0.1 mU per litre or, using the most recent third generation assays, even below 0.01 mU per litre in patients taking replacement therapy? The thyrotroph is sensitive to minor changes in thyroid hormone concentrations even within their respective normal ranges, but is not unique in this respect, as was once thought to be the case. There is now considerable evidence that doses of thyroxine which suppress TSH secretion, while maintaining thyroid hormone levels in the normal range, have more widespread effects. These include changes in nocturnal heart rate, systolic time intervals, urinary sodium excretion, liver and muscle enzyme activity, red cell sodium concentrations and plasma lipids similar to, but less marked than, those found in overt hyperthyroidism.

There are some who would question the relevance of these minor changes in target organ function in patients who are asymptomatic, the more so when a recent retrospective study failed to demonstrate an increase in morbidity or mortality in thyroxine treated patients with suppressed serum TSH concentrations compared to those with normal serum TSH [9]. There is also the clinical observation that some patients prefer taking a daily dose of thyroxine of 50 μg in excess of that required to normalize the serum TSH response to thyrotrophin-releasing hormone. In addition there is some evidence of tissue adaptation to thyroid hormone excess [10].

The greatest concern, however, is over the effect of thyroxine therapy on bone. There have been several studies which have shown a significant reduction in bone mineral density, assessed by densitometry, at one or more sites in patients whose serum TSH has been suppressed for many years. For example, in a recent longitudinal study of 15 premenopausal women, taking a mean thyroxine dose of 147 μg daily, following thyroidectomy for goitre or differentiated carcinoma, serum TSH was suppressed and was associated with a significantly greater rate of spinal bone mineral loss than in controls [11]. The changes tend to be more marked in postmenopausal women. These densitometric studies are supported by biochemical evidence. Using pyridinium crosslinks as specific urinary markers of bone resorption, it has been shown that bone collagen breakdown is increased not only in thyrotoxicosis but also in postmenopausal

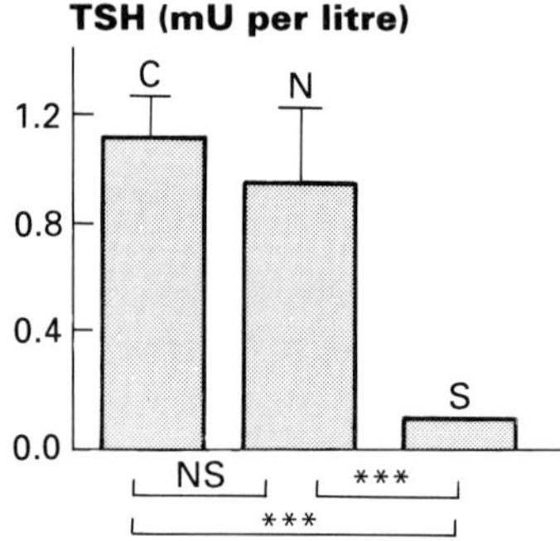

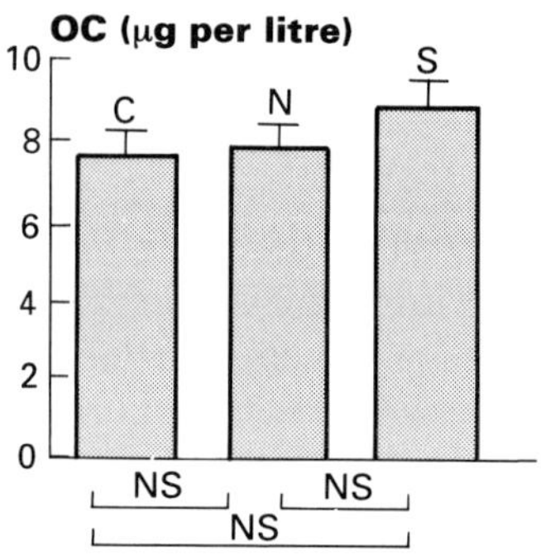

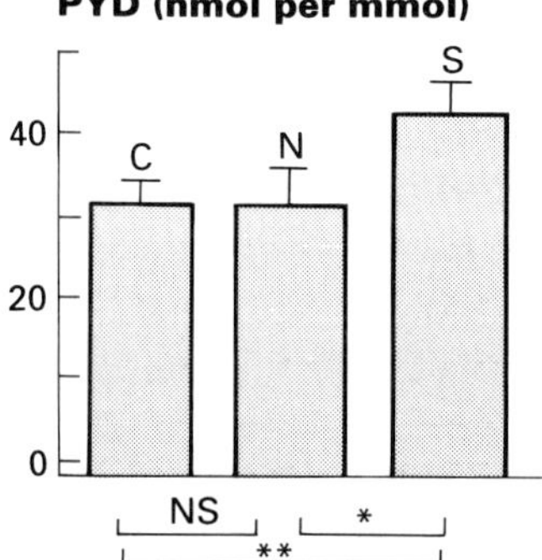

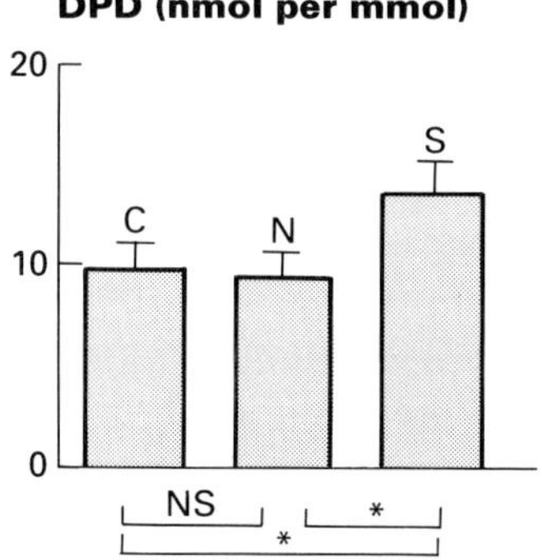

Fig. 2 Serum TSH, osteocalcin (OC) and pyridinium crosslink (PYD, pyridinoline; DPD, deoxypyridinoline), excretion (mean ± 1SD) in postmenopausal women according to T_4 treatment and serum TSH level. Controls (C); T_4-treated normal TSH (N); T_4-treated low TSH (S); ***, *P* less than 0.0001; **, *P* less than 0.01; *, *P* less than 0.05; NS, not significant. (Reproduced from Harvey *et al.* [12], by copyright permission of The Endocrine Society.)

women taking sufficient thyroxine to suppress TSH (Fig. 2) [12]. Also serum osteocalcin, a marker of bone turnover, is significantly increased in patients receiving suppressed doses of thyroxine following total thyroidectomy or iodine-131 treatment for differentiated thyroid carcinoma [13].

There would seem to be sufficient evidence to indicate that, whatever organ is examined, there is 'tissue thyrotoxicosis' if serum TSH is suppressed despite normal levels of thyroid hormones. It is therefore logical to follow, as far as possible, the advice of the American Thyroid Association in the management of primary hypothyroidism, namely that 'the goal of therapy is to restore most patients to the euthyroid state and to normalize serum T_4 and TSH concentrations'.

Once the correct dose of thyroxine has been established, it is good practice to undertake annual testing of thyroid function, not only to maximize compliance but also to identify those patients in whom an adjustment of dose may be necessary. For example, the mean dose of thyroxine required by patients developing hypothyroidism after iodine-131 therapy for Graves' disease is lower than in those with spontaneous primary hypothyroidism, and the dose may increase in later years [14]. The probable explanation is the continued presence of stimulating TSH-receptor antibodies in the early stages after iodine-131, resulting in non-suppressible function of the thyroid remnant. Rarely, patients with long-standing primary hypothyroidism may develop hyperthyroidism while taking thyroxine due to development of Graves' disease as a result of a change of production from blocking to stimulating TSH-receptor antibodies. There is a recent report of a patient undergoing three cycles of transition from hypothyroidism to hyperthyroidism and back to hypothyroidism during a period of 3 years [15].

Subclinical hypothyroidism

Subclinical hypothyroidism, developing spontaneously and due to autoimmune thyroid disease, is present in 3% of the population and in 10% of postmenopausal women. It is commonly found after treatment of hyperthyroidism by surgery, iodine-131, or antithyroid drugs but may also result from the use of medication such as lithium carbonate or amiodarone. There is some evidence that subclinical hypothyroidism is accompanied by reversible changes in target organ function, similar to, but less marked than, those recorded in overt hypothyroidism. These include impaired left ventricular function, reduced level of hearing, and increased capillary permeability to protein. However, it is the effect of thyroid hormones on lipid metabolism which has aroused the greatest interest, because of the increased frequency not only of hyperlipidaemia and coronary atherosclerosis in overt hypothyroidism but also of lymphocytic thyroiditis in patients with fatal myocardial infarction. It has even been claimed that a raised serum TSH is a risk factor for ischaemic heart disease. If it is, the link does not seem to be through hyperlipidaemia, as subclinical hypothyroidism is not associated with an increase in either total cholesterol or triglyceride concentrations, nor is there a consistent relationship with low-density lipoprotein cholesterol or high-density lipoprotein cholesterol [16–18].

Those favouring a pragmatic approach to the management of subclinical hypothyroidism will be most influenced by the knowledge that 50% of their patients will feel better when taking thyroxine, and by the fact that the annual rate of conversion to overt hypothyroidism is approximately 5% after iodine-131 or surgical treatment of hyperthyroidism and in those with circulating autoantibodies to thyroid peroxidase and/or thyroglobulin. It makes sense, having identified subclinical hypothyroidism, to prevent the progression to overt thyroid failure by prescribing thyroxine rather than to allow the insidious development of more severe hypothyroidism, particularly in those who might become lost to follow-up.

Temporary hypothyroidism

The great majority of patients with primary hypothyroidism require long-term thyroxine therapy but there are well-recognized situations such as subacute (de Quervain's) thyroiditis and postpartum thyroiditis in which thyroid failure is not only mild or asymptomatic but also temporary, lasting a few weeks only. Hypothyroidism due to Hashimoto's thyroiditis may remit spontaneously, particularly if excess iodine intake has been implicated. Transient neonatal hypothyroidism may follow the use of iodine-containing antiseptics applied vaginally during the last trimester or labour, or topically to the skin of the newborn. It may also occur in children born to mothers with autoimmune thyroid failure due to the transplacental passage of TSH-receptor blocking antibodies. Raised serum TSH concentrations of greater than 15 mU per litre are often recorded in patients with untreated or inadequately controlled Addison's disease but usually fall to the normal range with glucocorticoid replacement. Hypothyroidism may also be transient after subtotal thyroidectomy or iodine-131 therapy for Graves' disease and permanent hypothyroidism should not be diagnosed before 6 months have elapsed.

The recent finding that recovery from hypothyroidism may occur in patients with chronic autoimmune thyroiditis due to the disappearance of TSH-receptor blocking antibodies [19] raises the question of whether the need for thyroxine replacement therapy should not be reassessed from time to time in those with Hashimoto's disease or atrophic thyroid failure. However, only about 5% of such patients have a remission and identification of this small subset requires serial measurements of blocking antibody, the assay for which is not widely available. In its absence, routine discontinuation of thyroxine therapy for 4–6 weeks every 5 years or so in all patients with chronic autoimmune thyroiditis is not warranted.

REFERENCES

1 Franklyn J, Sheppard M. Radioiodine for hyperthyroidism. *Br Med J* 1992;305: 727–728.

2 Hashizume K, Ichikawa K, Sakurai A, *et al.* Administration of thyroxine in treated Graves' disease. Effects on the level of antibodies to thyroid stimulating hormone receptors and on the risk of recurrence of hyperthyroidism. *N Engl J Med* 1991;324: 947–953.

3 Tzanela M, Thalassinos NC, Nikou A, *et al.* Effect of ^{131}I treatment on the calcitonin response to calcium infusion in hyperthyroid patients. *Clin Endocrinol* 1993;38:25–28.

4 Hall P, Berg G, Bjelkengren G, *et al.* Cancer mortality after iodine-131 therapy for hyperthyroidism. *Int J Cancer* 1992;50:886–890.
5 Sridama V, DeGroot LJ. Treatment of Graves' disease and the course of ophthalmopathy. *Am J Med* 1989;87:70–73.
6 Tallstedt L, Lundell G, Tørring O, *et al.* Occurrence of ophthalmopathy after treatment for Graves' hyperthyroidism. *N Engl J Med* 1992;326:1733–1738.
7 Bartelena L, Marcocci C, Bogazzi F, *et al.* Use of corticosteroids to prevent progression of Graves' ophthalmopathy after radioiodine therapy for hyperthyroidism. *N Engl J Med* 1989;321:1349–1352.
8 Hashizume K, Ichikawa K, Nishii Y, *et al.* Effect of administration of thyroxine on the risk of postpartum recurrence of hyperthyroid Graves' disease. *J Clin Endocrinol Metab* 1992;75:6–10.
9 Leese GP, Jung RT, Guthrie C, *et al.* Morbidity in patients on L-thyroxine: comparison of those with a normal TSH to those with a suppressed TSH. *Clin Endocrinol* 1992;37: 500–503.
10 Nystrom E, Lundberg P-A, Petersen K, *et al.* Evidence for a slow tissue adaptation to circulating thyroxine in patients with chronic L-thyroxine treatment. *Clin Endocrinol* 1989;31:143–150.
11 Pioli G, Pedrazzoni M, Palummeri E, *et al.* Longitudinal study of bone loss after thyroidectomy and suppressive thyroxine therapy in premenopausal women. *Acta Endocrinol* 1992;126:238–242.
12 Harvey RD, McHardy KC, Reid IW, *et al.* Measurement of bone collagen degradation in hyperthyroidism and during thyroxine replacement therapy using pyridinium crosslinks as specific urinary markers. *J Clin Endocrinol Metab* 1991;72:1189–1194.
13 Diamond T, Nery L, Hales I. A therapeutic dilemma: suppressive doses of thyroxine significantly reduced bone mineral measurements in both premenopausal and postmenopausal women with thyroid carcinoma. *J Clin Endocrinol Metab* 1990;72:1184–1188.
14 Bearcroft CP, Toms GC, Williams SJ, *et al.* Thyroxine replacement in post-radioiodine hypothyroidism. *Clin Endocrinol* 1991;34:115–118.
15 Kraiem Z, Baron E, Kahana L, *et al.* Changes in stimulating and blocking TSH receptor antibodies in a patient undergoing three cycles of transition from hypo to hyperthyroidism and back to hypothyroidism. *Clin Endocrinol* 1992;36:211–214.
16 Lithell H, Boberg J, Hellsing K, *et al.* Serum lipoprotein and apolipoprotein concentrations and tissue lipoprotein-lipase activity in overt and subclinical hypothyroidism: the effect of substitution therapy. *Eur J Clin Invest* 1981;11:3–10.
17 Caron P, Calazel C, Parra HJ, *et al.* Decreased HDL cholesterol in subclinical hypothyroidism: the effect of L-thyroxine therapy. *Clin Endocrinol* 1990;33:519–523.
18 Arem R, Patsch W. Lipoprotein and apolipoprotein levels in subclinical hypothyroidism. Effects of levothyroxine therapy. *Arch Intern Med* 1990;150:2097–2100.
19 Takasu N, Yamada T, Takasu M, *et al.* Disappearance of thyrotropin-blocking antibodies and spontaneous recovery from hypothyroidism in autoimmune thyroiditis. *N Engl J Med* 1992;326:513–518.

PART 8
RESPIRATORY MEDICINE

T-lymphocyte/eosinophil interactions in the pathogenesis of asthma

C. J. CORRIGAN & A. B. KAY

SUMMARY

Persistent asthma is characterized by chronic inflammation of the bronchial mucosa. Many cell types are present but T cells and eosinophils are prominent. Here we summarize evidence that asthmatic bronchial inflammation is initiated and propagated by cytokines secreted by activated T cells and other cells, and describe how the release of specific cytokines could result in local preferential accumulation and activation of eosinophils. We also compare the role of atopy with non-immunoglobulin E (IgE)-mediated mechanisms and hypothesize from the available evidence that all asthma involves antigen-driven T cells. Thus, the underlying pathogenesis of the disease, despite its varied clinical associations, may be relatively uniform.

INTRODUCTION

Asthma is a disease characterized by reversible obstruction of the airways or bronchi. This is accompanied by non-specific bronchial hyperresponsiveness or 'irritability', which is the tendency of the bronchi in asthmatics to constrict in response to a wide range of pharmacological and irritant stimuli. It is now widely accepted that chronic inflammation of the bronchial mucosa lining plays a fundamental role in the genesis of these clinical manifestations. The most striking feature of the histopathology of asthma is the intense infiltration of the bronchial mucosa with eosinophils, macrophages and lymphocytes. In fact, the disease has many of the histopathological features of a chronic, cell-mediated hypersensitivity. The eosinophil appears to be a key cell in producing bronchial mucosal injury [1]. This in turn is believed to result in bronchial obstruction and irritability, although the precise mechanisms by which this occurs are not clear. Other important pathological features include destruction and desquamation of airway epithelial cells and collagen deposition below the basement membrane.

Asthma is often, though not invariably, associated with atopy, particularly in children. Atopy refers to the genetic predisposition of certain individuals to synthesize, inappropriately, IgE specific for certain external antigens, particularly inhaled aeroallergens such as grass pollen. This allergen-specific IgE sensitizes mast cells, and other cell types with high and low affinity IgE Fc receptors, causing an energy-dependent release of pre-formed, granule-derived and newly-formed, membrane-derived pharmacological agents on further allergen exposure. These atopic asthmatics experience an exacerbation of their disease on exposure to allergens to which they are sensitized. Such patients have traditionally been referred to as 'extrinsic' asthmatics, reflecting the relationship of their disease with external environmental factors. Non-atopic asthmatics, where IgE-mediated mechanisms do not obviously operate, have been labelled 'intrinsic' (Fig. 1). Some patients develop asthma after exposure to specific proteins or small molecular weight chemicals at work; these 'occupational' asthmatics form a third clinical category. It is not clear how far IgE-mediated or cell-mediated mechanisms (or both) can be implicated in the various forms of occupational asthma.

The extent to which IgE-mediated mechanisms play a role in asthma pathogenesis is uncertain. Insofar as some non-atopic individuals develop the disease whereas not all atopic individuals do, it would appear that IgE-mediated mechanisms are neither necessary nor sufficient for the development of asthma. IgE-mediated mechanisms are clearly important

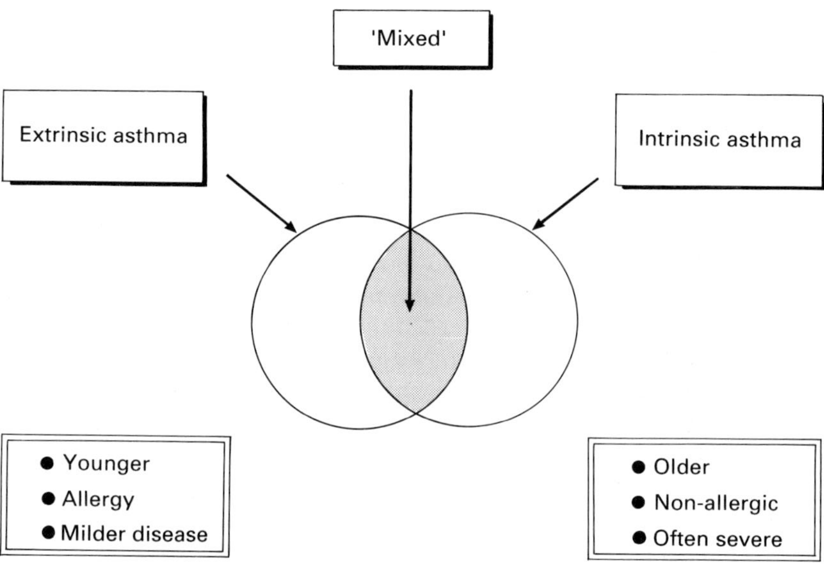

Fig. 1 Diagrammatic representation of extrinsic and intrinsic asthma. Most patients have a mixed picture.

in allergen-induced short-term exacerbations of asthma in atopic subjects, but the role of IgE in the pathogenesis of the ongoing chronic disease is less certain.

EVIDENCE FOR MUCOSAL INFLAMMATION IN ASTHMA

Many recent studies on the histology of asthma have compared mild asthmatic and normal volunteers, utilizing the techniques of bronchoalveolar lavage (BAL) and bronchial biopsy through the flexible fibreoptic bronchoscope. Elevated numbers of eosinophils, both in the bronchial mucosa and in BAL fluid, were constant features of mild asthma [2,3]. Similarly, elevated numbers of activated lymphocytes, identified either as irregular, atypical lymphocytes by transmission electron microscopy [4] or as CD25 bearing cells as shown by immunocytochemistry, were also demonstrated. Most of the CD25 expressing cells in these biopsies were shown to be T cells [5]. There is evidence that activation of selected T-cell populations with subsequent eosinophil recruitment and secretion may contribute both to epithelial damage and to bronchial hyperresponsiveness [6]. Although recent studies showed no significant changes in the numbers of mast cells and their subtypes, neutrophils or macrophages in the bronchial mucosa of mild asthmatics [7–9], this does not exclude the possible participation of these cell types in more severe disease; furthermore, cell numbers do not necessarily equate with function, and it has been shown, for example, that the spontaneous release of mediators from mast cells is increased in asthmatics [3].

The traditional clinical classification of asthma (intrinsic, extrinsic and occupational) implies variability in pathogenesis. One important question, therefore, relates to whether these clinical distinctions are apparent in histopathological terms. Preliminary studies that have addressed this question suggest that they are not: an autopsy study of the bronchial mucosa of a patient who had died with severe occupational asthma showed histological changes similar to those seen in fatal non-occupational asthma [8], whilst an immunocytochemical study [9] comparing bronchial biopsies from extrinsic and occupational asthmatics showed that these were indistinguishable in terms of their inflammatory cell infiltrate. A similar situation pertained with 'intrinsic' asthmatics, although there was in this case some evidence of an additional macrophage infiltrate [10]. Examination of BAL fluid obtained from a group of 'intrinsic' asthmatics [11] showed increased numbers of activated T cells, eosinophils and neutrophils as compared to normal controls. These observations suggest many similarities in the bronchial histopathology in patients with asthma, regardless of the nature of identifiable provoking agents, and lend support to the hypothesis that the pathogenesis of asthma is independent of coexisting atopy.

EOSINOPHILS AND ASTHMA PATHOGENESIS

Preferential accumulation of eosinophils in asthma

Eosinophils are non-dividing, granular cells that arise principally in the bone marrow. Eosinophil differentiation, like that of all leucocytes, is influenced by lymphokines. Interleukin 3 (IL-3), IL-5 and granulocyte/macrophage colony stimulating factor (GM-CSF) promote eosinophil differentiation [12]. Whereas IL-3 and GM-CSF act on the precursors of a number of leucocytes, IL-5 appears to be specific for eosinophils. IL-5 may be the most important cytokine for terminal differentiation of the committed eosinophil precursor, since it is released principally by T cells and the eosinophilia associated with parasitic infections is T-cell dependent [13]. This hypothesis is further supported by the observation that transgenic mice that constitutively express the gene for IL-5 develop a marked peripheral blood eosinophilia [14]. If IL-5 alone were sufficient to mediate the eosinophilia associated with asthma, this might explain why there is a consistent expansion of eosinophils and not other leucocyte lineages.

One of the fundamental problems in investigating the pathogenesis of asthma has been to explain why eosinophils preferentially accumulate in the inflamed mucosa. Established eosinophil chemoattractants, such as platelet activating factor (PAF) and C5a, whilst highly potent, are non-specific in the sense that they also attract neutrophils. On the other hand, IL-5 can specifically prime eosinophils for enhanced locomotor responses to PAF, leukotriene B_4 (LTB_4) and IL-8 [15]. Eosinophil migration from the vascular space into the tissues is initiated by an interaction between receptors on the cell surface and their ligands on the surface of vascular endothelial cells. Eosinophils and neutrophils both express the β_2 integrins LFA-1 (CD18/CD11a) and Mac-1 (CD18/CD11b) as well as the receptor for E-selectin. However, eosinophils appear to be unique insofar as: (i) IL-3 and IL-5 upregulated eosinophil, but not neutrophil, adhesion to unstimulated endothelial cells [16]; and (ii) eosinophils, but not neutrophils, express the β_1 integrin $\alpha_4\beta_1$ (CD49a/CD29, VLA-4), which is a ligand for vascular cell adhesion molecule 1 (VCAM-1) on the surface of stimulated endothelial cells [17]. These mechanisms, together with the properties of IL-3, IL-5 and GM-CSF in prolonging eosinophil survival, might offer a partial explanation as to how eosinophils accumulate preferentially in the asthmatic bronchial mucosa.

Pro-inflammatory properties of eosinophils

Eosinophils can secrete a number of lipid mediators and proteins which may have a role to play in the pathophysiology of asthma (Fig. 2). They elaborate eicosanoids derived from the 5- and 15-lipoxygenase pathways, especially LTC_4 and LTD_4, as well as substantial quantities of PAF [18,19]. Both LTC_4 and PAF cause bronchoconstriction whilst LTC_4 is a mucus secretagogue. PAF also increases vascular permeability. It has been difficult to demonstrate the presence of LTC_4 and LTD_4 and PAF in asthma, possibly because of their low concentrations and rapid metabolism, although clinical trials have suggested that LTD_4 receptor antagonists and 5-lipoxygenase inhibitors may be of some benefit for the therapy of chronic disease [20].

Eosinophils store four basic proteins in their granules: major basic protein (MBP), eosinophil-derived neurotoxin (EDN), eosinophil cationic protein (ECP) and eosinophil peroxidase (EPO). MBP is toxic for human respiratory epithelial cells and pneumocytes [21]. Inhalation of MBP, albeit at high concentrations, caused bronchial hyperresponsiveness in a primate model of asthma [22]. EPO is also toxic for respiratory epithelium and pneumocytes, particularly in combination with peroxide and halide ions [23]. Degranulation of eosinophils with release of these

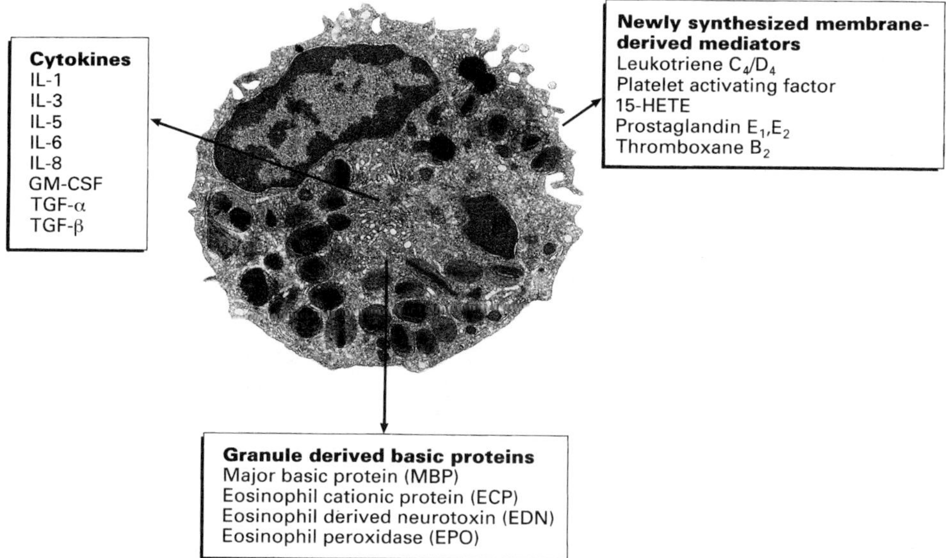

Fig. 2 A diagrammatic representation of the cytokines, mediators and basic proteins produced by human eosinophils. Many of these have pro-inflammatory properties relevant to the asthma process.

proteins follows engagement of their IgG, IgA and IgE receptors [24,25], and by direct stimulation with soluble mediators such as PAF and LTB_4 [26]. Despite these observations, it is not clear precisely what produces eosinophil degranulation *in vivo*, although the observation that adherence of eosinophils to fibronectin enhances LTC_4 production suggests that extracellular matrix protein may serve as one extravascular activating stimulus [27].

Eosinophils have the capacity to elaborate certain cytokines including transforming growth factor α (TGF-α) TGF-β, GM-CSF, IL-1, IL-3, IL-5, IL-6 and IL-8 [28–33]. The GM-CSF secreted by eosinophils was shown to exert an autocrine effect on cell survival [30]. These extensive pro-inflammatory properties of eosinophils, along with their abundance in the asthmatic bronchial mucosa, have strengthened the current consensus that eosinophils are prime inflammatory effector cells in this disease.

Eosinophils in asthma

It is well known that a blood and sputum eosinophilia is often, though not invariably, observed in association with asthma of diverse aetiology. Both longitudinal and cross-sectional studies of asthmatic patients suggest that blood eosinophil counts correlate with the degree of bronchial hyperresponsiveness. Immunostaining of the bronchial mucosa of patients who died with severe asthma revealed the presence of large numbers of activated eosinophils [34] and considerable amounts of MBP deposited in the airways [1]. In atopic asthmatics developing a late phase bronchoconstrictor response after allergen challenge, the degree of associated bronchial hyperresponsiveness correlated with the peripheral blood eosinophil count [35]. The numbers of eosinophils in peripheral blood, BAL fluid and bronchial biopsies in a group of asthmatics were elevated in comparison to normal controls, and it was possible to demonstrate an increasing degree of eosinophilia with clinical severity [36].

Increased concentrations of MBP were found in BAL fluid from atopic asthmatics compared to normal controls [3]. In this study, correlations were observed between the concentrations of MBP, the numbers of desquamated epithelial cells in BAL fluid and the degree of bronchial hyperresponsiveness. In two studies employing allergen bronchial challenge of atopic asthmatics with BAL 6 hours later, the late phase airways obstruction was accompanied by an influx of eosinophils and neutrophils into BAL fluid, which was not observed in subjects developing an isolated early phase response [37,38]. Similar observations were made in a study using local allergen challenge through the bronchoscope [39]. In subjects with red cedar asthma, plicatic acid inhalation elicited a BAL eosinophilia together with sloughing of bronchial epithelial cells [40].

In a placebo-controlled double-blind study of asthmatics, sodium cromoglycate therapy suppressed the accumulation of eosinophils in bronchial mucus and BAL fluid, coinciding with clinical improvement [41].

CD4+ T cells and asthma pathogenesis

CD4+ T cells and eosinophils

CD4+ T cells are clearly an important source of IL-5, IL-3 and GM-CSF. The roles of these agents in enhancing eosinophil maturation, survival, activation [42–44] and local eosinophil accumulation are well documented and have been discussed. In addition to T cells, other cell types, such as mast cells, macrophages, epithelial cells, fibroblasts and neutrophils as well as eosinophils themselves, are potential sources of cytokines which may influence eosinophil function [29,30,45–47]. Nevertheless, T cells are unique amongst inflammatory cells in the sense that they can recognize and respond to processed antigens directly (rather than through passively adsorbed surface immunoglobulins such as IgE), and it is our belief that they play a pivotal role in initiating and orchestrating ongoing immunologically driven chronic asthma, particularly in situations where the IgE response is absent or minimal.

T cells and asthmatic inflammation

Recent immunocytochemical studies of bronchial biopsies taken from patients with asthma have shown that activated (CD25+) T cells can be detected in the bronchial mucosa, and that their numbers correlate both with the numbers of local activated eosinophils and with disease severity. Activated (CD25+, HLA-DR+) CD4+, but not CD8+ T cells were also detected in the peripheral blood of patients with acute severe asthma [48,49] and their numbers were reduced following therapy to a degree which correlated with clinical improvement. Peripheral blood T cells from asthmatics clinically resistant to corticosteroid therapy were shown to express these activation markers *in vivo* [50] and to be refractory to the inhibitory effects of corticosteroids *in vitro* [51]. It was demonstrated in mild asthmatics that, while both CD4+ and CD8+ T cells in BAL fluid express activation markers, only the numbers of activated CD4+ T cells correlated with the numbers of BAL eosinophils and disease severity [52]. A selective increase in CD4+ T cells in BAL fluid was observed 48 hours after allergen challenge in those asthmatics who had previously been shown to develop a late phase reaction [53], suggesting that selective recruitment of CD4+ T cells to the lung may occur in association with this experimental model of asthma. These observations do not necessarily mean that CD4+ T cells and their products actually cause the late-phase asthmatic response (LPR), especially since the peak of this reaction usually occurs 6–9 hours after allergen challenge. However, they do suggest that the T-cell recruitment sets the scene for the intense inflammation and persistent airway narrowing that accompanies repeated allergen exposure. It should be mentioned, as an aside, that observations made from models of provoked asthma after a single challenge (i.e. LPRs) are not necessarily representative of ongoing chronic disease.

Measurement of lymphokines *in vivo* is problematical because of their low concentration, rapid metabolism and unquantifiable degree of dilution. Furthermore, 'physiological' concentrations of lymphokines have in general not been defined, and so it is often unknown whether a specific assay such as an enzyme-linked immunosorbent assay (ELISA) is sensitive enough. Bioassays are more relevant in this regard, provided it can be ensured that they are specific for the particular lymphokine being measured. The problem has been emphasized in a recent study of BAL fluid from asthmatics [54], where cytokines were detectable only after considerable concentration of the BAL fluid. Clearly, such a procedure might result in variable loss of specific proteins. One alternative to the direct measurement of lymphokines is the detection of their messenger RNA (mRNA) using the technique of *in situ* hybridization with lymphokine-specific complementary DNA (cDNA) probes or riboprobes. Although this is not a strictly quantitative technique, and with the proviso that mRNA synthesis does not always equate with secretion of the corresponding protein, it does have the advantage that it can localize the secretion of lymphokines within cells and tissues. Using this technique it was recently demonstrated that IL-5 mRNA was elaborated by cells in the bronchial mucosa of a majority of mild asthmatics but not normal controls (Fig. 3) [55]. The numbers of mRNA signals correlated broadly with the numbers of activated T cells and eosinophils in biopsies from the same subjects. In another study [56], it was shown that significantly higher numbers of BAL cells expressed mRNA encoding IL-2, IL-3, IL-4, IL-5 and GM-CSF but not interferon γ (IFN-γ) in mild atopic asthmatics as compared with non-atopic normal controls. Increased numbers of cells expressing mRNA encoding tumour necrosis factor α (TNF-α) were observed in BAL cells from asthmatics as compared with normal controls [57], reflecting the increased concentrations of the corresponding protein found in concentrated asthmatic BAL fluid [54]. Cultured peripheral blood CD4+ and CD8+ T cells from both atopic and non-atopic asthmatics were shown spontaneously to secrete factors which prolonged the life of eosinophils *in vitro* to an extent which correlated with the numbers of peripheral blood eosinophils in the same subjects [58]; antibody neutralization experiments suggested that this activity was attributable partly to GM-CSF and partly to IL-5. Taken together, these studies support the general hypothesis that, in atopic and

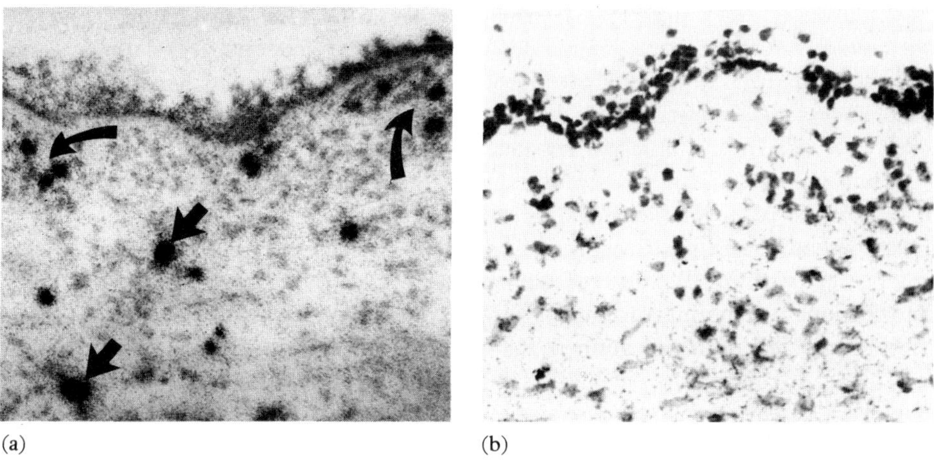

(a) (b)

Fig. 3 (a) Autoradiograph of bronchial mucosa from a patient with symptomatic asthma. *In situ* hybridization was performed under high stringency with phosphorus-32-labelled cRNA probe encoding for IL-5 mRNA. Arrows indicate the positive IL-5 mRNA cells. (Original magnification ×300.) (b) A control section was treated with RNase before hybridization with the radiolabelled IL-5 cRNA probe. No hybridization was detected. (Original magnification × 300.) (Courtesy of Dr Q. Hamid.)

non-atopic asthma, activated CD4+ T cells secrete lymphokines that are relevant to the accumulation and activation of eosinophils in the bronchial mucosa.

Are asthmatic CD4+ T cells of T_H2 phenotype?

There has been considerable interest recently in the classification of T cells according to their profiles of lymphokine secretion. Mouse T cells can be subdivided into T_H1 and T_H2 types, according to their selective secretion of IL-2 and IFN-γ or IL-4 and IL-5, respectively. T_H2 cells are of particular interest with regard to the pathogenesis of asthma because of the eosinophil-specific effects of IL-5 and because IL-4 enhances IgE synthesis. T_H1 cells, in contrast, appear to participate in delayed-type hypersensitivity reactions and inhibit IgE synthesis through their secretion of IFN-γ. In both atopic and non-atopic human subjects, T_H1 and T_H2 type T-cell clones can be distinguished *in vitro* [59]; furthermore, there is increasing evidence that these cell types may also be involved in inflammatory processes *in vivo*. For example, recent studies using *in situ* hybridization [60,61] demonstrated a T_H1-like pattern of cytokine mRNA expression in cutaneous tuberculin reactions and a T_H2-like pattern in allergen-induced late phase cutaneous reactions. T cells in the BAL fluid of mild, atopic asthmatics showed elevated expression of IL-4 and IL-5 mRNA compared with non-atopic controls, reflecting a T_H2-like pattern

[56]. However, it would appear that IL-4 and IL-5 expression need not always be coordinately regulated *in vivo*: T cells purified from the peripheral blood of non-atopic asthmatics spontaneously secreted elevated quantities of IL-5, but not IL-4, in comparison with normal controls, whereas those from atopic patients secreted elevated quantities of both IL-4 and IL-5 [62]. It is possible, therefore, that increased IL-4 synthesis is associated with the atopic state and is not a prerequisite for the development of asthma. Irrespective of whether or not T cells in asthma can be regarded as T_H2-like cells, characterization of their profiles of cytokine secretion in asthma in various clinical settings may allow a pathophysiological classification of the disease.

T cells, IgE and asthma

As stated, asthma and atopy are closely linked, and some investigators have suggested that all asthma is IgE-mediated thus casting doubt upon the concept of the 'intrinsic' form of the disease. For example, in a recent epidemiological survey [63] a direct correlation was observed in *all* asthmatics between serum IgE concentrations (corrected for age and sex) and clinical severity. On the other hand, some of the clinical and pathological distinctions between atopic and non-atopic asthma, such as the presence of both IL-4 and IL-5 in concentrated BAL fluid from atopic asthmatics but IL-5 and not IL-4 in fluid from non-atopic subjects [62], are impressive and indisputable. Similarly, in occupational asthma caused by sensitization to small chemicals such as toluene diisocyanate (see chapter on occupational asthma by P. S. Burge), subjects may be non-atopic with negative skin prick tests and yet have a profound peripheral blood eosinophilia with evidence of activated T cells and eosinophils in bronchial biopsies [10]. While it is possible that localized IgE-mediated reactions, which are not detectable systemically, may occur in such patients, a reasonable alternative hypothesis is that asthma is a chronic cell-mediated disease which may occur independently of the presence or absence of IgE or other antibody-mediated immune mechanisms. What then is the antigen(s) which drives T cells in the chronic non-atopic form of the disease? This is speculative but there are a number of suggestions. Viral antigens, particularly adeno- and rhinoviruses, are strong candidates, particularly as infections by these agents are common triggers in exacerbations of asthma. Autoantibodies formed from damaged bronchial mucosa is another possibility, although organ and tissue specific antibodies have been difficult to detect in this disease. The ability of common aeroallergens such as the house dust mite to elicit a T-cell (CD4+) response in non-atopics is well documented [64]. That such cells could escape normal control at damaged bronchial mucosal surfaces in non-atopic asthmatics is a testable hypothesis.

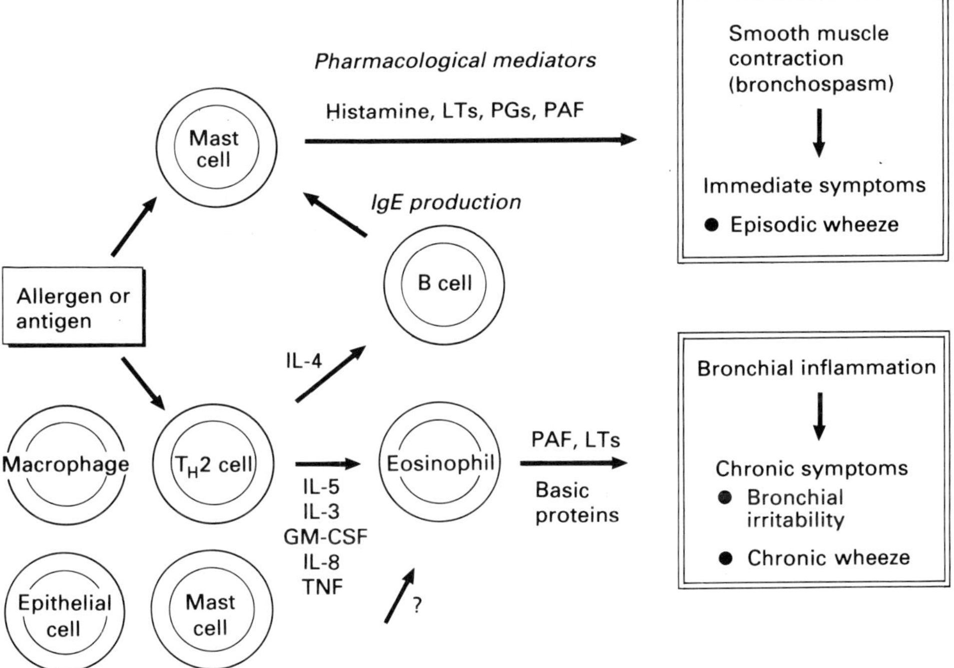

Fig. 4 Hypothesis for the pathogenesis of asthma. Eosinophils are believed to be prime pro-inflammatory effector cells causing bronchial damage, which in turn, leads to chronic asthma symptoms. Although many cells may secrete cytokines (i.e. mast cells, epithelial cells, macrophages) all of which influence eosinophil differentiation, survival and function, the T_H2 type T cell is seen as having a central role since it is capable of direct antigen recognition. The putative 'driving' antigen for asthmatic inflammation is suggested here to be allergen, although other antigens (viral, epithelial) are also possible candidates. Although T cells also influence the synthesis of IgE, IgE-mediated mechanisms are seen as playing a secondary role only in atopic subjects, where they may be responsible for acute, short-lived symptoms superimposed on the chronic, ongoing cell-mediated inflammatory disease.

CONCLUSION

Asthma is clearly a complex disorder with many variants and several possible mechanisms apart from the events associated with bronchial mucosal inflammation. For example, the influences of local neuronal and hormonal networks may be operative, but these are outside the scope of this article. Here we focus on T cells, eosinophils and mucosal damage in asthma and have summarized the evidence supporting the hypothesis that the disease is 'immunologically driven' even though in many instances the driving antigen(s) or allergen(s) are unknown. Asthma and atopy are closely linked but the disease can apparently occur in the absence of an abnormal IgE response or excessive local production of IL-4. The cytokine profile of cells in the bronchial mucosa of atopic asthmatics (who have been the most intensely studied) corresponds to that of T_H2 type T cells. IL-3, IL-5 and GM-CSF appear to be critical for eosinophil mobilization and activation, and eosinophil products may be responsible for the mucosal damage typical of the disease. IL-5 is possibly particularly important since it has several eosinophil-specific associated biological activities. It is equally clear that other inflammatory cells such as mast cells, fibroblasts, macrophages and epithelial cells may also produce cytokines, particularly GM-CSF, which are relevant to the asthma process. However, T cells, through their unique capacity for primary antigen recognition, may play a central role in orchestrating the asthmatic inflammatory response. These points have been summarized diagrammatically (Fig. 4).

REFERENCES

1 Filley WV, Holley KE, Kephart GM, Gleich GJ. Identification by immunofluorescence of eosinophil granule major basic protein in lung tissues of patients with bronchial asthma. *Lancet* 1982;ii:11–16.

2 Azzawi M, Bradley B, Jeffery PK, *et al.* Identification of activated T lymphocytes and eosinophils in bronchial biopsies in stable atopic asthma. *Am Rev Respir Dis* 1990;142: 1410–1413.

3 Wardlaw AJ, Dunnette S, Gleich GJ, *et al.* Eosinophils and mast cells in bronchoalveolar lavage in mild asthma: relationship to bronchial hyperreactivity. *Am Rev Respir Dis* 1988;137:62–69.

4 Jeffery PK, Wardlaw AJ, Nelson FC, *et al.* Bronchial biopsies in asthma: an ultrastructural, quantitative study and correlation with hyperreactivity. *Am Rev Respir Dis* 1989;140:1745–1753.

5 Hamid Q, Barkans J, Robinson DS, *et al.* Co-expression of CD25 and CD3 in atopic allergy and asthma. *Immunology* 1992;75:659–663.

6 Laitinen LA, Heino M, Laitinen A, *et al.* Damage of airway epithelium and bronchial reactivity in patients with asthma. *Am Rev Respir Dis* 1985;131:599–606.

7 Bradley BL, Azzawi M, Assoufi B, *et al.* Eosinophils, T lymphocytes, mast cells, neutrophils and macrophages in bronchial biopsy specimens from atopic subjects with asthma: Comparison with biopsy specimens from atopic subjects without asthma and normal control subjects and relationship to bronchial hyperresponsiveness. *J Allergy Clin Immunol* 1991;88:661–674.

8 Fabbri LM, Danielli D, Crescioli S, *et al.* Fatal asthma in a subject sensitized to toluene diisocyanate. *Am Rev Respir Dis* 1988;137:1494–1498.

9 Bentley AM, Maestrelli P, Saetta M, *et al.* Activated T-lymphocytes and eosinophils in the bronchial mucosa in isocyanate-induced asthma. *J Allergy Clin Immunol* 1992;89: 821–829.

10 Bentley AM, Menz G, Storz C, *et al.* Identification of T-lymphocytes, macrophages and activated eosinophils in the bronchial mucosa in intrinsic asthma: Relationship to symptoms and bronchial responsiveness. *Am Rev Respir Dis* 1992;146:500–506.

11 Mattoli S, Mattoso VL, Soloperto M, *et al.* Cellular and biochemical characteristics of bronchoalveolar lavage fluid in symptomatic nonallergic asthma. *J Allergy Clin Immunol* 1991;87:794–802.

12 Clutterbuck EJ, Hirst EMA, Sanderson CJ. Human interleukin-5 (IL-5) regulates the production of eosinophils in human bone marrow cultures: comparison and interaction with IL-1, IL-3, IL-6 and GM-CSF. *Blood* 1989;73:1504–1513.

13 Basten A, Beeson PB. Mechanism of eosinophilia. II. Role of the lymphocyte. *J Exp Med* 1970;131:1288–1305.

14 Dent LA, Strath M, Mellor AL, Sanderson CJ. Eosinophilia in transgenic mice expressing interleukin-5. *J Exp Med* 1990;172:1425–1431.

15 Sehmi R, Wardlaw AJ, Cromwell O, *et al.* Interleukin-5 (IL-5) selectively enhances the chemotactic response of eosinophils obtained from normal but not eosinophilic subjects. *Blood* 1992;79:2952–2959.
16 Walsh GM, Hartnell A, Wardlaw AJ, *et al.* IL-5 enhances the *in vitro* adhesion of human eosinophils, but not neutrophils, in a leucocyte integrin (CD11/18) dependent manner. *Immunology* 1990;71:258–265.
17 Walsh GM, Hartnell A, Mermod J-J, *et al.* Human eosinophil, but not neutrophil, adherence to IL-1 stimulated HUVEC is $\alpha_4\beta_1$ (VLA-4) dependent. *J Immunol* 1991; 146:3419–3423.
18 Shaw RJ, Walsh GM, Cromwell O, *et al.* Activated human eosinophils generate SRS-A leukotrienes following physiological (IgG-dependent) stimulation. *Nature* 1985;316: 150–152.
19 Cromwell O, Wardlaw AJ, Champion A, *et al.* IgG-dependent generation of platelet-activating factor by normal and low density human eosinophils. *J Immunol* 1990;145: 3862–3868.
20 Cloud ML, Enas GC, Kemp J, *et al.* A specific LTD_4/LTE_4-receptor antagonist improves pulmonary function in patients with mild, chronic asthma. *Am Rev Respir Dis* 1989;140:1336–1339.
21 Ayars GH, Altman LC, Gleich GJ, *et al.* Eosinophil and eosinophil granule mediated pneumocyte injury. *J Allergy Clin Immunol* 1985;76:595–604.
22 Gundel RH, Letts LG, Gleich GJ. Human eosinophil major basic protein induces airway constriction and airway hyperresponsiveness in primates. *J Clin Invest* 1991;87: 1470–1473.
23 Gleich GJ. The eosinophil and bronchial asthma: current understanding. *J Allergy Clin Immunol* 1990;85:422–436.
24 Abu-Ghazaleh RI, Fujisawa T, Mestecky J, *et al.* IgA-induced eosinophil degranulation. *J Immunol* 1989;142:2393–2400.
25 Khaliffe J, Capron M, Cesbron JY, *et al.* Role of specific IgE antibodies in peroxidase (EPO) release from human eosinophils. *J Immunol* 1986;137:1659–1664.
26 Kroegel C, Yukawa T, Dent G, *et al.* Stimulation of degranulation from human eosinophils by platelet-activating factor. *J Immunol* 1989;142:3518–3526.
27 Anwar ARE, Walsh GM, Cromwell O, *et al.* Adhesion to fibronectin primes eosinophils via $\alpha_4\beta_1$ (VLA-4). (Submitted.)
28 Wong DT, Weller PF, Galli SJ, *et al.* Human eosinophils express transforming growth factor alpha. *J Exp Med* 1990;172:673–681.
29 Moqbel R, Hamid Q, Ying S, *et al.* Expression of mRNA and immunoreactivity for the granulocyte/macrophage colony stimulating factor (GM-CSF) in activated human eosinophils. *J Exp Med* 1991;174:749–752.
30 Kita H, Ohnishi T, Okubo Y, *et al.* GM-CSF and interleukin-3 release from human peripheral blood eosinophils and neutrophils. *J Exp Med* 1991;17:745–748.
31 Del Pozo V, De Andres B, Martin E, *et al.* Murine eosinophils and IL-1: alpha IL-1 mRNA detection by in situ hybridization. *J Immunol* 1990;144:3117–3122.
32 Braun RK, Hansel TT, Erard F, *et al.* Human peripheral blood eosinophils produce and release IL-8 on stimulation with calcium ionophore. *Eur J Immunol* 1993;23: 956–960.
33 Desreumaux P, Janin A, Colombel JF, *et al.* Interleukin 5 messenger RNA expression by eosinophils in the intestinal mucosa of patients with coeliac disease. *J Exp Med* 1992; 175:293–296.
34 Azzawi M, Johnston PW, Majumdar S, *et al.* T lymphocytes and activated eosinophils in airway mucosa in fatal asthma and cystic fibrosis. *Am Rev Respir Dis* 1992;145: 1477–1482.
35 Durham SR, Kay AB. Eosinophil, bronchial hyperreactivity and late-phase asthmatic reactions. *Clin Allergy* 1985;15:411–418.
36 Bousquet J, Chanez P, Lacoste JY, *et al.* Eosinophilic inflammation in asthma. *N Engl J Med* 1990;323:1033–1039.
37 De Monchy JGR, Kauffman HF, Venge P, *et al.* Bronchoalveolar eosinophilia during allergen-induced late asthmatic reactions. *Am Rev Respir Dis* 1985;131:373–376.

38 Diaz P, Gonzalez MC, Galleguillos FR, *et al.* Leukocytes and lipid mediators in bronchoalveolar lavage during allergen-induced late-phase asthmatic reactions. *Am Rev Respir Dis* 1989;139:1383–1839.
39 Metzger WJ, Zavala D, Richerson HB, *et al.* Local allergen challenge and bronchoalveolar lavage of allergic asthmatic lungs: description of the model and local airway inflammation. *Am Rev Respir Dis* 1987;135:433–440.
40 Lam S, LeRiche J, Phillips D, Chan-Yeung M. Cellular and protein changes in bronchial lavage fluid after late asthmatic reaction in patients with red cedar asthma. *J Allergy Clin Immunol* 1987;80:44–50.
41 Diaz P, Galleguillos FR, Gonzalez MC, *et al.* Bronchoalveolar lavage in asthma: the effect of DSCG on leukocyte counts, immunoglobulins and complement. *J Allergy Clin Immunol* 1984;74:41–48.
42 Rothenberg ME, Petersen J, Stevens RL, *et al.* IL-5 dependent conversion of normodense human eosinophils to the hypodense phenotype uses 3T3 fibroblasts for enhanced viability, accelerated hypodensity and sustained antibody-dependent cytotoxicity. *J Immunol* 1989;143:2311–2316.
43 Rothenberg ME, Owen WF, Silberstein DS, *et al.* Human eosinophils have prolonged survival, enhanced functional properties and become hypodense when exposed to human interleukin-3. *J Clin Invest* 1988;81:1986–1992.
44 Lopez AF, Williamson DJ, Gamble JR, *et al.* Recombinant human granulocyte-macrophage colony stimulating factor stimulates *in vitro* mature human eosinophil and neutrophil function, surface receptor expression and survival. *J Clin Invest* 1986;78: 1220–1228.
45 Burd PR, Rogers HW, Gordon JR, *et al.* Interleukin-3-dependent and -independent mast cells stimulated with IgE and antigen express multiple cytokines. *J Exp Med* 1989;170:245–257.
46 Howell CJ, Pujol J-L, Crea AEG, *et al.* Identification of an alveolar macrophage-derived activity in bronchial asthma that enhances leukotriene C_4 generation by human eosinophils stimulated by ionophore A23187 as a granulocyte-macrophage colony-stimulating factor. *Am Rev Respir Dis* 1989;140:1340–1347.
47 Cromwell O, Hamid Q, Corrigan CJ, *et al.* Expression and generation of IL-6, IL-8 and GM-CSF by human bronchial epithelial cells and enhancement by IL-1β and TNFα. *Immunology* 1992;77:330–337.
48 Corrigan CJ, Hartnell A, Kay AB. T lymphocyte activation in acute severe asthma. *Lancet* 1988;i:1129–1131.
49 Corrigan CJ, Kay AB. CD4 T-lymphocyte activation in acute severe asthma: relationship to disease severity and atopic status. *Am Rev Respir Dis* 1990;141:970–977.
50 Corrigan CJ, Brown PH, Barnes NC, *et al.* Glucocorticoid resistance in chronic asthma. Peripheral blood T lymphocyte activation and comparison of the T lymphocyte inhibitory effects of glucocorticoids and cyclosporin A. *Am Rev Respir Dis* 1991;144: 1026–1032.
51 Corrigan CJ, Brown PH, Barnes NC, *et al.* Glucocorticoid resistance in chronic asthma. Glucocorticoid pharmacokinetics, glucocorticoid receptor characteristics and inhibition of peripheral blood T cell proliferation by glucocorticoids *in vitro*. *Am Rev Respir Dis* 1991;144:1016–1025.
52 Walker C, Kaegi MK, Braun MD, Blaser K. Activated T cells and eosinophils in bronchoalveolar lavages from subjects with asthma correlated with disease severity. *J Allergy Clin Immunol* 1991;88:935–942.
53 Gerblich AA, Campbell AE, Schuyler MR. Changes in T-lymphocyte subpopulations after antigenic bronchial provocation in asthmatics. *N Engl J Med* 1984;310:1349–1352.
54 Broide DH, Lotz M, Cuomo AJ, *et al.* Cytokines in symptomatic asthma airways. *J Allergy Clin Immunol* 1992;89:958–967.
55 Hamid Q, Azzawi M, Ying S, *et al.* Expression of mRNA for interleukin-5 in mucosal bronchial biopsies from asthma. *J Clin Invest* 1991;87:1541–1546.
56 Robinson DS, Hamid Q, Ying S, *et al.* Predominant T_{H2}-type bronchoalveolar lavage T-lymphocyte population in atopic asthma. *N Engl J Med* 1992;326:298–304.
57 Ying S, Robinson DS, Varney V, *et al.* TNFα mRNA expression in allergic inflammation. *Clin Exp Allergy* 1991;21:745–750.

58 Walker C, Virchow J-C, Bruijnzeel PLB, Blaser K. T cell subsets and their soluble products regulate eosinophilia in allergic and non-allergic asthma. *J Immunol* 1991;146: 1829–1835.
59 Wierenga EA, Snoek M, de Groot C, *et al.* Evidence for compartmentalisation of functional subsets of CD4+ T-lymphocytes in atopic patients. *J Immunol* 1990;144: 4651–4656.
60 Kay AB, Sun Ying, Varney V, *et al.* Messenger RNA expression of the cytokine gene cluster, IL-3, IL-4, IL-5 and GM-CSF in allergen-induced late-phase cutaneous reactions in atopic subjects. *J Exp Med* 1991;173:775–778.
61 Tsicopoulos A, Hamid Q, Varney V, *et al.* Interleukin-5 (IL-5) selectively enhances the chemotactic response of eosinophils obtained from normal but not eosinophilic subjects. *J Immunol* 1992;148:2058–2061.
62 Walker C, Bode E, Boer L, *et al.* Allergic and non-allergic asthmatics have distinct patterns of T cell activation and cytokine production in peripheral blood and bronchoalveolar lavage. *Am Rev Respir Dis* 1992;146:109–115.
63 Burrows B, Martinez FD, Halonen M, *et al.* Association of asthma with serum IgE levels and skin-test reactivity to allergens. *N Engl J Med* 1989;320:271–277.
64 O'Hehir RE, Bal V, Quint D, *et al.* An *in vitro* model of allergen-dependent IgE syntheses by human B lymphocytes: comparison of the response of an atopic and a non-atopic individual to *Dermatophagoides* spp. (house dust mite). *Immunology* 1989;66: 499–504.

Recent advances in sleep apnoea

J. R. STRADLING

The main area of advance in the last few years has been the realization that obstructive sleep apnoea is brought on by several risk factors and that there is a continuum between light, intermittent snorers and the severe patient with hundreds of obstructive apnoeas. Furthermore, this continuum of disease has a limited correlation with symptom severity, so that treatment should reflect this symptom severity rather than the severity measured from a sleep study using current techniques. Another area of recent interest arises from the observation that obstructive sleep apnoea has profound effects on the cardiovascular system with evidence of increased risk of stroke and myocardial infarction. It is also increasingly recognized that heart failure can produce a sleep apnoea syndrome with disabling symptoms, easily confused with those of heart failure itself.

NEW DEFINITIONS OF SLEEP APNOEA

When sleep apnoea was first properly described it was clear the authors understood that recurrent apnoeas were leading to repeated arousals from sleep with unrefreshing sleep and hence the daytime consequence of excessive sleepiness [1]. However, sleep laboratories at that time were staging sleep in 30 second epochs, largely ignoring the hundreds of very short (often less than 10 seconds) arousals so typical of obstructive sleep apnoea. Although the classic sleep staging based on 30 second epochs becomes progressively more abnormal as sleep apnoea worsens, the usual derivatives of sleep quality may be surprisingly normal in moderate sleep apnoea.

Because apnoeas, recorded from oronasal airflow thermistors, were the first abnormality to be noted, these became the basis of the condition's definition. Based on a few recordings in normal subjects, and the arbitrary definition of an apnoea (greater than 10 seconds), a definition of the sleep apnoea syndrome was produced: more than 5 per hour of greater than 10 second apnoeas or more than 35 such apnoeas per night [2]. Classical sleep staging was required to prove sleep. This definition with minor modifications (i.e. greater than 10 or greater than 15 per hour) persisted and dominated clinical practice. The inadequacy of this approach has been revealed by a number of developments.

Aetiology

Obstructive sleep apnoea (OSA) is due to sleep-induced passive narrowing of the pharynx. Disagreements still exist over whether this collapse of the pharynx is due to some specific failure of neuromuscular function or anatomical factors (or both). Because there is *normally* a withdrawal of tonic activation of postural muscles during sleep it has been difficult to prove that there is an *abnormal* fall in pharyngeal dilator tone in patients with OSA. In some neuromuscular diseases there can be associated OSA, but there is good evidence that in most patients with OSA some of the pharyngeal dilators may actually be receiving more phasic respiratory activity than normal, perhaps trying to combat the collapse [3].

There is more evidence that anatomical factors precipitate OSA. There are many case reports of pharyngeal anatomical problems (e.g. enlarged tonsils) leading to OSA, and the factor most predictive of OSA severity is obesity. Most of the available evidence points to neck obesity being more important than general obesity [4], suggesting that mass loading of the pharynx by external pressure is the aetiological mechanism. This would fit with the evidence of *increased* phasic respiratory pharyngeal dilator tone, trying to defend the airway, which becomes inadequate when the general tonic activity is withdrawn normally during sleep. Neck obesity is associated with the pattern of upper body (or central) obesity and it is possible that the good correlation between OSA severity and neck obesity is due to other factors such as fatty infiltration of pharyngeal muscles that reduces their mechanical efficiency.

Not all OSA is due to obesity and subtle degrees of retropositioning of the mandible may contribute [5]: this pattern of jaw development may be a legacy of mouth breathing due to adenoidal nasal obstruction as an infant [6]. Other contributory factors to OSA production are alcohol consumption and a long history of increased nasal obstruction. Both hypothyroidism and acromegaly can cause OSA.

Consequences of sleep-induced upper airway obstruction

All the above factors conspire to challenge the pharynx and its ability to maintain patency during the normal reduction of tonic muscular activity of sleep. The important point is that these factors are not 'all or none', they are fully variable over a large range. Thus it is not surprising that the influence on the upper airway is not 'all or none' either, but progressive. We all experience a degree of pharyngeal narrowing with sleep onset, and snoring is the first sign that this is producing a significant

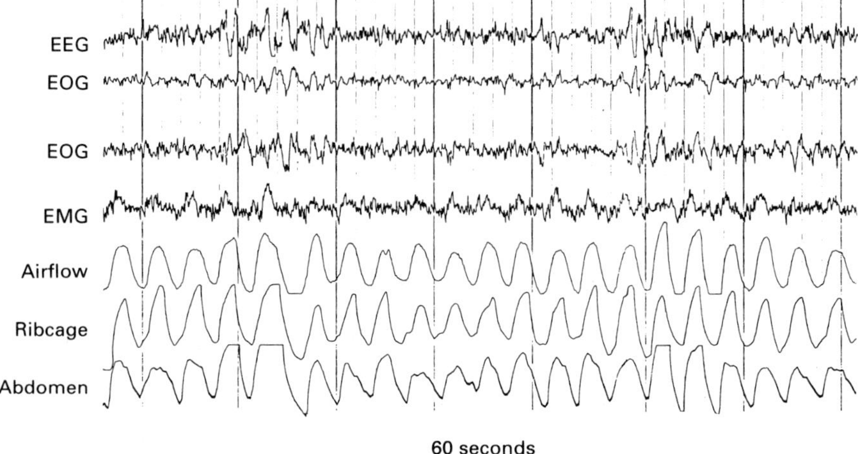

Fig. 1 Tracing from a patient with snoring-induced arousals, but no hypopnoea or apnoea (and no hypoxaemia – not shown here). A slight waxing and waning of the three respiratory traces is evident with the same cycle length as the arousals on the EEG.

increase in upper airway resistance. Initially there will be full respiratory compensation for this (at the expense of increased inspiratory effort), then hypoventilation when the compensation is inadequate, and finally complete collapse will produce apnoea. Factors such as body posture and current alcohol intake will alter the exact consequences of these longer-term underlying risk factors.

Recently it has been recognized that to generate an arousal from sleep it is not necessary to develop a full apnoea. First it was appreciated that reduced ventilation (hypopnoea) with hypoxaemia could occur and provoke recurrent arousals, and more recently that snoring alone (Fig. 1), without hypoventilation or hypoxaemia, could do the same [7,8]. This agrees with other data that the more important arousal stimulus in patients with OSA is the increased respiratory effort they make, rather than any consequential derangement of blood gases [9]. Thus snorers can generate enormous swings in pleural pressure (down to $-80\,cmH_2O$), much greater than the ventilatory effort required experimentally to arouse normal subjects. We and others have now treated patients demonstrating 'snoring-induced' arousals with nasal continuous positive airway pressure (CPAP) which abolishes their recurrent arousals and daytime sleepiness, just as it does in conventional OSA.

Because it is the recurrent sleep disruption that produces the symptoms in OSA it is now no longer appropriate simply to count apnoeas: some attempt to measure recurrent arousals and show they are due to upper airway narrowing is required.

Sleep studies in sleep-induced upper airway obstruction

From the above it will be clear that sleep studies that document apnoeas (or even apnoeas and hypopnoeas) and stage sleep using the classical, epoch-based, approach are not actually measuring the fundamental abnormality – multiple arousals due to sleep-induced upper airway narrowing. What then is the appropriate approach? The problem is that there are too many uncertainties over the relationship between the degree of sleep fragmentation and the daytime consequences. For example, following a sleep disrupting event (e.g. a noise) there are grades of arousal from nothing discernable on the electroencephalograph (EEG) (although changes in autonomic variables are present), to full wakefulness for more than 15 seconds [10]. There is evidence that recurrent arousals as short as 1.5 seconds may be important for daytime symptoms [11]. In addition, how many such events per night lead to daytime symptoms? At present one has to take a pragmatic approach to the diagnosis of OSA and its variants and use sleep study systems that somehow document the primary events of interest, recurrent brief arousals due to increases in upper airway resistance. It is likely that well over 50 such arousals per night are needed to produce symptoms.

Although full polysomnography measuring EEG, electromyograph (EMG) and eye movement, oxygen saturation and ribcage with abdominal movements can provide (if properly analysed) evidence of sleep fragmentation and upper airway obstruction, there are many other simpler ways [12]. For example, indices of sleep disruption can be derived from body movement, pulse rate changes, and blood pressure rises (Fig. 2): evidence of upper airway obstruction can be inferred from snoring, ribcage/abdominal phase angle changes (partial paradox), and blood pressure changes (pulsus paradoxus) (Fig. 2). Now the inadequacy of conventional sleep studies has been realized, the field has opened up for the use of innovative approaches to the diagnosis of OSA and its variants. The particular devices and approaches that are appropriate will also depend on the type of patient being investigated [12].

Epidemiology

This uncertainty over the definition of a 'sleep apnoea syndrome' has caused immense problems for epidemiologists. Most of the work on the epidemiology of OSA has used conventional definitions and thus the prevalence has varied with the definition (e.g. greater than 5 apnoeas per hour, greater than 10 apnoeas per hour, apnoeas plus hypopnoeas, or oxygen desaturation events) [13,14]. When the relationship between snoring and sleepiness is looked at [8] this suggests that there is much more significant pathology than when just hypoxic dips are considered

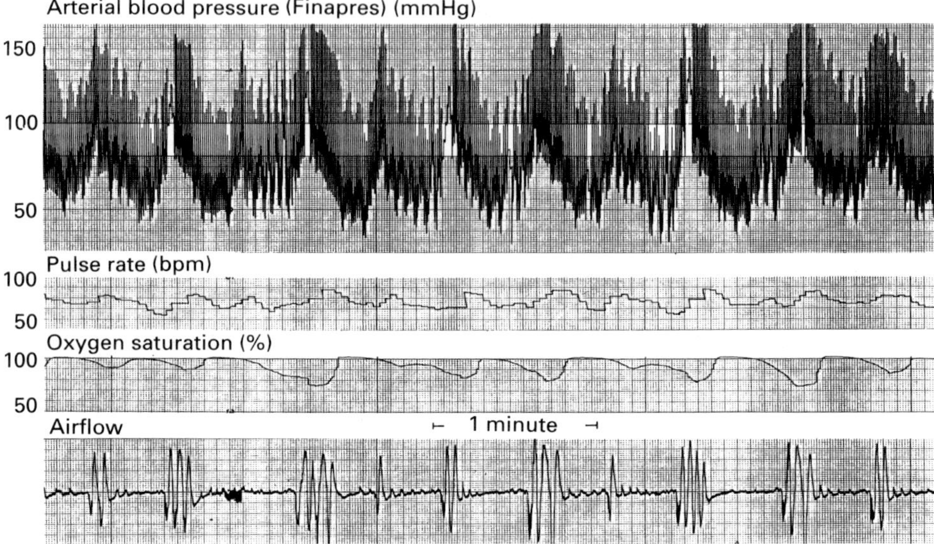

Fig. 2 Five minute tracing from a patient with obstructive sleep apnoea. The rises in blood pressure (top trace, recorded non-invasively by the Ohmeda Finapres device) and heart rate (second trace) coincide with the end of each apnoea and arousal. During each apnoea each frustrated inspiratory effort is accompanied by a fall in blood pressure (pulsus paradoxus).

(the latter suggesting a prevalence of about 3:1000 men aged 35–65 years) [14].

Conclusions

At present any unit investigating patients for possible sleep apnoea and its variants has to adopt a flexible approach. The history will reveal the impact of the symptoms on the patient's quality of life and the sleep study is used to answer the question 'is there enough sleep disruption due to upper airway problems that could explain the symptoms?' If this is the case, and the symptoms are bad enough, then a trial of nasal CPAP is warranted. Although starting a patient on nasal CPAP is currently labour intensive, there are new developments that may allow automatic titration of pressures to suit the patient.

The above decisions are qualitative and at present should not be based on unreliable indices derived from measuring the wrong variables.

CARDIOVASCULAR ASPECTS OF OBSTRUCTIVE SLEEP APNOEA

The primary reason for treating patients with OSA and its variants is the often overwhelming daytime hypersomnolence. Of particular importance is the increased rate of car accidents in these patients [15]. Recently the effects on the cardiovascular system have raised concern.

Cardiovascular mortality in obstructive sleep apnoea

There are very few long-term studies assessing any increased mortality in patients with OSA. Now that nasal CPAP is relatively easy to provide there is no longer a cohort of untreated patients. There are two retrospective studies that strongly suggest an increased mortality [16,17]. A group of patients accepting tracheostomy (the original definitive treatment) was compared with a group who refused such treatment. Thus, the groups were not matched. However, on average the tracheostomy patients had more severe OSA than those who did not and yet their cardiovascular mortality was less (Fig. 3).

The cause of this excess mortality is not clear because of problems with confounding variables. For example, obesity (particularly upper body, or central obesity) is a common risk factor for OSA and cardiovascular disease. It has been difficult to factor out these confounding variables when looking at possible links between OSA and cardiovascular death, such as hypertension, insulin resistance and lipid levels.

Although there are reasons why OSA might raise daytime blood pressures (e.g. increased catecholamine or steroid release, resetting of baroreceptors due to the nocturnal blood pressure surges), there is little evidence that this is the case, except perhaps for a short period after sleep, and in young, very obese males. Once other common variables

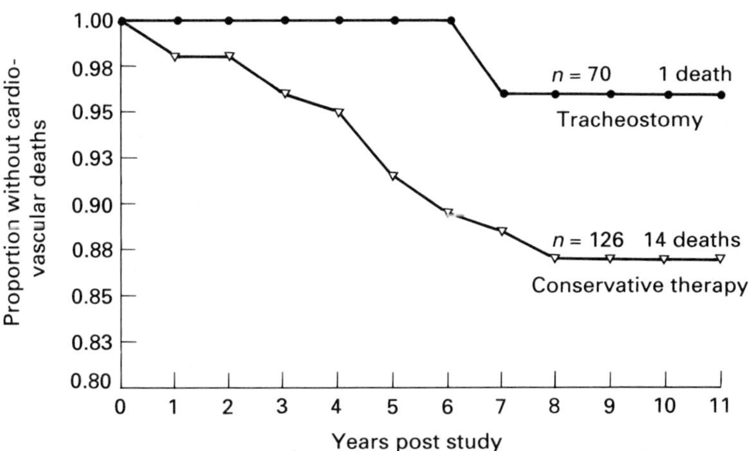

Fig. 3 Long-term survival without cardiovascular death of patients with obstructive sleep apnoea depending upon whether tracheostomy was accepted or refused by the patient. Patients not receiving tracheostomy had no specific therapy. (By permission from Partinen and Guilleminault [18].)

have been factored out, there is no good evidence that OSA is an independent risk factor for diurnal hypertension [19] or for insulin resistance or lipid levels (Stradling *et al.*, unpublished data).

It is more likely that any effect of OSA on cardiovascular mortality is through the very impressive surges in blood pressure that accompany the termination of each arousal (Fig. 2). The average rise in peak blood pressure is about 30 mmHg, but can be as large as 100 mmHg. Averaged out over the whole night this phenomenon raises *average* blood pressure compared to controls by about 8 mmHg, in itself likely to increase cardiovascular risk. It is possible, but unproven, that the hundreds of surges all night are more harmful to the cardiovascular system than the average rise of 8 mmHg would imply.

The cause of these surges in blood pressure is not clear. Initially they were thought to be due to the hypoxaemia provoking a sympathetic response. Subsequent evidence strongly suggests that they are due to the arousal itself [10,20] although other factors, such as pooling of blood in the thorax during the apnoea with release and a tachycardia on termination, may contribute.

During the obstructive apnoea there are repeated inspiratory efforts against the closed pharynx (Müller manoeuvre). These falls in intrathoracic pressure increase the preload and afterload on the heart because the heart is in the chest and subject to the same falls. Thus, the left ventricle 'sees' a higher aortic pressure and in the absence of a compensatory increase in transmyocardial pressure, the blood pressure will fall, less blood will be ejected, and end-systolic volume will increase. In conjunction with a small increase in venous return (due to the 'sucking in' effect of the subatmospheric pressures) there is pooling of blood within the thorax. The increase in venous return is not substantial because the great veins tend to collapse at the entrance to the thorax when the intrathoracic pressures fall much below the prevailing venous pressure. Overall, these increased loads on the left ventricle may be harmful, and one group has found an increased left ventricular wall thickness in patients with OSA [21] but this has not been confirmed using closely matched controls (Stradling *et al.*, unpublished data).

In conclusion it is likely that OSA does increase cardiovascular mortality and currently the most likely causes for this are the repeated surges in blood pressure associated with arousal at the end of each obstructive event.

Cheyne–Stokes respiration and heart failure

Periodic breathing as an accompaniment of left ventricular failure was recognized in the last century. More recently it has been shown to be accentuated by sleep and to produce hundreds of arousals (Fig. 4) and

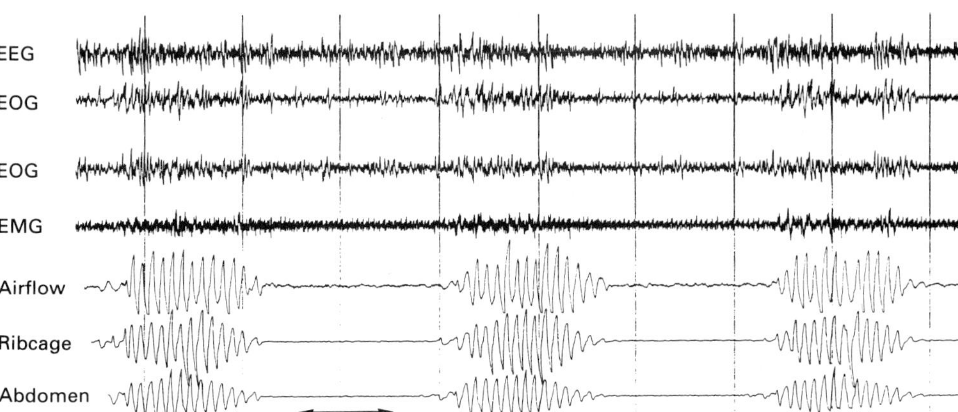

Fig. 4 Tracing of Cheyne–Stokes respiration from a patient with poor left ventricular function but no evidence of current pulmonary oedema. With each return of respiration there is arousal from sleep (not clearly visible with this compressed EEG tracing).

daytime symptoms similar to obstructive sleep apnoea [22]. The patient is sometimes aware of the hyperpnoea on arousal and this may be mistaken for paroxysmal nocturnal dyspnoea (PND). However, the hyperpnoea of Cheyne–Stokes passes within seconds whereas that of PND takes many minutes and usually the patient has to get up from bed. The daytime symptoms of sleepiness and lethargy may be blamed on the heart failure rather than sleep disruption. This may lead to an inappropriate increase in diuretic therapy, particularly so because Cheyne–Stokes respiration often occurs when there is no fluid overload.

The explanation of Cheyne–Stokes respiration in heart failure is not clear and cannot be solely explained by a prolonged circulation time. It is likely that there is extra respiratory drive from stimulation of both fast and slowly adapting lung receptors as well as bronchial C-fibres due to raised pulmonary venous pressures. There will usually be some additional hypoxaemia, and hypocapnia is usual. The interaction of these increased drives with the drive reductions of sleep onset allow bigger fluctuations in ventilation. The onset of arousal maintains the instability by constantly changing the degree of drive. There is evidence that suppressing arousal with benzodiazepines, for example, can remove periodic respiration. It is not clear if the return of ventilation produces arousal, or if arousal provokes the return of ventilation. Both situations can probably occur.

It has been suggested that this periodic breathing contributes to poor cardiac function and that abolishing it will improve function. Only one group has been able to show this by using nasal CPAP [23,24]. Most of the original patients probably had some additional obstructive component to their periodic respiration and resolution of this was probably the reason for their improvement. Other treatments that may abolish Cheyne–Stokes respiration in heart failure include acetazolamide, theophyllines and added oxygen, the latter being the more successful to date. The variability of response to these agents indicates that the exact pathogenesis probably varies from patient to patient. If treatment is successful in abolishing the nocturnal Cheyne–Stokes respiration and consequent sleep disruption, then the improvement in many of the symptoms can be dramatic.

REFERENCES

1 Gastaut H, Tassinari CA, Duron B. Etude polygraphique des manifestations episodiques (hypniques et repiratoires), diurnes et nocturnes, du syndrome de Pickwick. *Rev Neurol* 1965;112:568–579.

2 Guilleminault C, Tilkian A, Dement WC. The sleep apnoea syndromes. *Ann Rev Med* 1976;27:465–484.

3 Suratt PM, McTier RF, Wilhoit SC. Upper airway muscle activation is augmented in patients with obstructive sleep apnoea compared with that in normal subjects. *Am Rev Respir Dis* 1988;137:889–894.

4 Davies RJ, Stradling JR. The relationship between neck circumference, radiographic pharyngeal anatomy, and the obstructive sleep apnoea syndrome. *Eur Respir J* 1990; 3:509–514.

5 Riley R, Guilleminault C, Herran J, Powell N. Cephalometric analyses and flow-volume loops in obstructive sleep apnoea patients. *Sleep* 1983;6:303–311.

6 Guilleminault C, Quera-Salva MA. Obstructive sleep apnoea: is prevention ever possible? *Eur Respir J Suppl* 1990;11:539s–542s.

7 Guilleminault C, Stoohs R, Duncan S. Snoring (I). Daytime sleepiness in regular heavy snorers. *Chest* 1991;99:40–48.

8 Stradling JR, Crosby JH, Payne CD. Self-reported snoring and daytime sleepiness in men aged 35–65 years. *Thorax* 1991;46:807–810.

9 Gleeson K, Zwillich CW, White DP. The influence of increasing ventilatory effort on arousal from sleep. *Am Rev Respir Dis* 1990;142:295–300.

10 Davies RJO, Belt PJ, Robert SJ, *et al.* Arterial blood pressure responses to graded transient arousal from sleep in normal humans. *J Appl Physiol* 1993;74:1123–1130.

11 Cheshire K, Engleman H, Deary I, *et al.* Factors impairing daytime performance in patients with the sleep apnoea/hypopnoea syndrome. *Arch Intern Med* 1992;152:538–541.

12 Stradling JR. Sleep studies for sleep-related breathing disorders. A consensus report. *J Sleep Res* 1992;1:223–230.

13 Gislason T, Almqvist M, Eriksson G, *et al.* Prevalence of sleep apnea syndrome among Swedish men–an epidemiological study. *J Clin Epidemiol* 1988;41:571–576.

14 Stradling JR, Crosby JH. Predictors and prevalence of obstructive sleep apnoea and snoring in 1001 middle aged men. *Thorax* 1991;46:85–90.

15 Stradling JR. Obstructive sleep apnoea and driving. *Br Med J* 1989;298:904–905.

16 Partinen M, Guilleminault C. Daytime sleepiness and vascular morbidity at seven-year follow-up in obstructive sleep apnea patients. *Chest* 1990;97:27–32.

17 He J, Kryger MH, Zorick FJ, *et al.* Mortality and apnea index in obstructive sleep apnea. Experience in 385 male patients. *Chest* 1988;94:9–14.

18 Partinen M, Guilleminault C. Evalution of obstructive sleep apnea syndrome. In: Guilleminault C, Partinen M, eds. *Obstructive Sleep Apnea Syndrome*. New York: Raven Press, 1990:19 (Chapter 3).

19 Stradling JR. Systemic hypertension and sleep apnoea. In Gaultier C, Escourrou P, Curzi-Dascalova L, eds. *Sleep and Cardiorespiratory Control*. Montrouge: John Libbey Eurotext, 1991:115–122.

20 Ali NJ, Davies RJO, Fleetham JA, Stradling JR. The acute effects of continuous positive airway pressure and oxygen administration on blood pressure during obstructive sleep apnoea. *Chest* 1992;101:1526–1532.
21 Hedner J, Ejnell H, Caidahl K. Left ventricular hypertrophy independent of hypertension in patients with obstructive sleep apnoea. *J Hypertens* 1990;8:941–946.
22 Hanly PJ, Millar TW, Steljes DG, *et al.* Respiration and abnormal sleep in patients with congestive heart failure. *Chest* 1989;96:480–488.
23 Takasaki Y, Orr D, Popkin J, *et al.* Effect of nasal continuous positive airway pressure on sleep apnoea in congestive heart failure. *Am Rev Respir Dis* 1989;140:1578–1584.
24 Davies RJO, Harrington KJ, Ormerod OJM, Stradling JR. Nasal continuous positive airway pressure in chronic heart failure with sleep disordered breathing. *Am Rev Respir Dis* 1993;147:630–634.

Current status of lung transplantation

P. CORRIS

INTRODUCTION

The modern era for lung transplantation began in 1981 when Reitz *et al.* from Stanford University introduced heart lung transplantation for patients with pulmonary vascular disease [1]. Indications for combined heart and lung transplants (HLT) were subsequently widened to include various pulmonary conditions [2]. Survival rates were good and in marked contrast with results obtained for single lung transplantation over the preceding 25 years [3]. The success of HLT was based on reliable healing of the tracheal anastomosis compared with the bronchial anastomotic breakdown seen frequently following single lung transplantation (SLT). This reliable healing reflected a good blood supply to the proximal donor trachea via donor coronary artery/bronchial artery anastomoses, in contrast to the lack of blood supplied to the proximal donor bronchus following transplantation of a single lung. The initial lack of success with SLT was also based on both poor selection of potential recipients, many of whom were moribund with multiorgan failure, and the apparently insuperable problems of rejection and infection.

It was realized that many patients undergoing HLT, however, received a new heart unnecessarily. After a period of research success was achieved with SLT in patients with fibrosing lung disease by the Toronto Group in 1983 [4].

Success was related to careful patient selection, restoration of a viable blood supply to the bronchial anastomosis by wrapping it with a pedicle of greater omentum and the introduction of cyclosporin A as the principal immunosuppressant. It has been shown subsequently that the bronchial anastomosis does not require a wrap of omentum for reliable healing and very few centres now perform this procedure, although the Harefield Group are now carrying out bronchial artery anastomoses to ensure good blood supply to the donor bronchus.

In 1988 the double lung transplant operation (DLT) using an *en bloc* transplantation of both lungs with a tracheal anastomosis was introduced by Patterson *et al.* [5]. This procedure was, however, accompanied by much more frequent problems with airway healing than the HLT operation [6]. In addition, the operation was, if anything, more complex than HLT and the extensive mediastinal resection frequently led to denervation of the recipient's native heart. Bleeding was at least as great a problem as for HLT, and by 1989 the procedure as originally described had been largely abandoned. Noirclerc [7] provided the solution to the problem of airway healing by performing two separate bronchial anastomoses, since as in SLT, the donor bronchus is better vascularized with the anastomosis close to the lung parenchyma.

This concept was further developed by Pasque [8] with the bilateral sequential single lung transplant. As its name implies, two separated lungs are implanted with separate hilar anastomoses (each of bronchus, pulmonary artery and left atrial cuff). The heart and mediastinum are left largely undisturbed. The incision is a transverse bilateral thoracotomy, dividing the sternum horizontally.

PATIENT SELECTION

Indications (Figs 1 and 2)

Restrictive lung disease

Chronic fibrotic lung disease, especially idiopathic pulmonary fibrosis, provides an ideal indication for SLT [4]. The transplanted lung receives preferential perfusion and ventilation, because it is more compliant and has a lower vascular resistance than the native lung. By the time of assessment for transplantation most patients are hypoxic and dependent upon supplemental oxygen. Lung function in the first 40 patients accepted for transplantation in Newcastle had a mean FEV_1 (forced expiratory volume in 1 second) of 38% predicted, mean vital capacity (VC) of 35%

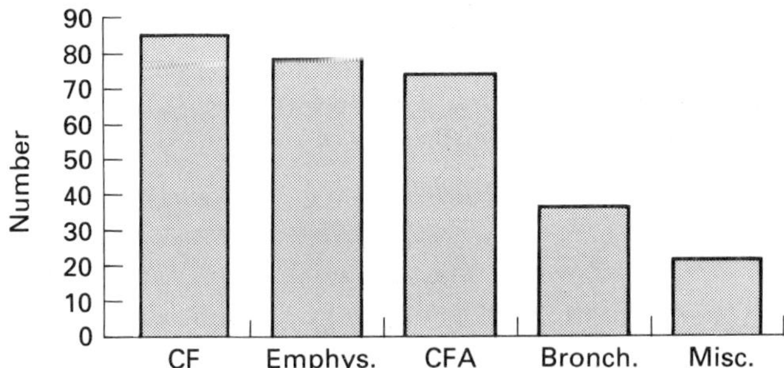

Fig. 1 Diagnoses of patients with lung disease assessed for pulmonary transplantation, Freeman Hospital 1987–92. CF, Cystic fibrosis; CFA, chronic fibrosing alveolitis; Emphys., emphysema; Bronch., bronchiectasis; Misc., miscellaneous.

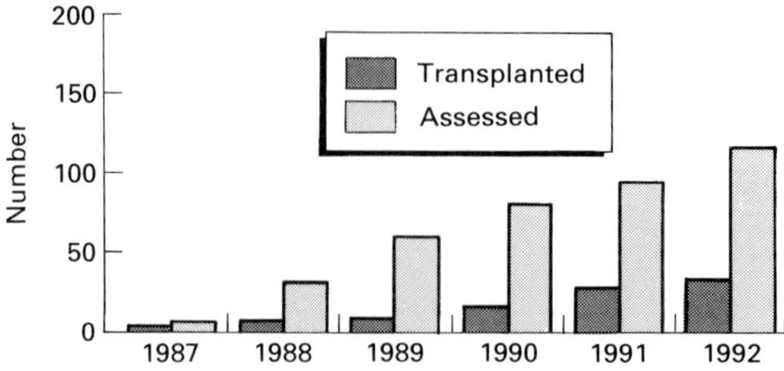

Fig. 2 Pulmonary transplantation, Freeman Hospital. Patients assessed and transplanted.

predicted and a mean diffusing capacity using the single breath method of 30% predicted.

Other restrictive lung diseases such as fibrotic sarcoidosis may also be successfully treated using SLT.

Obstructive lung disease

Patients with emphysema form an important group requiring lung transplantation. These patients are usually ex-smokers and approximately 40% are homozygous for α-1-antitrypsin deficiency. α-1-Antitrypsin is the polymorphic glycoprotein responsible for the majority of anti-protease activity in the serum. This deficiency leads to a lack of protection against neutrophil elastase in the lung. Homozygous transmission (PiZZ) is characterized by the onset of dyspnoea in the third or fourth decade with the development of progressive, predominantly basal emphysema. Earlier reports of SLT in patients with emphysema suggested that such patients were not suitable for this operation, since the native lung developed marked over-expansion leading to compression of the transplanted lung during positive pressure ventilation in the early post-operative period. With careful patient selection, ensuring that one does not leave a native lung with a large ventilated bulla, and with improved methods of lung preservation SLT can now be undertaken for patients with emphysema, which has become the most frequent indication for this operation [9].

Suppurative lung disease

With improvements in the management of cystic fibrosis, 80% of children with this disease reach adulthood. Because of the bilateral sepsis both lungs need replacement. Combined heart lung transplantation has been undertaken for this disease, using the 'domino procedure' when a standard heart lung transplant is combined with the donation of the recipient's heart for transplantation in another recipient [10]. More recently most patients with cystic fibrosis have been transplanted using the bilateral sequential single lung transplant since concomitant cardiac replacement is unnecessary in these patients. Patients with bronchiectasis form a small but significant further group who benefit from lung transplantation.

Pulmonary vascular disease

This category includes patients with primary pulmonary hypertension (PPH) and secondary pulmonary hypertension as a consequence of congenital heart disease. PPH is a disease predominantly affecting females of the third and fourth decades of life. Prognosis is variable but most patients are dead within 5 years of diagnosis. The initial approach has been to carry out HLT. However, recent clinical and laboratory experiences suggested that right ventricular function recovers following isolated lung transplantation and SLT has been successfully carried out in these patients [11]. Patients with PPH due to volume overload from left to right shunt form a large group of patients requiring lung transplantation. These patients are usually recognized once Eisenmenger's syndrome has developed. Some patients have had previous palliative or corrective surgery and usually require HLT. Patients with correctable congenital defects like patent ductus arteriosus have undergone SLT with simultaneous correction of the defect [12].

Indications and general selection criteria for lung transplantation

The shortfall in suitable donor organs leads to an upper age limit of 50 years for transplantation for heart and lungs or both lungs alone, and an upper age limit of 60 years for transplantation for single lung. Transplantation is usually considered for a patient when estimated life expectancy is less than 18 months. Since a majority of patients with lung disease lack features which permit accurate prediction of survival, estimates are based on the current lung function, the rate of decline over previous years and the date of onset of cor pulmonale.

Lung function in patients with different lung diseases who have been accepted for transplantation in Newcastle is shown in Table 1.

In patients with cystic fibrosis or bronchiectasis, an increased number of hospital admissions for infective exacerbations or progressive weight loss is a further guide to deterioration which may predate an accelerated loss of lung function. The early unsuccessful transplant recipients were all bed bound and the majority of transplant centres now require recipients to be capable of self-care and able to participate in gentle exercise rehabilitation to maintain muscle bulk and physical fitness. Ideally recipients should be within 15 kg of ideal body weight and there

Table 1 Lung function in patients accepted for transplantation in Newcastle (results for group expressed as mean)

	FEV_1 per cent predicted	VC	Diffusing capacity (single breath)
Pulmonary fibrosis	38	35	30
Emphysema	22	48	29
Cystic fibrosis	20	33	39
Bronchiectasis	23	39	47

is an increased mortality in adult patients whose body weight is less than 40 kg. Systemic diseases especially with involvement of hepatic and renal systems are contraindications for surgery. Renal dysfunction limits the use of cyclosporin. It is important to be aware of hepatic dysfunction in patients with cystic fibrosis and α-1-antitrypsin deficiency. Diabetes mellitus is not a contraindication. The presence of a subpleural aspergilloma remains a contraindication due to the risk of developing a fungal empyema post-transplant. Previous surgery is a relative contraindication as mortality due to significant haemorrhage is higher. However, the use of aprotinin and the development of bilateral sequential lung transplantation via the transverse bilateral thoracotomy has reduced this risk and made surgery safer for patients who have had previous thoracotomies.

Selection criteria for lung transplantation are given in Table 2.

Matching donor to recipient

Donor matching is based on ABO compatibility and lung size using the predicted total lung capacity of both donor and recipient. The screening lymphocytotoxic crossmatch using recipient serum and a bank pool of lymphocytes is carried out in all potential recipients accepted for transplantation to exclude the presence of preformed antibodies. A direct crossmatch using lymphocytes from the potential donor is only carried

Table 2 Selection criteria for lung transplant recipients

Age less than 50 years for HLT and DLT
less than 60 years for SLT
Life expectancy less than 18 months
No significant impairment of renal or hepatic function
No significant coronary artery disease (SLT and bilateral sequential lung transplantation only)
Psychological stability and ability to comply with medication
No evidence of other progressive systemic disease
Preserved nutritional state when patients not moribund

out prospectively when the screening test is positive. Wherever possible donor and recipient are matched for cytomegalovirus (CMV) status. If a CMV negative recipient receives a CMV positive organ, serious CMV infection can be ameliorated by giving prophylactic CMV hyperimmune globulin.

Immunosuppression

No HLA matching of donor and recipient is possible and hence all patients require immunosuppression for life. At present patients receive azathioprine, rabbit antithymocyte globulin, methylprednisolone and cyclosporin during the immediate postoperative period. Antithymocyte globulin is stopped after 3 days and methylprednisolone substituted by oral prednisolone in a rapidly tailing-off dose to a maintenance of 0.1–0.2 mg per kg. If patients are well at 6 months maintenance steroids are withdrawn. Rejection episodes are treated with pulsed methylprednisolone 10 mg per kg for 3 days followed by augmented oral prednisolone for 1 month. Patients who do not respond to methylprednisolone may be given murine monoclonal antibody directed against T cells (OKT3) intravenously over 7–10 days.

RESULTS OF TRANSPLANTATION

Rehabilitation of patients following successful surgery is excellent with restoration of a normal lifestyle with little or no functional restriction. Maximum exercise performance as measured by maximum oxygen consumption, however, is generally reduced compared with the predicted values. The overall 1 year survival following lung transplantation lies between 60 and 70% at 1 year falling to 40% at 5 years. Figure 3 shows actuarial survival for the first 100 patients receiving lung transplantation at Freeman Hospital.

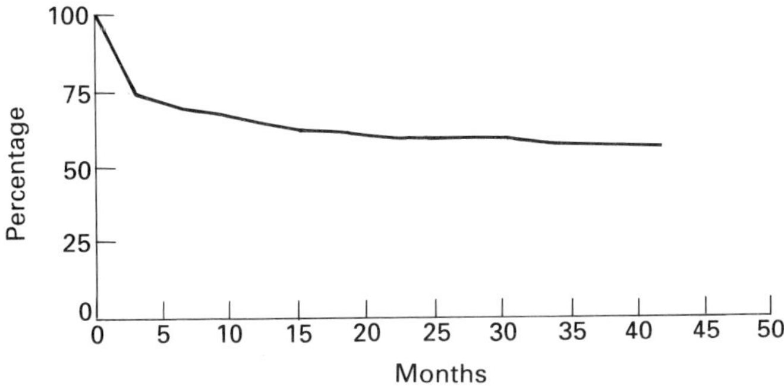

Fig. 3 Pulmonary transplant survival curve, Freeman Hospital (n = 100).

Although recurrence of disease in transplanted lungs remains a worry, there is to date no published evidence to suggest that this has caused clinical problems. Granulomas have developed in the transplanted lungs of patients with sarcoidosis. There have been no reports of recurrent fibrosing alveolitis, emphysema or primary pulmonary hypertension. The abnormally high bioelectric mucosal potential difference, which is a characteristic abnormality in the respiratory mucosa of patients with cystic fibrosis, is not seen in the lungs following heart–lung transplantation for this condition.

Medical complications post transplantation

The main medical complications following lung transplantation comprise opportunistic pneumonia, acute and chronic lung rejection. Acute lung rejection and opportunistic pneumonia may present with identical clinical features. The development of breathlessness, fever, radiological infiltrates or sustained falls in pulmonary function indicate the need for fibreoptic bronchoscopy with transbronchial lung biopsy and bronchoalveolar lavage to enable a definitive diagnosis. The characteristic histological features of acute lung rejection comprise perivascular T-lymphocyte infiltrates which may extend into adjacent alveolar walls [12].

Chronic rejection and obliterative bronchiolitis (OB)

Obliterative bronchiolitis is the probable manifestation of chronic rejection in pulmonary transplants. This is the commonest cause of morbidity and mortality in late survivors and occurs in 20–40% of patients. The symptoms are increasing shortness of breath and recurrent productive cough. There is a progressive fall in FEV_1. Transbronchial biopsy demonstrates a peribronchial infiltrate of mononuclear cells accompanied by plugging of internal bronchioles with granulation tissue. Frequent episodes of acute rejection which persist are linked to the development of OB [13]. The early identification of patients at risk of OB is the subject of much intense research and we have recently shown that those patients who experience episodes of organizing pneumonia are at subsequent risk of OB.

Post-transplant lymphoproliferative disease

Lymphoproliferative disease is the third commonest cause of death in heart–lung transplant recipients with an incidence of 8% [14]. The aetiology of most lymphoproliferative disease is Epstein–Barr virus related oncogenesis. Two forms of this disease exist. An early form presents within the first year of transplantation with a nodal or localized disease. This carries a better prognosis as it responds to lowering of immunosuppression and acyclovir. The late form usually presents with disseminated disease and is resistant to treatment.

CONCLUSION

Lung transplantation now offers an effective therapy for patients with end-stage pulmonary disease. Debate remains as to which procedure should be offered to each disease entity. The major problems facing lung transplantation at this time comprise a shortfall in suitable donor organs compared with the number of potential recipients and for this reason we do not advocate that patients on an active waiting list should be intubated with a view to chronic ventilation. In the early postoperative period, opportunist infection and graft rejection remain major problems.

REFERENCES

1 Reitz BA, Wallwork J, Hunter SA, *et al.* Heart lung transplantation: A successful therapy for patients with pulmonary vascular disease. *N Engl J Med* 1982;306:557–563.
2 Penketh A, Higgenbottam T, Hakim M, Wallwork J. Heart and lung transplantation for patients with end-stage lung disease. *Br Med J* 1987;295:311–314.
3 Wildevwer COH, Benfield JR. A review of 23 lung transplantations by 20 surgeons. *An Thorac Surg* 1972;9:489–515.
4 Cooper JD, Ginsberg RJ, Goldbrough M. Toronto Lung Transplant Group 1986– Unilateral lung transplantation for pulmonary fibrosis. *N Engl J Med* 1986;314:1140–1145.
5 Patterson GA, Cooper JD, Dark JH, *et al.* Experimental and clinical double lung transplantation. *J Thorac Cardiovasc Surg* 1988;95:70–74.
6 Patterson GA, Todd TR, Cooper JD, *et al.* Airway complications after double lung transplantation. *J Thorac Cardiovasc Surg* 1990;99:14–21.
7 Noirclerc M, Chazalette JP, Metra D. Les transplantations bi-pulmonaire; rapport de la première observation Français; et commentaires des cinq suivantes. *Annal Chirugeri* 1989;43:497–600.
8 Pasque M, Cooper JD, Kaiser LR, *et al.* Improved technique for bilateral lung transplantation: rationale and initial clinical experience. *An Thorac Surg* 1990;49: 785–791.
9 Cooper JD. Current status of lung transplantation. *Transplant Proc* 1991;23:2107–2114.
10 Yacoub MH, Bonner NR, Khaghani A, *et al.* Heart lung transplantation for cystic fibrosis and subsequent domino heart transplantation. *J Heart Transplant* 1990;9(5): 459–467.
11 Freems SD, Patterson GA, Williams WG, *et al.* Single lung transplantation and closure of patent ductus arteriosis for Eisenmenger's syndrome. *J Thorac Cardiovasc Surg* 1990;1001:1–5.
12 Billingham ME, Carey NRB, Hammond ME, *et al.* A working formulation for the standardisation of nomenclature in the diagnosis of heart and lung rejection. *J Heart Transplant* 1990;9(6):587–593.
13 Scott JP, Higgenbottam TW, Sharple L, *et al.* Risk factors for obliterative bronchiolitis in heart lung transplant recipients. *Transplantation* 1991;51:813–817.
14 Armitage JM, Kormos RL, Scott J, *et al.* Post transplant lymphoproliferative disease in thoracic organ transplantations: 10 years of cyclosporin based immunosuppression. *J Heart Transplant* 1991;10(6):877–887.

Occupational asthma, clinical and epidemiological features

P. S. BURGE

DEFINITION AND DIAGNOSIS OF OCCUPATIONAL ASTHMA

Different groups define occupational asthma in substantially different ways. The differences mainly relate to restrictions on the mechanism involved and the presence of pre-existing asthma. The most restrictive definition requires an allergic mechanism and no pre-existing asthma. This excludes many small molecular weight chemicals in which the specific immunoglobulin E (IgE) antibodies have not been found but where the disease appears identical to those where antibodies have been found (i.e. the acid anhydrides). This applies for instance to colophony, the principal cause of occupational asthma in electronic soldering flux. Colophony is one of the most commonly recognized causes of occupational asthma in the UK. It affects only a proportion of similarly exposed workers, some of whom exhibit extreme sensitivity to very small exposures. These are the usual features of an allergic reaction. Some groups exclude individuals with pre-existing asthma. Around 20% of children in the UK can be diagnosed prospectively as having asthma. This, however, is recalled by less than 5% at a pre-employment medical. The exclusion of those who may have pre-existing asthma is not therefore useful clinically. Even in those workers who have asthma at the time of first employment, a worker with no disability can be turned into a worker whose health and livelihood is threatened by the development of sensitization to an occupational allergen. The disease in those with pre-existing asthma is identical to those who have developed occupational asthma for the first time. The steps necessary to control the disease in the affected worker, and the steps necessary to prevent further cases in work colleagues, are also the same. It is, however, less easy to attribute residual disability, which is largely a legal rather than a clinical problem.

Most groups exclude chemicals which are thought to act principally as irritants from agents responsible for occupational asthma. Sulphur dioxide is one example. However, it can induce an asthmatic attack which is clinically identical to that induced by a sensitizing agent. It should, however, be much easier to control, as subsequent reactions should not occur at very low concentrations. Some definitions require a minimum fall in lung function following exposure, such as a 20% fall in the forced expiratory volume in 1 second (FEV_1) [1]. This definition will exclude those with smaller irritant reactions. There are, however, a group of symptomatic workers who improve away from the workplace, but whose fall in FEV_1 is smaller than 20%. There is no agreement as to the diagnosis in this situation, for which there may be several causes. Some have true occupational sensitization, but their exposure to the offending agent is very small, because good respiratory protection is used [2]. In some individuals with severe occupational asthma, repeated exposures have led to a state of relatively fixed airways obstruction, with little further deterioration on exposure. If such workers are removed from exposure for some weeks, considerable improvement (such as a doubling in FEV_1) can occur [3,4]. Subsequent re-exposure often results in large reactions, typical of 'ordinary' occupational asthma. Some workers with smoking related chronic obstructive airways disease have small decreases in lung function at work, which may be due to irritation in a susceptible group [5]. Finally there are some workers who have large falls in lung function over a period of days or weeks at work, but very small decreases on any one day. Some of these are exposed to agents such as formaldehyde, which is both an irritant and a sensitizer [6].

Definition

In Great Britain the Industrial Injuries Advisory Council defines occupational asthma as asthma which develops after a variable period of symptomless exposure to a sensitizing agent at work [7], and defines a limited list of sensitizing agents which can be compensated. Some limited occupational groups can be compensated; i.e. colophony asthma, when the colophony is inhaled as part of an electronic soldering flux but not when it is inhaled as part of a hot melt glue. The justification for this is obscure. Any other agent is potentially able to be compensated under the recent revision, but requires individual proof.

In practice, the mechanism for an individual's occupational asthma is often speculative. Indeed the agent is often not clearly defined although the circumstances of exposure can usually be defined more precisely. The Shield surveillance scheme for occupational asthma [8] asks doctors reporting cases to identify the mechanism which they think is responsible. The mechanism was thought to be allergic in 56%, irritant in 18%, pharmacological in 1% and unknown in the remaining 25%.

Diagnosis

The diagnosis of occupational asthma should be considered in all workers with symptoms suggestive of airways obstruction. As the disease is common in elderly smokers, bronchitis rather than asthma is often the first diagnosis. All workers should be asked whether their symptoms improve on days away from work or on holiday; those with occupational asthma will be found amongst the positive responders. The more severe occupational asthmas take longer than a weekend away from work to show improvement. However, holiday improvement is less specific as domestic causes of airways obstruction may also be avoided at this time. Once occupational asthma is suspected a full occupational history should be taken. Those still at work should have serial measurements of peak expiratory flow measured 2 hourly for a period of 4 weeks in the first instance, with the daily maximum, mean and minimum peak flow plotted in a standard manner [3,9,10]. The precise cause can sometimes be inferred by making readings in various parts of a workplace, or, when the agent is suitable, by finding specific IgE antibodies to the offending agents (such as acid anhydrides, flour, enzymes, etc.). Bronchial provocation testing is the gold standard test [11].

EPIDEMIOLOGY

The prevalence and incidence of occupational asthma has usually been studied in individual work forces when problems have been identified. There are several industries where an incidence of at least 5% is found, such as workers exposed to western red cedar or isocyanates [12,13]. There are a few industries where more than 50% of the exposed workers develop occupational asthma. This particularly applies to platinum salts [14] and in workers exposed to high concentrations of detergent enzymes [15]. These latter groups show that given the right levels of exposure to the right materials the majority of the working population are predisposed to develop asthma. There is substantially more doubt about how common occupational asthma is in general. It has been estimated at 2–15% of the adult asthmatic population [16,17]. Population data have improved in the last 2 years in Finland and in the UK. In Finland, occupational asthma is now a prescribed disease based on clinical diagnosis of the reporting doctor. They have an annual incidence of 1:27 500 of the general working population [18].

The Shield surveillance scheme has been run by the Midlands Thoracic Society for the last 4 years, in a region of 5.1 million total population, and a working population of 2.2 million [8]. Cases are notified by chest physicians, medical boarding centre (Respiratory Diseases) assessors and some occupational physicians on the basis of

Table 1 Incidence of occupational asthma by occupational group from Shield

	Incidence per million per year
General working population	43
Paint sprayers	1833
Rubber and plastics	1054
Electroplaters	1000
Foundry core makers and moulders	467
Bakery workers	445
Chemical processing workers	143
Machine tool operators	140
Carpenters	130
Solderers	112
Farmers	44
Clerks	8

most likely diagnosis. An annual incidence of 43 per million of the general working population was found. Surveillance of Work and Occupational Respiratory Diseases (SWORD) is a national (UK) reporting scheme organized by the British Thoracic Society and the Society of Occupational Medicine [19]. All types of occupational lung disease are reported, but occupational asthma is the most commonly recognized. It has been shown that the incidence of occupational asthma varies widely over the country and appears to be related to the presence of a trained occupational respiratory allergist rather than to the nature of the local industry. The incidence varies widely between the different occupations. Some examples in the West Midlands are shown in Table 1.

Causes

Isocyanates are the usual cause for occupational asthma in paint sprayers. Two pack polyurethane paints, which are widely used in small garages for car body repairs, and also for spraying aircraft which do not fit into spray booths, are a particular problem. Control is difficult and involves attention to detail, particularly the wearing of air-fed respiratory protection with an inlet well removed from the extract of the spray booth. Respiratory protection is also needed for paint mixing. Some become sensitized from incidental exposure, such as from touching up done in an open workshop.

Rubber and plastics workers are a mixed occupational group, where isocyanates are again the most common sensitizing agent. Isocyanates are released during the moulding of polyurethanes and foam production and cutting. Other responsible agents in this group include epoxy resin curing agents, acrylics and latex, as well as less clearly defined mould releasing agents.

The electroplating industry has its origins in the West Midlands, which also accounts for the number of cases (but not the incidence) seen in Shield. Electroplaters are commonly exposed to a variety of agents including strong acids, chrome, nickel, copper, cadmium and silver. Chrome sensitization seems to be the principal problem in this group.

Castings in foundries have an outer case of compressed sand. If the casting is to be hollow a more firmly bound sand core must be fixed into the mould before molten metal is poured in. These cores are bound by a variety of different resins including furanes and formaldehyde (hot box), and isocyanates with amines (cold box). All are capable of causing occupational asthma. Again the isocyanates appear to cause the most problems.

Bakery workers are the group most often diagnosed as having occupational asthma in most European countries. Flour is the most common allergen. Some workers are additionally sensitized to amylase, a natural constituent but sometimes also an added constituent of flour [20]. A few bakers are sensitized to amylase but not to flour. There has been controversy about the role of storage mites in bakers' asthma, but positive radio-allergosorbent tests (RASTs) or skin tests to them probably mainly represent cross-reactions to the common house-dust mite, *Dermatophagoides pteronyssinus* [21]. The storage mites are likely to be a specific sensitizing agent in some farmers and grain handlers. Bread is very different in different countries. It is unclear whether the lower incidence in the UK is due to different methods of bread making, to our greater reliance on mass-production large bakeries where environmental control is more organized, or to our failure to provide good medical care to a group who mostly work during the night.

Machine tool workers are exposed to aerosols of coolant oils. These are not a very potent cause of asthma, but exposure levels (and the occupational exposure standard) are often relatively high. Reactions may be to constituents of the clean oil, or to contaminants in used oil, which often contain significant amounts of microorganisms and endotoxins, as well as dissolved metals [22]. The use of coolant oils necessitates the production of an aerosol to cool and lubricate the cutting tool.

The risk for carpenters varies greatly with the type of work and the type of wood used. Western red cedar is one of the world's most commonly recognized causes of occupational asthma [12]. It is relatively uncommon in the UK as little is processed here. Hardwoods cause more problems than softwoods. To gain access to the lungs the particle size must be small. It is therefore more of a problem for carpenters working in workshops with sanding machines than those sawing on building sites.

The risk for solderers is relatively small, which is surprising since colophony, in electronic soldering flux, is the third most commonly identified cause of occupational asthma [23]. Many of those sensitized to colophony are not solderers themselves, but are incidentally exposed from nearby flow solder machines, or from extractors from soldering irons which return the extracted air through filters into the general factory air. Acid fluxes used in plumbing are a much rarer cause of occupational asthma [24].

Farmers are rarely identified as having occupational asthma in the UK, although they are the group most commonly affected in Finland [18]. It is likely that occupational asthma in farmers is particularly underreported. Some of the differences between Finland and the UK may be due to different agricultural practices, particularly the large-scale farming often practised in the UK. There are many possible causes. Pig farmers have more asthma than dairy farmers [25], but the causative agent has not yet been clearly identified. Asthma during harvest, particularly due to harvest mould such as *Didymella* and *Alternaria*, may affect up to 30% of harvesters [26,27]. Mites in stored grain, and those infesting chicken, can cause problems [28,29]. The role of agrochemicals is unclear.

There are now over 300 recognized causes of occupational asthma divided into two main groups: those that are complete antigens and small molecular weight chemicals. The most important feature of both is that they should be in a form capable of inhalation; whether they only need to reach the nose or whether they need to reach the bronchi is not clear. There are groups of substances amongst the small molecular weight chemicals which seem to be particularly liable to cause occupational asthma. Many of these bind to body proteins and often alter their tertiary structure so that there is carrier specificity of the antigen. This particularly applies to the acid anhydrides and isocyanates, where there is some cross-reactivity between chemically dissimilar haptens [30,31]. Both of these are adhesives; several other adhesives, such as colophony [23] and acrylics [32] also cause occupational asthma, but their mechanisms have so far not been determined. Some agents bind to proteins such as reactive dyes [33], whilst others denature proteins. This applies particularly to a wide range of chemically unrelated sterilizing agents, i.e. formaldehyde [34], glutaraldehyde [35], chloramine T [36], ethylene oxide [37], isothiazolinone [38] and chlorhexidine [39]. A number of metals are also responsible for occupational asthma; they may also bind to proteins and alter their tertiary structure. Amongst these are chrome, nickel, zinc, cobalt and possibly vanadium, where some cross-reactivity may occur [40]. Platinum salts, which must be charged to cause sensitization, are some of the most potent causes of occupational asthma known [41].

SMOKING AND OCCUPATIONAL ASTHMA

One of the 'surprises' from SWORD and Shield is the finding that occupational asthma is principally recognized in older men. There is now substantial evidence that smoking enhances the production of specific IgE in an occupational setting, and smoking also increases the prevalence of occupational asthma. The enhancement of specific IgE production was first shown in pharmaceutical workers exposed to ispaghula and in a coffee roastery (where green coffee beans are the principal allergen) [42]. In this study a relative risk of 3–4 was found for smokers against non-smokers. Similar results have been found with workers exposed to prawn antigens [43], humidifier antigens [44], and acid anhydrides [45]. There is a suggestion that the cigarette smoking must take place at the time of occupational exposure and that workers who have given up smoking before they are occupationally exposed are not at an increased risk, whereas those who start smoking during occupational exposure are at an increased risk. Smoking may act in many ways, including increasing exposure to an occupational agent. For instance, nickel absorption is greater in electroplater smokers compared with non-smokers.

Cigarette smoking may also shorten the latent interval between first exposure and the onset of sensitization. This has been demonstrated with ethylene diamine [46]. Cigarette smoking has been found to be a more potent risk factor than atopy in platinum asthma, both in the production of a positive skin prick test to the complex platinum salts and in the onset of symptoms. Thus, work-related respiratory symptoms were present in 50% of those smoking more than 11 cigarettes daily within 4 months of the first exposure, whereas the time taken for 50% of non-smokers to develop work-related respiratory symptoms was over a year. After 4 years, 80% of smokers and 40% of non-smokers had developed positive skin prick tests to platinum salts [14]. Smoking has also been shown to be a risk factor for work-related respiratory symptoms in electronic workers exposed to colophony where no known specific IgE mechanism has been found, and where skin prick tests are negative [47].

PROGNOSIS OF WORKERS DEVELOPING OCCUPATIONAL ASTHMA

It is often assumed that removing a single cause for asthma will result in complete recovery. Most studies, however, have shown persisting asthma, particularly related to exercise and infections, in workers who have been removed from exposure [48]. There is now increasing evidence that the longer exposure persists after symptoms have developed the poorer the prognosis. This has been shown for workers exposed to western red cedar for which the largest number of workers followed up to date have been reported. Few studies have shown any improvement in FEV_1 following cessation of exposure, suggesting that some permanent decrement in FEV_1 has occurred. The reasons for continuing symptoms are not completely clear. It may be that antigen inhaled at work persists for a long time, particularly if that antigen is combined with body proteins or has entered lymph nodes. The half-life for IgE antibodies to acid anhydrides is longer than the biological half-life of IgE and has been shown to be in the order of a year [49]. The underlying pathophysiology of continuing symptoms in occupational asthma is continuing inflammation. This has been shown in six workers sensitized to western red cedar, who had persistent symptoms after removal from exposure and when investigated by bronchial lavage showed sloughing of the epithelium and increased eosinophils, an appearance similar to that seen in the patients with intrinsic asthma [50].

There are some groups who do particularly well after cessation of exposure. This particularly applies to platinum refiners in the UK who are removed from exposure very soon after their first symptoms develop, and to laboratory animal workers. Platinum refiners in the USA, however, have a less good prognosis, which may be due to reluctance to identify workers with occupational asthma at an early stage and remove them from exposure [51].

The diagnosis of occupational asthma threatens not only the health but also the livelihood of the affected worker. An individual is often faced with the decision of remaining exposed to an agent causing his disease, or of leaving work and probable unemployment. This dilemma is clearly shown in those formally followed up from the Birmingham clinic [52], where those removed from exposure had fewer symptoms and had improved at follow-up, but lost on average 54% of their total income (this included any compensation). Those staying at work had more symptoms, a reduction in their lung function, and a 35% loss of income.

PREVENTION OF OCCUPATIONAL ASTHMA

The principal cause of occupational asthma is exposure to a sensitizing agent. Increasing levels of exposure lead to an increased incidence of occupational asthma. The aim, therefore, is to identify the precise cause and either remove it or reduce exposure substantially. The best results come from removing a sensitizing agent from the workplace completely and substituting it with a material which does not result in sensitization. Clearly substantial confidence in the precise diagnosis is necessary before this can take place. One of the earliest examples of substitution was the removal of aminoethylethanolamine as a flux for soldering aluminium. An attempt has been made to substitute colophony used in electronics soldering [53]. There is a workable replacement. However, it does not work as quickly as colophony and, therefore, it is not as industrially economic. However, substitution does not necessarily solve the problem. A switch from toluene diisocyanate (TDI), which is more volatile, to diphenylmethane diisocyanate (MDI), which is less volatile, was promoted partly to reduce sensitization as at that time TDI was a well-recognized cause of occupational asthma and MDI was not. It is now more common to see workers sensitized to MDI than TDI. Alternative forms of substitution include working with tissue cultures instead of live animals in laboratories and ventilating buildings without humidifiers to prevent humidifier asthma.

If the offending material cannot be withdrawn completely, the levels of exposure can nearly always be reduced, and in particular the number of exposed workers can be reduced by confining the sensitizing agent to a small part of a workplace. This often involves changing the layout of a factory, which can be very expensive. An occupational health input in the factory design stage is, therefore, very important. Examples where substantial reductions in sensitization have been achieved by these methods have included the manufacture of biological detergents using the enzymes alcalase and maxtilase [54]. This process has involved changing the form of the enzyme from a slurry into a pelletized format, which is much less dusty, by enclosing the process, producing good local exhaust extraction and confining the process to a small part of the works. Workers are also protected with personal respiratory protection.

Working with sensitizing agents involves a risk of developing occupational asthma, but this risk should be accepted both by the management and the worker and plans made in advance about the management of a sensitized worker. Under such circumstances it is easier to educate the workers about the safe handling of materials and thereby reduce occupational exposures. There are now guidelines for the management of workers exposed to potential respiratory sensitizing agents [55]. An assessment of the risks of sensitization is the first stage. All workers with exposure to any agent which might possibly cause occupational asthma need education about the risks and symptoms of occupational asthma. When any risk of sensitization is present, worker surveillance is recommended, which should be more intense when the risk is higher. These recommendations put several groups of hospital workers into the at-risk group, including endoscopist (glutaraldehyde), X-ray dark room staff (amines and glutaraldehyde), orthopaedic surgeons (acrylics), pharmacists and nurses handling bulk drugs such as ispaghula, and groups preparing sterile surfaces (formaldehyde, chlorhexidine, etc.).

Personal protective equipment is the least useful form of prevention but is theoretically easier to institute. It may be easier to prevent sensitization than to prevent symptoms once sensitization has occurred. The studies involving personal protective equipment in highly sensitized workers have usually shown some continuing asthma, despite wearing such equipment [2], which needs to be handled obsessionally to prevent exposure during gowning up and degowning.

Once occupational asthma is diagnosed in an individual, it is important that the clinician recommends that the affected worker is no longer exposed to the offending agent, rather than advised to leave work. It is up to the occupational health service (or the employment medical advisory service in the absence of occupational health), to recommend how this can be achieved. In this way it is more likely that the affected worker is left in employment, and that the original cause is recognized and steps taken to prevent further cases developing.

REFERENCES

1 Smith DD. Medical-legal definition of occupational asthma. *Chest* 1990;98:1007–1011.
2 Slovak AJM, Orr RG, Teasdale EL. Efficacy of the helmet respirator in occupational asthma due to laboratory animal allergy (LAA). *Am Ind Hyg Assoc J* 1985;46:411–415.
3 Burge PS, O'Brien IM, Harries MG. Peak flow rate records in the diagnosis of occupational asthma due to isocyanates. *Thorax* 1979;34:317–323.
4 Hendy MS, Beattie B, Burge PS. Occupational asthma due to soluble oil mists. *Br J Industr Med* 1983;42:51–54.
5 Kongerud J, Soyseth V, Burge PS. Serial measurements of peak expiratory flow and responsiveness to methacholine in the diagnosis of aluminium potroom asthma. *Thorax* 1992;47:292–297.
6 Burge PS, Harries MG, Lam WK, *et al.* Occupational asthma due to formaldehyde. *Thorax* 1985;40:255–260.
7 Department of Health and Social Security. *Occupational Asthma*. London: HMSO, 1985;Cmnd 9717:5–13.
8 Gannon PFG, Burge PS. A preliminary report of a surveillance scheme of occupational asthma in the West Midlands. *Br J Industr Med* 1991;48:579–582.
9 Burge PS, O'Brien IM, Harries MG. Peak flow rates in the diagnosis of occupational asthma due to colophony. *Thorax* 1979;34:308–316.
10 Burge PS. Single and serial measurements of lung function in the diagnosis of occupational asthma. *Eur J Respir Dis* 1982;63(Suppl 123):47–59.
11 Cartier A, Bernstein IL, Burge PS, *et al.* Guidelines for bronchoprovocation on the investigation of occupational asthma. *J Allergy Clin Immunol* 1989;84:823–829.
12 Vedal S, Chan-Yeung M, Enarson D, *et al.* Symptoms and pulmonary function in Western Red Cedar workers related to duration of employment and dust exposure. *Arch Environ Health* 1986;41:179–183.
13 Diem JE, Jones RN, Hendrick DJ, *et al.* Five year longitudinal study of workers employed in a new toluene diisocyanate manufacturing plant. *Am Rev Respir Dis* 1982;126:420–428.
14 Venables KM, Dally MB, Nunn AJ, *et al.* Smoking and occupational allergy in workers in a platinum refinery. *Br Med J* 1989;299:939–942.
15 Greenberg M, Milne JF, Watt A. Survey of workers exposed to dusts containing derivatives of Bacillus subtilis. *Br Med J* 1970;ii:629–633.
16 Kobayashi S. Occupational asthma due to inhalation of pharmacological dusts and other chemical agents with some reference to other occupational asthmas in Japan. In: Yamamura Y, ed. *Allergology*. Amsterdam: Exerpta Medica, 1974:124–132.
17 Salvaggio J. Occupational and environmental respiratory disease. In: *NIAID Task Force Report, Asthma and Other Allergic Diseases*. NIH publications no 79–387, 1979.
18 Keskinen H, Alanko K, Saarinen L. Occupational asthma in Finland. *Clin Allergy* 1978;8:569–579.
19 Meridith SK, Taylor VM, McDonald JC. Occupational respiratory disease in the United Kingdom 1989: a report to the British Thoracic Society and the Society of Occupational Medicine by the SWORD project group. *Br J Industr Med* 1991;48: 292–298.

20 Baur X, Fruhmann G, Haug B, *et al.* Role of Aspergillus amylase in bakers asthma. *Lancet* 1986;i:43.
21 Tee RD, Gordon DJ, Gordon S, *et al.* Immune response to flour and dust mites in a United Kingdom bakery. *Br J Industr Med* 1992;49:581–587.
22 Robertson AS, Weir DC, Burge PS. Occupational asthma due to oil mists. *Thorax* 1988;43:200–205.
23 Burge PS. Occupational asthma, rhinitis and alveolitis due to colophony. *Clin Immunol Allergy* 1984;4:55–82.
24 Weir DC, Robertson AS, Jones S, Burge PS. Occupational asthma due to soft soldering fluxes containing zinc chloride and ammonium chloride. *Thorax* 1989;44:220–223.
25 Iversen M, Dahl R, Korsgaard J, *et al.* Respiratory symptoms in Danish farmers: an epidemiological study of risk factors. *Thorax* 1988;43:872–877.
26 Darke CS, Knowelden J, Lacey J. Respiratory disease of workers harvesting grain. *Thorax* 1976;31:294–302.
27 Harries MG, Lacey J, Tee TD, *et al.* Didymella exitialis and late summer asthma. *Lancet* 1985;i:1063–1066.
28 Cuthbert OD, Brostoff J, Wraith DG, Brighton WD. Barn allergy, asthma and rhinitis due to storage mites. *Clin Allergy* 1979;9:229–236.
29 Lutsky I, Bar-Sela S. Northern fowl mite (Ornithonyssus sylviarum) in occupational asthma in poultry workers. *Lancet* 1982;ii:874–875.
30 Howe W, Topping MD, Hawkins R, Newman Taylor AJ. Tetrachlorphthalic anhydride asthma: evidence for specific IgE antibody. *J Allergy Clin Immunol* 1983;71:5–11.
31 Baur X. New aspects of isocyanate asthma. *Lung* 1990;168(Suppl):606–613.
32 Lozewicz S, Davison AG, Hopkirk A, *et al.* Occupational asthma due to methyl methacrylate and cyanoacrylates. *Thorax* 1985;40:836–839.
33 Luczynska CM, Topping MD. Specific IgE antibodies to reactive dye-albumin conjugates. *J Immunol Methods* 1986;95:177–186.
34 Hendrick DJ, Lane DJ. Formalin asthma in hospital staff. *Br Med J* 1975;i:607–608.
35 Burge PS. Occupational risks of glutaraldehyde. *Br Med J* 1989;299:342.
36 Bourne MS, Flindt MLH, Walker JM. Asthma due to industrial use of chloramine. *Br Med J* 1979;ii:10–12.
37 Marshall CP, Pearson FC, Sagona MA, *et al.* Reactions during haemodialysis caused by allergy to ethylene oxide gas sterilisation. *J Allergy Clin Immunol* 1985;75:563–567.
38 Clark EG. Risk of isothiazolinones. *J Soc Occup Med* 1987;37:30–31.
39 Waclawski ER, McAlpine LG, Thomson NC. Occupational asthma in nurses due to chlorhexidine and alcohol aerosols. *Br Med J* 1989;298:929–930.
40 Shirakawa T, Kusaka Y, Morimoto K. Specific IgE antibodies to nickel in workers with known reactivity to cobalt. *Clin Exp Allergy* 1992;22:213–218.
41 Cromwell O, Pepys J, Parish WE, Hughes EG. Specific IgE antibody to platinum salts in sensitised workers. *Clin Allergy* 1979;9:109–117.
42 Zetterstro'm O, Osterman K, Machado L, Johansson SGO. Another smoking hazard: raised serum IgE concentration and increased risk of occupational allergy. *Br Med J* 1981;283:1215–1217.
43 McSharry C, Wilkinson PC. Cigarette smoking and the antibody response to inhaled antigens. *Immunology Today* 1986;7:98.
44 Finnegan MJ, Little S, Gordon DJ, *et al.* The effect of smoking on the development of allergic disease and specific immunological responses in a factory workforce exposed to humidifier contaminants. *Br J Industr Med* 1991;48:30–33.
45 Venables KM, Topping MD, Howe W, *et al.* Interaction of smoking and atopy in producing specific IgE antibody against a hapten protein conjugate. *Br Med J* 1985; 290:201–204.
46 Aldrich FD, Strange AW, Geesaman RE. Smoking and ethylene diamine sensitisation in an industrial population. *J Occup Med* 1987;29:311–314.
47 Burge PS, Perks WH, O'Brien IM, *et al.* Occupational asthma in an electronics factory; a case control study to evaluate aetiological factors. *Thorax* 1979;34:300–307.
48 Chan-Yeung M, MacLean L, Paggiaro PL. Follow-up study of 232 patients with occupational asthma caused by western red cedar (Thuja plicata). *J Allergy Clin Immunol* 1987;79:792–796.

49 Venables KM, Topping MD, Nunn AJ, *et al*. Immunologic and functional consequences of chemical (tetrachlorphthalic anhydride)-induced asthma after four years of avoidance of exposure. *J Allergy Clin Immunol* 1987;80:212–218.

50 Chan-Yeung M, Leriche J, MacLean L, Lam S. Comparison of cellular and protein changes in bronchial lavage fluid of symptomatic and asymptomatic patients with red cedar asthma on follow-up examination. *Clin Allergy* 1988;18:359–365.

51 Baker DB, Gann PH, Brooks SM, *et al*. Cross-sectional study of platinum salts sensitization among precious metals refinery workers. *Am J Industr Med* 1990;18: 653–664.

52 Gannon PFG, Weir DC, Robertson AS, Burge PS. Health, employment and financial outcomes in workers with occupational asthma. *Br J Industr Med* 1993;50:491–496.

53 Burge PS, Harries MG, O'Brien IM, Pepys J. Bronchial provocation studies in workers exposed to the fumes of electronic soldering fluxes. *Clin Allergy* 1980;10:137–149.

54 Juniper CP, How MJ, Goodwin BFJ, Kinshott AK. Bacillus subtilis enzymes: a 7 year clinical, epidemiological and immunological study of an industrial allergen. *J Soc Occup Med* 1977;27:3–12.

55 Health and Safety Executive. *Medical Aspects of Occupational Asthma*. London: HMSO, MS 25, 1990.

PART 9
COLLAGEN VASCULAR DISEASE

Raynaud's and scleroderma syndromes

C. M. BLACK

Systemic sclerosis (SSc) or scleroderma is an uncommon heterogeneous disorder of the connective tissue. Its clinical expression ranges from the 'presclerotic' state – that is, patients with Raynaud's phenomenon, abnormal capillaries and circulating autoantibodies – through to limited cutaneous systemic sclerosis (lcSSc), diffuse cutaneous systemic sclerosis (dcSSc) and scleroderma *sine* scleroderma. The extent of skin involvement and the accompanying pattern of internal organ involvement formed the basis for the current classification into limited and diffuse disease (Table 1) [1]. The spectrum also includes localized scleroderma (morphoea), juvenile scleroderma, and the environmentally-induced scleroderma-like disorders (Table 2) [2]. The characteristic hallmarks of the disease are over-production of extracellular matrix by fibroblasts, damage to the endothelium of small blood vessels with resultant intimal proliferation and tissue ischaemia, and activation of the immune system [3].

AETIOPATHOGENESIS

The immune inflammatory component is best seen in the puffy stage of diffuse scleroderma and may be one of the earliest events in disease evolution. The vascular abnormalities are most obviously expressed in the limited form of the disorder, where there may be a long history of Raynaud's phenomenon, digital scars, ulcers, telangiectasiae and late-onset pulmonary hypertension; in the diffuse disease there may be hypertensive renal crisis. The fibrotic component is most evident in the diffuse form where there are rapidly spreading skin sclerosis, tendon friction rubs and joint contractures. Involvement of the lungs, kidneys, heart, gut or skin may cause considerable morbidity and mortality [4]. SSc is the most deadly of the connective tissue diseases: in a recent report, although scleroderma accounted for only 12.7% of a cohort of 410 patients with connective tissue disease of less than one year's duration, these same SSc patients accounted for about 50% of all the early deaths in the group [5].

Table 1 Subsets of SSc. (By permission from LeRoy *et al.* [1])

*Diffuse cutaneous SSC (dcSSc)**
Onset of Raynaud's phenomenon within 1 year of onset of skin changes (puffy or hidebound)
Truncal and acral skin involvement
Presence of tendon friction rubs
Early and significant incidence of interstitial lung disease, oliguric renal failure, diffuse gastrointestinal disease, and myocardial involvement
Absence of anti-centromere antibodies (ACA)
Nailfold capillary dilatation and capillary destruction†
Anti-topoisomerase antibodies (30% of patients)

Limited cutaneous SSc (lcSSc)
Raynaud's phenomenon for years (occasionally decades)
Skin involvement limited to hands, face, feet and forearms (acral) or absent
A significant late incidence of pulmonary hypertension, with or without interstitial lung disease, trigeminal neuralgia, skin calcifications, telangiectasiae
A high incidence of ACA (70–80%)
Dilated nailfold capillary loops, usually without capillary dropout

* Experienced observers note some patients with dcSSc who do not develop organ insufficiency and suggest the term chronic dcSSc for these patients.
† Nailfold capillary dilatation and destruction may also be seen in patients with dermatomyositis, overlap syndromes, and undifferentiated connective tissue disease. These syndromes may be considered as part of the spectrum of scleroderma-associated disorders.

Table 2 Spectrum of scleroderma and scleroderma-like syndromes

Scleroderma – localized	Morphoea (plaque, guttate, generalized) Linear *En coup de sabre*
Raynaud's phenomenon	Raynaud's disease (idiopathic) Raynaud's syndrome (secondary) including a 'pre-sclerotic' state
Scleroderma – systemic	Limited cutaneous systemic sclerosis (lcSSc) Diffuse cutaneous systemic sclerosis (dcSSc) Scleroderma *sine* scleroderma
Scleroderma – juvenile	Localized disease (Morphoea, linear, *en coup de sabre*) lcSSc dcSSc
Scleroderma – chemically induced	Environmental/occupational e.g. Silica, vinyl chloride, epoxy resin Drugs, e.g. bleomycin, cocaine, carbidopa
Scleroderma-like (1) Immunological/inflammatory	Chronic graft-versus-host disease Eosinophilic fasciitis Overlap syndromes (SSc with rheumatoid arthritis, systemic lupus erythematosus, etc.)
Scleroderma-like (2) Metabolic/ inherited	Phenylketonuria Amyloidosis
Localized systemic sclerosis and visceral diseases	Idiopathic pulmonary fibrosis, infiltrating cardiomyopathy and others

The cause of SSc is almost certainly multifactorial with genetic, environmental and immune factors playing a role at some stage in its evolution [6–8]. Although there are few data to support a generalized derangement of the immune system in scleroderma, there is a growing body of evidence in support of a more specific defect. Based on the following observations, it is possible that activated cells of the immune system may help drive the vascular damage or the fibrotic response, either through direct effector mechanisms or through the production of soluble factors.

1 Many patients produce antibodies with well-defined target epitopes, some of which are directed against antigens performing essential cell functions. These antibodies also appear to delineate separate subsets of the disease (Table 3).

2 T cells are activated in the circulation and tissues. The activated subset has been identified as T-helper CD4+ cells, and recently it has been shown that CD4+ T cells from patients with scleroderma are stimulated by human type-l collagen. Increased numbers of $\gamma\delta$ and activated CD4+ T cells are also present in the uninvolved skin of line-200 chickens, an animal model of SSc.

3 Elevated levels of interleukin 2 (IL-2), IL-2 receptor, IL-4 and IL-6 have been reported in the blood.

4 Immunoglobulins from some patients with SSc bind the terminal galactosyl (α1–3)-galactose disaccharide of laminin, the 138 amino acid region of the Pm-Scl antigen or retroviral proteins.

Table 3 Serum autoantibodies in SSc with clinical and laboratory correlates

Antigen	ANA staining pattern	HLA associations	Frequency in all patients (%)	Clinical associations	Organ involvement
Scl-70 topoisomerase 1	Speckled	DR5 (DR11) DR3/DR52a DQ7 DQB1	15–20	Diffuse	Lung fibrosis
ACA centromere	Centromere (kinetochore)	DR1 (DQ5) DQB1 DR4 (D13 subtypes)	25–30	Limited	Pulmonary hypertension
RNA I and III	Speckled/ nucleolar	?	20	Diffuse	Renal, skin
U_3 RNP	Nucleolar	?	5	Overlap mixed	Pulmonary hypertension, muscle
U_1 RNP	Speckled	?	10	Limited overlap blacks	Muscle
Th (To)	Nucleolar	?	5	Limited	Pulmonary hypertension, small bowel
PM-Scl	Nucleolar	DR3 DR52	3–5	Overlap mixed	Muscle

5 There is a well-recognized association with genes of the immune system including the histocompatibility antigen (HLA) class II (DR1, DR3, DR5) and class III (C4 null) genes [6,9].

The development of an anticentromere antibody response in patients with SSc seems to need the presence of a polar amino acid at position 26 in the antigen binding cleft of the HLA-DQB1 molecule and there may also be a similar requirement for a topoisomerase-1 (Scl-70) response [10,11]. The presence of Scl-70 antibodies plus a DR52a gene appears to mark off a subset of Caucasoid SSc patients destined to develop pulmonary fibrosis [12]. There would also appear to be global differences not only in the autoantibodies found in scleroderma subsets but also in the HLA associations, and transracial gene mapping may be required to sort out these complex associations. Other current areas of genetic interest which may extend our understanding are the immunoglobulin and T-cell receptor genes and chromosomal instability.

The stimuli which could produce an immune response in the idiopathic disease are unknown (although the activation of certain proto-oncogenes in lymphocytes of scleroderma patients has aroused some interest). In the environmentally-induced disease the situation is different and well-known stimuli include vinyl chloride, epoxy resin, toxic oil, silica and bleomycin.

The mechanisms by which the cells in the immune system or their products damage the connective tissue is a rapidly growing area of research in scleroderma. Several soluble factors, such as IL-2, IL-4, IL-6, transforming growth factor β (TGF-β) and platelet-derived growth factor, and adhesion molecules (β_1, β_2 integrins, intercellular adhesion molecule 1 (ICAM-1), endothelial leucocyte adhesion molecule 1 (ELAM-1)) are thought to facilitate the interaction between cells of the immune system and the connective tissue. The prime targets for this attack would appear to be the endothelial cell and the fibroblast. The relationship between endothelial damage and fibroblast activation is unknown. They may represent two entirely separate processes, different target responses to a common process, or a sequential event with the initial target being the endothelial cell and the resultant factors acting on the fibroblasts. Activation of these two cell types may in addition provide micro-environments in which extracellular matrix (ECM) epitopes could provide further stimulations to the immune system.

The mechanisms of vascular injury still elude us. An endothelial cytotoxic factor was first observed in scleroderma serum and plasma in the late 1970s. This is now thought to be granzyme-1, a serine proteinase present in the granules of activated T cells. Free-granzyme-1 has been identified in the serum of scleroderma patients, and monoclonal antibodies to granzyme-1 destroy the endothelial cytotoxicity of scleroderma serum samples [13]. Other agents which can damage the endothelial cell include endothelial cell antibodies, free radicals and activated adhesion molecules. In normal tissue, endothelial cell interactions with leucocytes are site-specific and transient, but in inflamed tissues the leucocytes adhere to the endothelium and migrate across the vessel wall into the tissues. These events are heavily dependent upon cytokine activation of appropriate adhesion molecules on endothelial cells and leucocytes. Recent work has shown positive immunostaining with monoclonal antibodies for the ELAM-1 and ICAM-1 on endothelial cells in scleroderma skin but not in control skin, and there is also enhanced adhesion of lymphocytes to endothelial cells in this condition [14,15]. The demonstration of ELAM-1 and ICAM-1 on scleroderma endothelial cells suggests that these molecules may be responsible for the adhesion of the pathogenetic lymphocytes to the activated endothelial cells. This is an area obviously worthy of further investigation and one which is currently receiving much attention.

One possible link between the vascular abnormalities and connective tissue deposition in scleroderma could be provided by the endothelins. These are a recently described family of potent vasoconstrictor peptides synthesized and secreted by endothelial cells. High basal and stimulated levels of endothelin-1 have been reported in both scleroderma and primary Raynaud's phenomenon. Kahaleh also recently reported that endothelin-1 has a significant mitogenic and collagen-enhancing effect on normal fibroblasts [16], and it is therefore possible that endothelins may be important in the development of the fibrotic lesion, either alone or acting in synergy with other cytokines and growth factors known to stimulate fibroblasts.

There are many other possible stimuli to collagen synthesis. For example, increased expression of ICAM-1 on SSc fibroblasts is responsible for increased binding of T cells to those fibroblasts, through ICAM-1/lymphocyte-function-associated-antigen-1 interactions [17]. Other stimuli may be found within the family of integrins. The integrins perform the essential function of integrating the intracellular cytoskeleton with the extracellular environment. The integrins are known to participate in cell transduction events. An alteration in integrin expression may therefore influence cell behaviour. Cutaneous perivascular lymphocytic infiltrates in patients with scleroderma show increased expression of β_1 and β_2 integrins, and β_1 integrins can also be identified in scleroderma skin between collagen bundles, and close to resident fibroblasts [15]. In addition, it has recently been shown that the expression of one of the collagen-binding integrins, $\alpha_1\beta_1$, is changed in some scleroderma fibroblasts, there being a lower relative expression of the α_1 chain than in matched normal cells [18].

Cytokines may also induce fibroblast activation and be responsible for the establishment of autocrine loops which result in continued extracellular matrix synthesis. For example, fibroblasts exposed but briefly to TGF-β exhibit persistent activity that lasts for days. This may occur because TGF-β induces expression of its own messenger RNA and receptor. There may also be communication between cytokines and a cascade set in motion which continues to stimulate the apparatus (cytoplasmic or nuclear) necessary for cellular activity [19].

The possibilities for cell–cell, cytokine–cell, cell–matrix interaction are numerous. Once the scleroderma process is initiated and is gathering momentum, there are so many potential interactions and deranged functions that it is as yet impossible to know the ordering of events which leads to widespread and often ongoing vascular damage and extracellular matrix (ECM) proliferation. However, with modern technology and the ever-increasing interest in the subject, the next few years should see many of these questions unravelled, the pathogenesis better explained and the benefits of this understanding translated into clinical practice.

'PRE-SCLERODERMA'

If the damaging effects of scleroderma, particularly in its diffuse form, are to be modified or halted, the disease must be recognized as early as possible. Unfortunately, the early puffy stage of diffuse scleroderma, the stage of maximum immunological activity and the presumed reversible stage of the disease, is often missed; by the time the patient presents there is a rapidly spreading fibrotic lesion and widespread vascular injury. A need exists for early warning signs, 'a pre-sclerotic state', in which screening tests can be performed and evolving connective tissue disease recognized. The nearest we can get to this state at the present time is Raynaud's phenomenon. This condition often harbours individuals who have symptoms, signs or serology suggestive of a systemic undifferentiated connective tissue disease.

Raynaud's phenomenon occurs in 5–10% of the adult population. It has a predilection for females and most individuals do not seek medical advice for the condition. For those whose symptoms are sufficient to seek help, a basic screening programme should be undertaken to determine if the vasospasm is primary or secondary. Based on current information (the figure is probably inflated due to the large referral bias in reported series), up to 20% of patients with primary Raynaud's phenomenon will progress to a defined disease, usually rheumatic, of which systemic sclerosis is the most common. Klippel [20] reviewed five studies in which 20% of the 220 primary Raynaud's patients developed a specific disease when followed for between 2 and 8.8 years. Of those whose condition evolved, 71% developed systemic sclerosis [21].

In view of such reports, it is recommended that all patients with Raynaud's phenomenon have a complete clinical evaluation, a comprehensive antinuclear antibody analysis and nailfold capillary microscopy. The nailfold capillaries can be examined with an ophthalmoscope and some workers regard this method as having a sensitivity equal to that of the microscope method. However, I would rather regard it as an adjunct to more sensitive techniques. Microscopic examination of the proximal nailfold capillary network is a simple semi-quantitative reproducible method of determining microvascular pathology in a patient with Raynaud's phenomenon. The relative risk of developing SSc for a Raynaud's patient with a systemic sclerosis capillary pattern on microscopy, compared with that of Raynaud's patients with a normal pattern, is about 13.

The prognostic yield for evolution of a connective tissue disease is considerably improved when combined with analysis of 'disease-specific' autoantibody profiles. Most useful has been the ability of anti-centromere antibodies (ACA) and anti-scleroderma 70 (anti-topoisomerase-1) antibodies to predict the development of scleroderma. Anti-topoisomerase-1 was found to have 100% specificity for scleroderma and ACA a 98% sensitivity for lcSSc [22,23]. In a recent study by Weiner *et al.* [24], the presence of either anti-scleroderma 70 antibodies or ACA was more sensitive but less specific than abnormal *in vivo* capillary microscopy in predicting subsequent clinical progression. It should, however, be remembered that only a small proportion of cases of primary Raynaud's phenomenon will evolve into a specific connective tissue disease even when followed up for more than 10 years. More longitudinal information is required and is being currently collected in a cooperative study in the USA. There are patients presenting with Raynaud's phenomenon only, or Raynaud's phenomenon/undifferentiated connective tissue disease, who will have minor nailfold capillary abnormalities and non-specific antinuclear antibodies whose disease does not evolve. The case for a 'presclerotic state' must not be overstated.

CLINICAL DISEASE

The suggestion made in 1988 of dividing scleroderma into two main subsets is useful, not only because of its simplicity, but also because these patients have different patterns of disease and different autoantibody profiles, and they progress in different ways (Table 1). Patients with limited disease have an early phase which lasts 10 years. During this time there are few, if any, constitutional symptoms. Skin involvement is limited to the extremities and face with no, or minimal progression. Raynaud's phenomenon, pitting scars, digital ulcers, calcinosis and telangiectasiae can all be troublesome and oesophageal symptoms are prominent. In the late stage of this subset there may be worsening of the vascular disease with widespread telangiectasia, digital tip ulcers, widespread calcinosis and pulmonary hypertension. Pulmonary interstitial disease can also occur as a late complication. The gut involvement can worsen with oesophageal strictures, malabsorption, pseudo-obstruction and anal incontinence.

Diffuse disease is quite different. The first 5 years is the early phase and the patient is fatigued and loses weight. There is rapid progression of skin disease with an increased risk of renal failure and early cardiac, pulmonary (interstitial) and gastrointestinal disease. Arthritis, myositis and tendon involvement are prominent. After 5 years, which is the late stage of diffuse disease, the constitutional symptoms tend to disappear and the skin becomes stable and atrophic with some regression. The musculoskeletal problems are less active, but lead to deformity and wasting. There is, however, continued progression of existing visceral disease in many patients, but reduced risk of new organ involvement.

Recent improvements in the management of hypertensive renal crisis mean that renal disease is no longer the major cause of death in scleroderma, an unenviable role now assumed by pulmonary disease, which may affect either the interstitium, resulting in pulmonary fibrosis, or the vasculature, causing pulmonary hypertension, or both. Pulmonary hypertension is impossible to diagnose early by non-invasive techniques and is invariably fatal. However, pulmonary fibrosis is increasingly amenable to early diagnosis with new techniques. The combination of bronchoalveolar lavage, high resolution computerized tomography (CT) and technetium-99m diethylene-triamine-pentacetate (DTPA) scans is beginning to provide much earlier diagnosis and indicators of progression. Using high resolution CT it is apparent that the earliest detectable abnormality is usually a narrow, often ill-defined, subpleural crescent of increased attenuation in the posterior segment of the lower lobe. The early CT changes may have an amorphous ground-glass pattern of parenchymal opacification or alternatively a more reticular appearance. The relative extent of each pattern is important because there is good correlation between these appearances and histological findings at open lung biopsy, i.e. an inflammatory biopsy equating to an amorphous pattern and fibrosis to a reticular one. Such information may reduce the need for an invasive biopsy [25,26].

Evaluation of SSc is difficult. We do not have available tools that permit very early accurate diagnosis of internal organ involvement or sufficiently sensitive indices of progression. There are as yet no internationally agreed standards for activity and severity, although work towards these two aims is in progress on an international scale. The frequency with which monitoring is repeated depends on subset and the length of the disease.

TREATMENT

Although there is no cure for scleroderma at the present time, management should be as skilful as possible to maximize quality of life, and should be tailored to the stage and subset of the disease (Tables 4 and 5). There are many possible therapies for Raynaud's phenomenon, ranging from a conservative approach with advice concerning lifestyle, through to calcium channel blockers, ketanserin (a serotonin antagonist), captopril (an angiotensin converting enzyme (ACE) inhibitor), or intravenous prostacyclin, with digital sympathectomy as a useful agent for the critically ischaemic finger (Table 6). Because of the risk of pulmonary hypertension, consideration should also be given to long-term vascular protection with drugs such as captopril or nifedipine.

If the diffuse form of the disease is caught in its very early stage, then consideration may be given to immunosuppression with drugs such as cyclophosphamide, methotrexate, antithymocyte globulin or cyclosporin followed by an antifibrotic drug such as D-penicillamine or α- and γ-interferon (Table 7). The presence in the lungs, heart and gut of fibrosis, which may progress after the skin disease has plateaued, would argue for the long-term use of an antifibrotic agent and this should not be tailed off until the disease has been quiescent for at least 1 year [27]. The complications arising from internal organ involvement such as oesophageal reflux, bacterial overgrowth, cardiac arrhythmias and hypertensive renal

Table 4 Diffuse cutaneous SSc: characteristic findings in the early and late stages

Diffuse cutaneous	Early (less than 5 years after onset)	Therapeutic approach	Late (greater than 5 years after onset)	Therapeutic approach
Constitutional	Fatigue, weight loss	Immunosuppression, antifibrotic therapy, vascular therapy	None	Treatment of complications, reduction of antifibrotic therapy
Skin thickening	Rapid progression		Stable or regression	? Continued vascular therapy
Organ involvement	Increased risk of renal, cardiac, pulmonary (fibrosis), gastrointestinal, articular and muscular involvement		Musculoskeletal deformities, progression of existing (but reduced risk of new) visceral involvement	

Main therapeutic message
Early disease: intensive regimen, multiple therapy.
Late disease: less therapy needed.

Table 5 Limited cutaneous SSc: characteristic findings in the early and late stages

Limited cutaneous	Early (less than 10 years after onset)	Therapeutic approach	Late (greater than 10 years after onset)	Therapeutic approach
Constitutional	None		Only secondary to below complications	
Skin thickening	No or minimal progression	Vascular therapy, oral or intravenous (± digital sympathectomy)	No progression	Vascular therapy, oral or intravenous (± digital sympathectomy)
Organ involvement	Raynaud's phenomenon, digital tip scars, ulcers, oesophageal symptoms	Removal of calcinosis Particular attention to oesophagus	Raynaud's phenomenon, digital tip scars, ulcers, calcinosis, oesophageal stricture, malabsorption, anal incontinence, pulmonary hypertension and indolent pulmonary fibrosis	Removal of calcinosis Therapy for oesophageal and mid-gut problems

Main message: mostly vascular therapy.

Table 6 Treatment of Raynaud's phenomenon

Stages of Raynaud's phenomenon	Recommended treatment	
Simple short attacks	Warmth, heating appliances No smoking or β-blockers Fish oil and evening primrose oil: increase prostaglandin I_3 (PGI_3) levels with vasodilatory and anti-aggregatory effects	
Frequent prolonged attacks interfering with daily living often accompanied by digital infarcts	Nifedipine, diltiazem, felodipine, isradipine, nicardipine – calcium channel blockers causing relaxation of vascular smooth muscle	
	Transdermal glyceryl trinitrate, smooth muscle relaxant Ketanserin – selective 5-hydroxytryptamine ($5HT_2$) receptor antagonist reducing 5HT-induced vasospasm and platelet aggregation	
	Captopril – angiotensin converting enzyme (ACE) inhibitor causing vasodilatation? by accumulation of vasodilator kinins	
Severe, prolonged Raynaud's: attacks with ulceration and incipient gangrene	Prostaglandin/PGE_1 Prostacyclin (iloprost)	Direct vasodilatation inhibits platelet aggregation, increases red blood cell deformability and decreases blood viscosity
Secondary infection	Antibiotics, surgery (e.g. débridement, nail removal, nail bed removal)	
Gangrene	Amputation – auto, surgical	
Surgical approach to Raynaud's phenomenon	Cervical sympathectomy – should be avoided Lumbar sympathectomy – still has a place for Raynaud's of the lower limb Digital sympathectomy for severe pain and ulceration of fingers or toes: may be used in conjunction with intravenous prostacyclin	

Table 7 Drug procedures currently used in treatment of scleroderma

Drug	Mechanism of action	Efficacy in trials	
		Uncontrolled	Controlled (double blind)
D-Penicillamine	Forms a complex with hydroxylysine aldehyde and lysine groups needed for formation of stable collagen crosslinks, so reducing collagen production	Yes/lung, skin renal	?
Interferon-α and -γ	Specific inhibitory effect on collagen production by fibroblasts, possibly by elimination of a sub-population of high-collagen-producing fibroblasts, or by inhibiting procollagen mRNA synthesis	Yes	?
Cyclosporin A	Alters early immune response by reducing IL-2 production? via reduced mRNA transcription. Also reduction in IL-1 from monocytes	Yes	?
Methotrexate	Folic acid antagonist	Yes	?
Azathioprine	Purine antagonist reducing DNA synthesis	?	?
Cyclophosphamide + prednisolone	Alkylating agent Immunosuppressant	+ Yes for arthralgia, myositis	?
Plasmapheresis + prednisolone and cyclosporin	Removes immune complexes and vasoactive substances	Alone no good – ? in combination	
Pentoxifylline	Reduces fibroblast proliferation and synthesis of collagen glycosaminoglycans and fibronectin	Yes	?
Antithymocyte globulin	Disruption of T-cell activity early in disease may reduce cytokine production and hence fibroblast activation	Yes	?
Photopheresis	Extracorporeal exposure of blood to photoactivated 8-methoxypsoralen to reduce activity of aberrant T cells	Yes	?
Factor XIII	Inhibits collagen synthesis	Yes	?

crisis must each be treated individually. Fortunately, in recent years new drugs such as omeprazole for oesophageal disease and ACE inhibitors for renal disease have greatly increased the skill with which we manage these problems. Scleroderma is usually a life-long and, at times, potentially disfiguring and life-threatening disease. It requires accurate staging and suitable therapy and sympathetic management, with emotional and physical support for the patients and their families.

REFERENCES

1 LeRoy EC, Black CM, Fleischmajer R, *et al*. Scleroderma (systemic sclerosis): classification, subsets and pathogenesis. *J Rheumatol* 1988;15:202–205.
2 Medsger Jr TA. Systemic sclerosis (scleroderma), eosinophilic fasciitis, and calcinosis. In: McCarty DJ, ed. *Arthritis and Allied Conditions*. Philadelphia: Lea & Febiger, 1989:118–165.
3 Black CM (ed.). Systemic sclerosis (scleroderma). *Ann Rheum Dis, Heberden Papers* 1991;50(Suppl 4):837–838.
4 Silman AJ. Mortality from scleroderma in England and Wales 1968–1985. *Ann Rheum Dis* 1991;50:95–96.
5 Bulpitt K, Clements PJ, Lachenbruch PA, Paulus HE. Co-operative systemic studies on the rheumatic diseases: Prospective study of early systemic sclerosis (SSc): Outcome and prognostic indications. *Arthritis Rheum* 1990;33(Suppl 5):R6.
6 Briggs D, Black C, Welsh K. Genetic factors in scleroderma. *Rheum Dis Clin N Am* 1990;16:31–51.
7 Korn JH. Immunological aspects of scleroderma. *Curr Op Rheumatol* 1989;1:479–485; 1990;2:922–928; 1991;3:947–952.
8 Needleman B. The immunologic aspects of scleroderma. *Curr Op Rheumatol* 1992; 4:862–868.
9 Fox RI, Kang HI. Genetic and environmental factors in systemic sclerosis. *Curr Op Rheumatol* 1992;4:857–861.
10 Reveille JD, Owerbach D, Goldstein R, *et al*. Association of polar amino acids at position 26 of the HLA-DQB1 first domain with the anticentromere autoantibody response in systemic sclerosis (scleroderma). *J Clin Invest* 1992;89:1208–1213.
11 Reveille JD, Durgan E, MacLeod-St Clair MJ, *et al*. Association of amino acid sequences in the HLA-DQB1 first domain with the antitopoisomerase I autoantibody response in scleroderma (progressive systemic sclerosis). *J Clin Invest* 1992;90:1–9.
12 Briggs DC, Vaughan RW, Welsh KI, *et al*. Immunogenetic prediction of pulmonary fibrosis in systemic sclerosis. *Lancet* 1991;338:661–662.
13 Kahaleh MB. Vascular disease in scleroderma. Endothelial T-lymphocyte fibroblast interactions. *Rheum Dis Clin N Am* 1990;16:53–73.
14 Claman HN, Giorno RC, Siebold JR. Endothelial and fibroblastic activation in scleroderma: the myth of the 'uninvolved skin'. *Arthritis Rheum* 1991;34:1495–1501.
15 Sollberg S, Peltonen J, Uitto J, Jimenez SA. Elevated expression of β_1 and β_2 integrins, intercellular adhesion molecule-1, and endothelial leukocyte adhesion molecule-1 in the skin of patients with systemic sclerosis of recent onset. *Arthritis Rheum* 1992; 35:290–298.
16 Kahaleh MB. Endothelin an endothelial-dependent vasoconstrictor in scleroderma. *Arthritis Rheum* 1991;34(8):978–983.
17 Abraham D, Lupoli S, McWhirter A, *et al*. Expression and function of surface antigens on scleroderma fibroblasts. *Arthritis Rheum* 1991;34:1164–1172.
18 Ivarsson M, McWhirter A, Black CM, Rubin K. Impaired regulation of collagen pro-α_1(I) mRNA and change in pattern of collagen binding integrins on scleroderma fibroblasts. *J Invest Dermatol* 1993;101:216–221.
19 Smith EA. Connective tissue metabolism including cytokines in scleroderma. *Curr Op Rheumatol* 1992;4:869–877.
20 Klippel JH. Raynaud's phenomenon: the French tricolor. *Arch Intern Med* 1991;151: 2389–2393.
21 Lally EV. Raynaud's phenomenon. *Curr Op Rheumatol* 1992;4:825–836.
22 Fitzgerald O, Hess EV, O'Connor GT, Spencer-Green G. Prospective study of the evolution of Raynaud's phenomenon. *Am J Med* 1988;84:718–726.
23 Kallenberg CGM, Wonda AA, Hoet MH, Van Venrooij WJ. Development of connective tissue disease in patients presenting with Raynaud's phenomenon: A six-year follow-up with emphasis on the predictive value of antinuclear antibodies as detected by immunoblotting. *Ann Rheum Dis* 1988;47:634–641.
24 Weiner ES, Earnshaw WC, Senecal JL, *et al*. Clinical associations of anticentromere

antibodies and antibodies to topoisomerase I: a study of 355 patients. *Arthritis Rheum* 1988;31:378–385.
25 Harrison NK, Glanville AR, Strickland B, *et al.* Pulmonary involvement in systemic sclerosis: the detection of early changes by thin section CT scan, bronchoalveolar laveage and ^{99m}Tc-DTPA clearance. *Resp Med* 1989;83:403–414.
26 Harrison NK, Myers AR, Corrin B, *et al.* Structural features of interstitial lung disease in systemic sclerosis. *Am Rev Resp Dis* 1991;144:706–713.
27 Medsger Jr TA. Treatment of systemic sclerosis. *Ann Rheum Dis* 1991;50:877–886.

Developments in the treatment of systemic lupus erythematosus

M. J. WALPORT

INTRODUCTION

The reported survival of patients with systemic lupus erythematosus (SLE) has progressively improved during the past 40 years. The explanation for this change is not absolutely clear. It is easy to assume that the improval in survival is due to better treatment of disease but other explanations should be considered, and these have been the subject of a recent critical review [1]. The single major advance contributing to classification of patients with SLE and related diseases has been the identification of an increasing spectrum of autoantibodies associated with the presence of disease. The description of LE cells in 1948, antinuclear factor in 1957, followed successively by antibodies to double-stranded DNA (dsDNA), extractable nuclear antigens and, most recently, cardiolipin, has facilitated the early identification of patients with SLE. These tests simplify the identification of patients with milder disease and inclusion of such patients in clinical series is likely to produce an improval in survival figures. It has been argued that this hypothesis may be tested by examining prevalence surveys published at different times during the last 40 years to see if prevalence has risen – an observation that could be explained by increased identification of milder cases of disease. Review of such data [1] shows that the reported prevalence rates did rise between 1950 and 1965, but since then have remained static. However, the methods of acquisition of prevalence data by community surveys are very different to the processes involved in the formation of a clinical practice that subsequently acts as the basis of a clinical series.

Despite this caveat, successive publications of series of patients with nephritis show improved survival figures during the last 40 years and there is now controlled evidence, reviewed below, that specific combination treatment regimens of prednisolone with cytotoxic drugs do improve outcome in patients with severe nephritis, both in terms of survival and prevention of renal failure. A second major factor is the improved treatment of hypertension, an important determinant of outcome in nephritis, and obsessive attention to blood pressure control is crucial in the management of patients with glomerulonephritis. In this review I will focus on recent studies, the results of which have contributed to the effective management of patients with SLE. Treatment of the clinical features associated with the presence of antiphospholipid antibodies has been omitted, as the following chapter in this volume (by G.R.V. Hughes) deals with this controversial subject.

PRINCIPLES

There is enormous heterogeneity in the clinical manifestations of SLE between different patients. The key to management of individual patients is the definition of the affected target organs. Wherever possible, objective measures of disease activity in each affected organ should then be defined, e.g. for renal disease: urinary sediment, 24 hour proteinuria, creatinine clearance, blood pressure. These should be recorded sequentially on flow charts. Most patients also learn subjective criteria to assess their own disease activity, such as increased hair loss, arthralgia and malaise. Although the pattern of organ involvement in any given patient often becomes established early in the course of disease, it is essential to remain alert to the onset of new organ involvement, particularly the development of renal disease, which is an adverse prognostic factor.

Having defined the extent of target organ involvement, the next step is to form an overall assessment of disease activity. There are three broad categories of disease, each of which has different treatment implications, considered below: (i) mild: cutaneous or joint involvement in the absence of significant constitutional symptoms; (ii) moderate: inflammatory involvement of other organs plus or minus constitutional symptoms – this category would include patients with mesangial nephritis (WHO grade II); and (iii) severe: severe inflammatory involvement of vital organs, e.g. patients with neuropsychiatric disease, cardiac, severe pulmonary or severe renal involvement (focal or diffuse proliferative nephritis, WHO grades III and IV).

TREATMENT OF MILD DISEASE AND CUTANEOUS DISEASE

Mild disease

Antimalarial drugs, particularly hydroxychloroquine, are widely prescribed for the treatment of mild to moderate manifestations of SLE, including rash, arthralgia and mild constitutional symptoms. Until recently there was little objective evidence of effectiveness. This has now been provided by a placebo-controlled trial of withdrawal of hydroxychloroquine in a group of patients with stable mild SLE who had been using the drug for a mean of 3 years [2]. Amongst the 47 patients studied, just over 40% were also taking prednisolone at a mean dose of approximately 6 mg daily. The patients were followed for 6 months and amongst the 25 patients remaining on hydroxychloroquine there were 9 flares of disease compared with 16 clinical flares amongst the 22 patients assigned to placebo.

There is a consensus that hydroxychloroquine dosage should be less than 400 mg per day and less than 6.5 mg per kg ideal body weight per day in order to minimize the risks of ocular toxicity. However, ocular toxicity has been seen rarely in patients treated according to these guidelines [3] and ocular monitoring should be performed by: (i) counselling patients to report development of scotomata, loss of colour vision or dark adaptation; and (ii) regular screening for scotomata using an Amsler grid [3]. The data sheet for hydroxychloroquine recommends formal ophthalmological screening at 6 monthly intervals. It may be possible to discontinue hydroxychloroquine therapy during the winter months in patients in whom photosensitivity is a major feature in exacerbation of rash.

Treatment of the more severe manifestations of cutaneous disease

Photosensitivity may provide an important contribution to the rash of SLE and patients should be counselled about ultraviolet light (UV) avoidance and the use of UV-blocking creams and ointments. Judicious use of topical steroids and intralesional steroids may also prove effective. A range of drugs have been used in patients with severe cutaneous LE, unresponsive to topical therapy, but without evidence of severe systemic disease, in whom there is a need to avoid the toxicity of high dose prednisolone and cytotoxic drugs. These include other antimalarial drugs such as mepacrine, which causes skin yellowing and may cause mood disturbance, and chloroquine, which probably carries a greater risk than hydroxychloroquine of retinal toxicity. Combinations of hydroxychloroquine and mepacrine may be useful in severe cutaneous LE.

Other drugs that are currently in fashion, but for which formal trial data are lacking, are dapsone and thalidomide. Dapsone is usually given in a dose of 50–100 mg daily, and is thought to be of particular value in urticarial vasculitis [4]. Use of this drug is reviewed elsewhere [5]. The major side-effect of dapsone is microangiopathic haemolytic anaemia, which is common, dose-related and needs to be monitored by regular measurement of haemoglobin, inspection of blood film, and bilirubin levels. It is contraindicated in glucose-6-phosphate dehydrogenase deficiency. Neuropathies, rashes and blood dyscrasias are other side-effects.

There are several reports of the use of thalidomide in small series of patients with discoid lupus [6], lupus panniculitis [7] and subacute cutaneous LE [8]. Thalidomide carries the risk of foetal malformation, sedation and peripheral neuropathy. For obvious reasons, patients need to be carefully counselled before prescription of this drug, and recent correspondence has highlighted the arguments for and against the prescription of thalidomide [9–11]. It is not widely appreciated that the neuropathy associated with thalidomide appears to be related to cumulative dosage of the drug and the dose should be minimized to delay the onset of this side-effect which needs to be monitored by regular electrophysiological testing [12].

TREATMENT OF MODERATE DISEASE

Steroids

Although dosage regimens for prednisolone in SLE have arisen through art rather than science, a number of generally accepted principles have emerged. The starting dose should be chosen according to the disease severity. Mild to moderate inflammatory disease is generally treated initially with doses of 0.5 mg per kg per day, severe with 1–1.5 mg per kg. Wherever possible, escalating doses of steroids should be avoided. At the start of therapy, treatment is usually given as a once daily dose.

Having started treatment the aim should be to control disease activity before reducing prednisolone and most clinicians would maintain the starting prednisolone dose for approximately 4 weeks. Treatment should then be tapered to a maintenance regimen and here clinical practice is diverse. Some groups use alternate day steroid therapy, others maintain a daily dose. Our own practice is to taper treatment over 2–3 months to 10 mg prednisolone daily and below this dose to not reduce treatment by more than 1 mg each month. More rapid withdrawal of treatment may be associated with development of a flare of disease leading to rebound prescription of high doses of prednisolone. We frequently maintain patients on doses of 5–7 mg of prednisolone for many months, until there is clinical and serological evidence of remission of disease, before attempting to tail prednisolone completely. There is much empiricism in this approach to steroid use and many opportunities for clinical trials to test the validity of our prejudices.

Azathioprine

Azathioprine, at a dose of approximately 2.5 mg per kg, has an important role as a steroid-sparing agent in patients with moderate to severe SLE. There is an important genetic polymorphism of one of the enzymes, thiopurine methyltransferase, involved in the metabolism of this drug. Approximately 0.3% of the population show virtually absent activity of this enzyme and these individuals develop profound marrow suppression after taking azathioprine [13]. For this reason, it is essential to monitor the haematological response to azathioprine extremely closely for the first 6 weeks after starting the drug. A further drug-metabolizing enzyme of azathioprine is xanthine oxidase. This paves the way to a lethal drug interaction between azathioprine and allopurinol; fortunately the coexistence of gout with SLE is extremely rare.

TREATMENT OF SEVERE DISEASE

Cytotoxic agents

The use of cytotoxic drugs such as azathioprine or cyclophosphamide is almost universal in patients with life-threatening internal organ involvement. The two commonest indications for this treatment are severe nephritis with impaired renal function and active cerebral disease. Focal and diffuse proliferative nephritis (WHO grades III and IV) accompanied by the presence of crescents, sclerosis and tubular interstitial changes are all indicators of poor renal prognosis and have been used as entry criteria into trials of pulsed cyclophosphamide [14].

The most prolonged studies using pulse cyclophosphamide are those conducted by workers at the National Institutes of Health (NIH) [15,16]. Entry criteria were the presence of SLE with severe nephritis. Five different treatments were compared: (i) prednisolone alone; (ii) azathioprine + prednisolone; (iii) oral cyclophosphamide + prednisolone; (iv) oral azathioprine + oral cyclophosphamide + prednisolone; and (v) intravenous pulse cyclophosphamide + prednisolone. Numbers of patients in each group varied from 18 to 30 patients and the follow-up on 19 of the patients now extends to 15 years or more. The end-points measured were progression to end-stage renal failure and death. Three groups of treatment that were significantly better than prednisolone alone were intravenous pulse cyclophosphamide, oral cyclophosphamide and combined oral cyclophosphamide and azathioprine. In terms of survival there were no significant differences between any of the groups, although there was a trend to shorter survival in the group receiving steroids alone [16].

Pulsed cyclophosphamide has been used in other settings in SLE. The NIH group have published an uncontrolled study of nine patients with severe neuropsychiatric lupus, six of whom had continuing disease despite administration of high dose prednisolone, who received the pulsed intravenous cyclophosphamide regimen [17]. Eight of these patients made good or excellent recovery. A similar regimen for children with diffuse proliferative nephritis is also in use [18]. Aplastic anaemia as a feature of lupus disease activity may also respond to pulsed cyclophosphamide [19,20].

For how long should pulse cyclophosphamide be administered? There are limited data to answer this question. Investigators at NIH randomized 65 patients with severe lupus nephritis to three groups: (i) 6 pulses of methylprednisolone at monthly intervals; (ii) 6 pulses of cyclophosphamide at monthly intervals; and (iii) 6 pulses of cyclophosphamide at monthly intervals followed by 8 pulses at intervals of 3 months [21]. The end-point was a doubling of serum creatinine and patients were withdrawn if they became pregnant or required additional pulse therapy before they met the renal outcome criteria. The number of patients receiving long-course cyclophosphamide who had doubling of their serum creatinine over 5 years of follow-up was significantly fewer than in the group treated with pulse methylprednisolone. After completion of the first 6 months of the study the probability of development of an exacerbation was significantly lower amongst the group receiving long-course cyclophosphamide compared with that receiving short-course cyclophosphamide [21].

The optimal dose and interval between pulses of cyclophosphamide is unknown. Two groups have published extensively on the use of this agent. The NIH group titrate the dose from 500 mg to 1 g per m^2 of body surface area, aiming to maintain the leucocyte count between 1.5×10^9 and 3.0×10^9 per litre at the nadir of the leucopenia, which occurs between 10 and 14 days after drug administration [21]. The Ann Arbor group titrate to higher doses if necessary, with the aim of achieving a nadir of $2.0–3.0 \times 10^9$ leucocytes per litre at 7 or 14 days after treatment (the lymphocyte nadir is at 7 days, the neutrophil at approximately 14 days) (a detailed protocol is given elsewhere [22]). The administration of cyclophosphamide should be accompanied by a high fluid intake to minimize bladder toxicity. Some also co-administer mesna (sodium 2-mercaptoethane sulphonate), which inactivates acrolein, a toxic metabolite of cyclophosphamide which causes the bladder urothelial injury [23]. It has recently been appreciated that allergic reactions to mesna are rather common [24].

An important aspect of the use of these drugs is obtaining informed consent from patients before their prescription. For cyclophosphamide it is necessary to warn patients of the risks of acute haematological and bladder toxicity and of the possibilities of long-term induction of infertility, bladder and lymphoid neoplasia. This may seem unpalatable when faced with an acutely ill young woman with nephritis but the success of treatment of the severe inflammatory manifestation of SLE means that the late complications of treatment are now much commoner and it is too late to inform patients after the event.

Plasma exchange

The place of plasmapheresis in SLE has been uncertain since the introduction of the technique. The results of a controlled study of plasma exchange in patients with severe lupus nephritis have recently been published [25]. Eighty-six patients with focal proliferative, diffuse proliferative or membranous plus diffuse proliferative changes on renal biopsy were randomized to receive oral cyclophosphamide and high dose prednisolone plus or minus 4 weeks of plasma exchange carried out three times each week. There were no significant differences between the two groups in any of the outcome measures, including death and renal failure. The plasmapheresis was associated with a significant early reduction in IgG, anti-dsDNA antibody and cryoglobulin levels during the first few weeks of treatment, confirming the effectiveness of the procedure in the exchange of plasma. It was of interest that the risk of infection was not increased in the group receiving plasma exchange compared with the control group [26].

It is perhaps premature to entirely reject plasma exchange as a treatment option in SLE. There is a multicentre international trial of plasma exchange currently in progress in which plasma exchange is being synchronized with administration of pulsed cyclophosphamide. The principle of this combined treatment is that plasma exchange causes a fall in antibody levels which is followed by a compensatory increase in antibody production by B cells. During this rebound synthesis B cells may divide and mature into new plasma cells and be especially sensitive to the cytotoxic actions of cyclophosphamide. This concept is supported by limited pilot data [27,28] and the results of this trial will be of great interest.

TREATMENT OF HYPERTENSION

It has been speculated that some of the improved survival of patients with SLE during the past 30 years may be attributed not to the specific treatment of the disease but to treatment for specific complications of disease. A recent survey of variables associated with mortality in SLE identified elevated systolic blood pressure as the most significant correlate of early mortality [29]. It could be argued that this is explained by hypertension acting as a surrogate marker of the presence of nephritis, though this is not always the case [30]. There is a correlation between the presence of hypertension and renal disease and a study in children has shown that hypertension may precede overt nephritis [31]. The vigorous treatment of hypertension is extremely important – amongst a group of patients with nephritis, those with hypertension showed a much worse renal prognosis [32]. Steinberg *et al.* have argued vigorously that aggressive management of hypertension may be as important as immunosuppressive treatment itself [32]. The rate of progression of renal failure in other diseases, such as diabetic nephropathy, is slowed by effective antihypertensive treatment [33].

DO PATIENTS DIE OF TREATMENT RATHER THAN DISEASE?

The management protocols outlined above are effective in controlling the inflammatory manifestations of SLE but to what extent do they cause iatrogenic morbidity? What are the causes of death in patients with SLE? Two studies by Urowitz *et al.* some years ago [34,35] showed a bimodal pattern of deaths in SLE. Deaths occurring during the first 2 years of disease were caused approximately equally by infection or by the effects of the SLE itself, mainly cerebral and renal disease. There was a second cluster of deaths occurring after more than 5 years of SLE and this was found to be caused either by active SLE or by cardiovascular disease, particularly disease of the coronary arteries, occurring in the context of inactive SLE. These findings have stimulated several studies into the factors which may predispose to death caused by infection or coronary artery disease.

Infections in SLE

A retrospective study by Ginzler *et al.* [36] attempted to identify risk factors for sepsis in SLE. Significant factors which emerged were increasing steroid dosage, active lupus nephritis, uraemia and bone marrow toxicity secondary to azathioprine therapy. Azathioprine treatment was associated with an increased incidence of herpes zoster infection. Other factors that may contribute to sepsis in SLE are: (i) severe hypocomplementaemia, which is a well characterized risk factor for the development of pyogenic sepsis, particularly meningococcal disease [37]; and (ii) hyposplenism, either surgical, for treatment of idiopathic thrombocytopenic purpura, or occurring as part of the disease process [38], which is a risk factor for the development of pyogenic infections, particularly overwhelming pneumococcal septicaemia.

Accelerated cardiovascular disease

There are many factors which may play a role in the causation of accelerated cardiovascular disease in patients with SLE. These include: (i) damage to the coronary arteries by vasculitis; (ii) hyperlipidaemia secondary to the nephrotic syndrome and/or corticosteroid therapy; (iii) hypertension secondary to nephritis and/or corticosteroids, and (iv) coronary artery thrombosis associated with the presence of anticardiolipin antibodies. A number of recent studies have examined risk factors for cardiovascular disease in SLE patients. The cohort of patients attending Johns Hopkins Hospital have been studied particularly carefully in this respect [39,40]. Important risk factors in this group were hypertension, hypercholesterolaemia, and obesity, coupled with age and duration of prednisolone usage.

There appear to be two important contributing factors to hyperlipidaemia in SLE, corticosteroid therapy and the nephrotic syndrome. There is evidence for a relationship between steroid dose and cholesterol levels [41,42]. The place of lovastatin or simvastatin in the management of hypercholesterolaemia in this context has not been established, and both drugs may cause myositis which may be difficult to disentangle in the face of SLE. This is an area where a clinical trial is needed.

THE FUTURE?

Although much is understood about the mechanisms of inflammation in SLE, the aetiology of the disease is not known. New treatments are therefore directed against effector pathways of disease. The advent of monoclonal antibodies has allowed targeting of particular subsets of lymphocytes and individual mediators of inflammation, including cytokines and adhesion molecules. Experimental therapies in rheumatic diseases have been directed mainly against lymphocytes and there are reports of treatment with anti-CD4 antibodies [43] and using extracorporeal photochemotherapy [44]. Because of the evidence that suggests a role for female sex hormones in promoting disease, androgenic hormone therapy has been tried in both males and females, without much success so far [45,46].

CONCLUSION

It is apparent from this review that there are many areas of ignorance and too few trials of high quality. The hallmark of the current era of clinical practice is measurement and audit. It is no longer acceptable to manage our patients empirically in isolated units. Wherever possible patients should be included in protocols asking precise questions about optimal methods of clinical management. There is good evidence that the clinical outcome of patients participating in clinical trials is better than those managed in routine clinical practice. Surely we should give this benefit to all patients with SLE.

REFERENCES

1 Swaak AJ, Nossent JC, Smeenk RJ. Prognostic factors in systemic lupus erythematosus. *Rheumatol Int* 1991;11:127–132.
2 The Canadian Hydroxychloroquine Study Group. A randomized study of the effect of withdrawing hydroxychloroquine sulfate in systemic lupus erythematosus. *N Engl J Med* 1991;324:150–154.
3 Easterbrook M. Ocular effects and safety of antimalarial agents. *Am J Med* 1988;85: 23–29.
4 Ruzicka T, Goerz G. Dapsone in the treatment of lupus erythematosus. *Br J Dermatol* 1981;104:53–56.
5 Fredenberg MF, Malkinson FD. Sulfone therapy in the treatment of leukocytoclastic vasculitis. Report of three cases. *J Am Acad Dermatol* 1987;16:772–778.
6 Knop J, Bonsmann G, Happle R, *et al.* Thalidomide in the treatment of sixty cases of chronic discoid lupus erythematosus. *Br J Dermatol* 1983;108:461–466.
7 Burrows NP, Walport MJ, Hammond AH, *et al.* Lupus erythematosus profundus with partial C4 deficiency responding to thalidomide. *Br J Dermatol* 1991;125:62–67.
8 Naafs B, Bakkers EJ, Flinterman J, Faber WR. Thalidomide treatment of subacute cutaneous lupus erythematosus. *Br J Dermatol* 1982;107:83–86.
9 Bessis D, Guillot B, Monpoint S, *et al.* Thalidomide for systemic lupus erythematosus [letter]. *Lancet* 1992;339:549–550.
10 Hawkins DF. Thalidomide for systemic lupus erythematosus [letter]. *Lancet* 1992; 339:1057.
11 Carmichael AJ, Knight A. Thalidomide: a restricted role [letter]. *Lancet* 1992;339:1362.
12 Wulff CH, Hoyer H, Asboe Hansen G, Brodthagen H. Development of polyneuropathy during thalidomide therapy. *Br J Dermatol* 1985;112:475–480.
13 Lennard L, Van Loon JA, Weinshilboum RM. Pharmacogenetics of acute azathioprine toxicity: relationship to thiopurine methyltransferase genetic polymorphism. *Clin Pharmacol Ther* 1989;46:149–154.
14 Austin HA, Muenz LR, Joyce KM, *et al.* Prognostic factors in lupus nephritis. Contribution of renal histologic data. *Am J Med* 1983;75:382–391.
15 Austin HA, Klippel JH, Balow JE, *et al.* Therapy of lupus nephritis. Controlled trial of prednisone and cytotoxic drugs. *N Engl J Med* 1986;314:614–619.
16 Steinberg AD, Steinberg SC. Long-term preservation of renal function in patients with lupus nephritis receiving treatment that includes cyclophosphamide versus those treated with prednisone only. *Arthritis Rheum* 1991;34:945–950.
17 Boumpas DT, Yamada H, Patronas NJ, *et al.* Pulse cyclophosphamide for severe neuropsychiatric lupus. *Q J Med* 1991;81:975–984.
18 Lehman TJ. Current concepts in immunosuppressive drug therapy of systemic lupus erythematosus. *J Rheumatol Suppl* 1992;33:20–22.
19 Walport MJ, Hubbard WN, Hughes GRV. Reversal of aplastic anaemia secondary to systemic lupus erythematosus by high-dose intravenous cyclophosphamide. *Br Med J* 1982;285:769–770.
20 Winkler A, Jackson RW, Kay DS, *et al.* High-dose intravenous cyclophosphamide treatment of systemic lupus erythematosus-associated aplastic anemia [letter]. *Arthritis Rheum* 1988;31:693–694.
21 Boumpas DT, Austin HA, Vaughn EM, *et al.* Controlled trial of pulse methylprednisolone versus two regimens of pulse cyclophosphamide in severe lupus nephritis. *Lancet* 1992;340:741–745.
22 McCune WJ, Golbus J, Zeldes W, *et al.* Clinical and immunologic effects of monthly administration of intravenous cyclophosphamide in severe systemic lupus erythematosus. *N Engl J Med* 1988;318:1423–1431.
23 Habs MR, Schmahl D. Prevention of urinary bladder tumors in cyclophosphamide-treated rats by additional medication with the uroprotectors sodium 2-mercaptoethane sulfonate (mesna) and disodium 2,2′-dithio-bis-ethane sulfonate (dimesna). *Cancer* 1983;51:606–609.
24 Zonzits E, Aberer W, Tappeiner G. Drug eruptions from mesna after cyclophosphamide

treatment of patients with systemic lupus erythematosus and dermatomyositis. *Arch Dermatol* 1992;128:80–82.

25 Lewis EJ, Hunsicker LG, Lan SP, *et al.* A controlled trial of plasmapheresis therapy in severe lupus nephritis. *N Engl J Med* 1992;326:1373–1379.

26 Pohl MA, Lan SP, Berl T. Plasmapheresis does not increase the risk for infection in immunosuppressed patients with severe lupus nephritis. *Ann Intern Med* 1991;114: 924–929.

27 Dau PC, Callahan J, Parker R, Golbus J. Immunologic effects of plasmapheresis synchronized with pulse cyclophosphamide in systemic lupus erythematosus. *J Rheumatol* 1991;18:270–276.

28 Schroeder JO, Euler HH, Loffler H. Synchronization of plasmapheresis and pulse cyclophosphamide in severe systemic lupus erythematosus. *Ann Intern Med* 1987;107: 344–346.

29 Seleznick MJ, Fries JF. Variables associated with decreased survival in systemic lupus erythematosus. *Semin Arthritis Rheum* 1991;21:73–80.

30 Budman DR, Steinberg AD. Hypertension and renal disease in systemic lupus erythematosus. *Arch Intern Med* 1976;136:1003–1007.

31 Ostrov BE, Min W, Eichenfield AH, *et al.* Hypertension in children with systemic lupus erythematosus. *Semin Arthritis Rheum* 1989;19:90–98.

32 Dinant HJ, Decker JL, Klippel JH, *et al.* Alternative modes of cyclophosphamide and azathioprine therapy in lupus nephritis. *Ann Intern Med* 1982;96:728–736.

33 Mogensen CE. Long-term anti-hypertensive treatment inhibits progress of diabetic retinopathy. *Br Med J* 1982;285:685–688.

34 Urowitz MB, Bookman AAM, Koehler BE, *et al.* The bimodal mortality of systemic lupus erythematosus. *Am J Med* 1976;60:221–225.

35 Rubin LA, Urowitz MB, Gladman DD. Mortality in systemic lupus erythematosus: the bimodal pattern revisited. *Q J Med* 1985;216:87–98.

36 Ginzler E, Diamond H, Kaplan D, *et al.* Computer analysis of factors influencing frequency of infection in systemic lupus erythematosus. *Arthritis Rheum* 1978;21:37–44.

37 Morgan BP, Walport MJ. Complement deficiency and disease. *Immunol Today* 1991; 12:301–306.

38 Dillon AM, Stein HB, English RA. Splenic atrophy in systemic lupus erythematosus. *Ann Intern Med* 1982;96:40–43.

39 Petri M, Spence D, Bone LR, Hochberg MC. Coronary artery disease risk factors in the Johns Hopkins Lupus Cohort: prevalence, recognition by patients, and preventive practices. *Medicine (Baltimore)* 1992;71:291–302.

40 Petri M, Perez-Gutthann S, Spence D, Hochberg MC. Risk factors for coronary artery disease in patients with systemic lupus erythematosus. *Am J Med* 1992;93:513–519.

41 Ettinger WH, Goldberg AP, Applebaum Bowden D, Hazzard WR. Dyslipoproteinemia in systemic lupus erythematosus. Effect of corticosteroids. *Am J Med* 1987;83:503–508.

42 Blum RL. Computer-assisted design of studies using routine clinical data. Analyzing the association of prednisone and cholesterol. *Ann Intern Med* 1986;104:858–868.

43 Hiepe F, Volk HD, Apostoloff E, *et al.* Treatment of severe systemic lupus erythematosus with anti-CD4 monoclonal antibody [letter]. *Lancet* 1991;338:1529–1530.

44 Knobler RM, Graninger W, Lindmaier A, *et al.* Extracorporeal photochemotherapy for the treatment of systemic lupus erythematosus. A pilot study. *Arthritis Rheum* 1992; 35:319–324.

45 Lahita RG, Cheng CY, Monder C, Bardin CW. Experience with 19-nortestosterone in the therapy of systemic lupus erythematosus: worsened disease after treatment with 19-nortestosterone in men and lack of improvement in women. *J Rheumatol* 1992;19: 547–555.

46 Asherson RA, Lahita RG. Sex hormone modulation in systemic lupus erythematosus: still a therapeutic option? *Ann Rheum Dis* 1991;50:897–898.

The antiphospholipid antibody syndrome

G. R. V. HUGHES

This syndrome, a prothrombotic state, is a major cause of strokes and other organ thrombosis, recurrent abortion, and a constellation of other features making it an important disease, crossing almost all 'specialist' boundaries.

HISTORY

During the 1970s we began detailed studies of a group of patients with systemic lupus erythematosus (SLE) who had a clotting disorder leading to both venous and arterial thrombosis. This led to the description of a syndrome which we called the anticardiolipin syndrome and in a series of publications in the 1980s, we described not only the association with thrombosis, but the broader features of the illness (Table 1), including recurrent strokes [1,2], livedo reticularis [3], pulmonary hypertension [4], recurrent abortion [5], labile hypertension, migraine, epilepsy, transverse myelitis [6] and heart valve disorders [7,8].

The work started in 1975 in Jamaica where, carrying on our interest in central nervous system lupus and antineuronal antibodies [9], we had become interested in Jamaican neuropathy – a viral-induced myelopathy with false positive VDRL. We wondered whether some of the features resembled lupoid sclerosis, and began to explore the possibility that antiphospholipid antibodies (APA), e.g. the VDRL, could possibly cross-react with neuronal phospholipids [10]. In the event, these studies quickly led to the recognition of the more generalized thrombotic syndrome now called the antiphospholipid syndrome.

The early clinical studies were led by Dr Byron and subsequently by Drs Colaco, Englert, Derue, Asherson and others. In the laboratory, we felt that the rather indirect 'lupus anticoagulant' test was cumbersome, and it was the work of Dr Nigel Harris and Dr Aziz Gharavi which developed the more acceptable anticardiolipin antibody (ACA) test – firstly a radio-immunoassay [11] and subsequently the enzyme-linked immunosorbent assay (ELISA) which is now widely used [12].

The development of these assays has allowed routine standard tests of

Table 1 The antiphospholipid syndrome

Arterial thrombosis
Strokes and transient ischaemic attacks
Multi-infarct dementia
Myocardial infarction
Peripheral arterial thrombosis
Ocular thrombosis
Venous thrombosis
Recurrent deep venous thromboses
Pulmonary emboli (including pulmonary hypertension)
Liver vein thrombosis (e.g. Budd–Chiari)
Adrenal vein thrombosis (Addison's disease)
Retinal vein thrombosis
Axillary vein thrombosis
Renal vein (and glomerular) thrombosis
Other
Livedo reticularis
Labile hypertension
Leg ulcers
Heart valve disorders
Thrombocytopenia
Avascular necrosis
Acute catastrophic syndrome
Heamolytic anaemia
Pregnancy
Recurrent (early) miscarriage

huge numbers of serum samples. They also challenged the then-accepted wisdom that APAs were simply crossreactive anti-DNA antibodies [13]. Most important, following a number of international workshops, we have developed standardized method protocols and standard serums to ensure reasonable cross-laboratory consistency [14].

CLINICAL FEATURES

The thrombotic features may affect major arteries (including aortic arch syndrome, strokes, carotid stenosis, limb ischaemia, etc.) as well as veins (recurrent deep venous thrombosis, retinal vein thrombosis, hepatic vein occlusion etc.). Although we now know that the antibody may persist for years, the onset of thrombosis may be dramatic. As the manifestations of the syndrome touch on many specialties, I have chosen to list them by specialty.

Neurology

At the present time, the majority of presentations are to the neurologist, with transient ischaemic attacks and strokes being far the commonest (Table 2) [15]. In an unknown number of undiagnosed patients, progres-

Table 2 The antiphospholipid syndrome – neurological manifestations

Strokes
Transient ischaemic attack
Widespread cerebral infarction
Epilepsy
Chorea and movement disorders
Migraine
Visual disturbances
Transverse myelopathy

sive cerebral infarction leads to dementia. A number of our patients have presented with progressive psychiatric or affective disorders, subsequently being found to have multiple ischaemic lesions on magnetic resonance imaging.

Migraine is common in our experience, often historically starting in the teens. Movement disorders, such as chorea, although rare, are often features that have been present in the past history of our patients.

Transverse myelopathy, although an unusual manifestation, is of great interest to me personally as, rightly or wrongly, it was the possible association of APAs with myelopathy which started this research. Alarcon-Segovia *et al.* [16], nevertheless, find that, statistically, this is one of the strongest associations.

Cardiology

A number of patients have developed myocardial infarction. The number of patients with myocardial infarction who have this aetiology is not yet known, though one study reported 20% of all young patients with myocardial infarction as having the disorder [17]. More interesting is the development of valvular (particularly mitral valve) lesions in some patients. In these patients, the development of valvular pathology may be dramatic, echocardiography showing a combination of valvular degeneration and endocardial thrombosis. Rare patients develop intracardiac thrombus so large as to suggest a diagnosis of atrial myxoma. These patients, with their cardiac and valvular failure, splinter haemorrhages and even clubbing, pose major diagnostic difficulties in the differential diagnosis from bacterial endocarditis [7,8]. Another association with APA now widely accepted is that with pulmonary hypertension, and it may be that this syndrome will throw new light on the aetiopathogenesis of some cases of this mysterious disorder [4].

Nephrology

Renal vein thrombosis may occur, and we have seen bilateral renal vein thrombosis following miscarriage in an APA-positive woman. It might be reasonably expected that glomerular thrombosis and renal ischaemia would be major associations with APA, but at the present time there is, rather surprisingly, little in the way of literature on this aspect of the syndrome.

Endocrinology

One of the most interesting associations has been with the development of Addison's disease, almost certainly from adrenal thrombosis. After our initial acute case – a man in whom anticoagulants had been stopped and who developed widespread thrombosis, subsequently becoming comatose with acute adrenal insufficiency – Asherson in my unit collected several other cases and reviewed the literature [18].

Dermatology

Recurrent skin ulcers, especially in the hip, have been seen in some patients, presumably as a result of small and large vein thrombosis. One of the most striking associations is with livedo reticularis [3]. This may be subtle, e.g. as a solitary area on the back of the wrist under the watch strap, or widespread. Sneddon's syndrome, the association of livedo with strokes, is clearly related to the antiphospholipid syndrome, although when we looked at series of patients with Sneddon's syndrome, APAs were by no means detectable in the majority – either the antibodies had disappeared in the APA-negative group, or, perhaps more likely, Sneddon's syndrome has multiple aetiologies.

Rheumatology

We first described the syndrome in association with SLE, and clearly the two are, in many patients, closely related. Between 5 and 30% of SLE patients have APAs, and this subgroup are undoubtedly at more risk. However, as different specialties recognize the importance of the syndrome, more cases of 'primary' antiphospholipid syndrome appear, in whom, over as long a period of follow-up as 10 years, no features of SLE develop [19]. In addition to SLE, the antiphospholipid antibody syndrome is seen in lupus variants such as discoid LE, subacute LE and Sjögren's syndrome, but is notably rare in rheumatoid arthritis.

Surgery

Clearly, postoperative risk of thrombosis is higher in APA-positive patients, although no formal studies have been reported. In vascular surgery, it is clear that a number of APA-positive individuals present with carotid, brachial and leg ischaemia. The bland and often widespread intimal hyperplasia seen in these patients may well prove an important lead in studies of atheroma development. In orthopaedic surgery, APA may prove an additional risk factor for avascular necrosis, possibly in contributing to arterial ischaemia, e.g. in the head of the femur [20].

Haematology

Thrombocytopenia is seen in some patients [21]. Normally this is borderline (frequently in the range of $90-100 \times 10^9$ per litre) though some patients may develop severe thrombocytopenia.

Intensive care

One of the most serious and potentially fatal aspects of the syndrome is the occasional acute collapse, with thrombocytopenia, hypotension, jaundice, widespread organ failure, disseminated intravascular coagulation, adult respiratory distress syndrome and death. In the few autopsies carried out, there has been widespread thrombosis. The aetiology of what we have chosen to call the 'catastrophic antiphospholipid syndrome' [22] is unknown, though in some cases, infection appears to have played a part.

Obstetrics

ACA-positive women becoming pregnant have a higher chance of spontaneous miscarriage [5]. The pathology is thought to be a progressive thrombosis of the microvasculature of the placenta, and in pregnancies going beyond mid-term, a progressive fall-off in foetal circulation can be demonstrated using Doppler flow studies [23].

The rate of miscarriage in APA patients is still uncertain, though the epidemiology is being studied and, increasingly, ACA testing is becoming a routine investigation in the women with miscarriage.

PATHOGENESIS

The reasons for the clotting tendency are unknown, though evidence for a number of mechanisms exists. These have been fully reviewed elsewhere [24]. The tests used to measure APA now generally include the ELISA APA test and the more quirky lupus anticoagulant. The two tests essentially measure the same family of antibodies and, when positive, essentially indicate the same risks. There are some discrepancies, however, of great interest to those working in this area. Patients have been described with antibodies directed apparently against one particular phospholipid [25] and hybridoma studies demonstrate the importance not only of the antigen, but of its structural presentation [26]. Phospholipid can, for example, exist in lamellar and hexagonal form, with antibodies recognizing one and not the other. During the past 3 years, considerable interest has been generated in the 'cofactor', and now clearly defined molecule apolipoprotein-H which has natural anticoagulant properties and which is critical in the binding of APAs to phospholipids. This cofactor has been the subject of a number of workshops and clearly plays an important role in the clotting mechanisms [27].

TREATMENT

The treatment is anticoagulation and, whether with warfarin, heparin or aspirin (or combinations), is not the subject of intense investigation. Some patients re-thrombose with seemingly adequate anticoagulation, and in these patients the international normalized ratio (INR) has to be kept at a value of around 3.0. Steroids or immunosuppressives to reduce antibody levels have not proved beneficial in the long term.

CONCLUSION

The recognition that APAs are associated with a distinct syndrome including arterial and venous thrombosis has opened new avenues for treatment and research. It has been suggested that in the USA alone, there are almost 9000 young people per year who suffer an episode of cerebral ischaemia (500 000 new strokes per year) associated with the antiphospholipid antibody syndrome – a recognizable and potentially treatable condition.

REFERENCES

1 Hughes GRV. Thrombosis, abortion, cerebral disease and lupus anticoagulant. *Br Med J* 1983;287:1088–1089.
2 Harris EN, Gharavi AE, Asherson RA, *et al.* Cerebral infarction in SLE. Association with anticardiolipin antibodies. *Clin Exp Rheumatol* 1984;2:47–51.
3 Hughes GRV. Connective tissue disease and the skin. *Clin Exp Dermatol* 1984;9:535–544.
4 Asherson RA, Mackworth-Young CG, Boey ML, *et al.* Pulmonary hypertension in SLE; a report of 3 cases. *J Rheumatol* 1986;12:416–418.
5 Derue GJ, Englert JH, Harris EN, *et al.* Fetal loss in systemic lupus: association with anticardiolipin antibodies. *J Obstet Gynaecol* 1985;5:207–209.
6 Alarcon-Segovia D, Delize M, Oria CV, *et al.* Antiphospholipid antibodies and the antiphospholipid syndrome in SLE. A prospective analysis of 500 consecutive patients. *Medicine (Baltimore)* 1989;68:353–356.
7 Khamashta MA, Cervera R, Asherson RA, *et al.* Association of antibodies against phospholipids with heart valve disease in SLE. *Lancet* 1990;335:1541–1542.
8 Cervera R, Khamashta MA, Font J, *et al.* High prevalence of significant heart valve lesions in patients with the 'primary' antiphospholipid syndrome. *Lupus* 1991;1:43–48.

9 Bresnihan B, Oliver M, Grigor R, Hughes GRV. Brain reactivity of lymphocytotoxic antibodies in SLE with and without cerebral involvement. *Clin Exp Immunol* 1977; 30:333–337.

10 Wilson WA, Hughes GRV. Aetiology of Jamaican neuropathy. *Lancet* 1975;i:240.

11 Harris EN, Gharavi AE, Boey ML, *et al.* Anticardiolipin antibodies: Detection by radioimmunoassay and association with thrombosis in SLE. *Lancet* 1983;ii:1211–1214.

12 Gharavi AE, Harris EN, Asherson RA, Hughes GRV. Isotype distribution and phospholipid specificity. *Ann Rheum Dis* 1987;46:1–6.

13 Harris EN, Gharavi AE, Loizou S, Hughes GRV. Cross-reactivity of antiphospholipid antibodies. *J Lab Clin Immunol* 1985;16:1–6.

14 Khamashta MA, Hughes GRV. Detection and importance of anticardiolipin antibodies. *J Clin Pathol* 1993;46:104–107.

15 Montalban J, Codina A, Ordi J, *et al.* Antiphospholipid antibodies in cerebral ischaemia. *Stroke* 1991;22:750–753.

16 Alarcon-Segovia D. Pathogenetic potential of antiphospholipid antibodies. *J Rheumatol* 1988;15:390–393.

17 Hamsten A, Norberg R, Bjorkholm M. Antibodies to cardiolipin in young survivors of myocardial infarction. *J Clin Pathol* 1993;46:104–107.

18 Asherson RA, Hughes GRV. Addison's disease and primary antiphospholipid syndrome. *Lancet* 1989;ii:874.

19 Asherson RA, Khamashta MA, Ordi-Ros J, *et al.* The 'primary' antiphospholipid syndrome: major clinical and serological features. *Medicine (Baltimore)* 1989;68:366–374.

20 Asherson RA, Liote SE, Page B, *et al.* Avascular necrosis of bone and aPL in SLE. *J Rheumatol* 1993;20:284–288.

21 Harris EN, Gharavi AE, Hegde U, Hughes GRV. Anticardiolipin antibodies in autoimmune thrombocytopenia purpura. *Br J Haematol* 1985;59:231–234.

22 Asherson RA. The catastrophic antiphospholipid syndrome. *J Rheumatol* 1992;19: 508–512.

23 Kerslake S, Morton KE, Versi E, *et al.* Early Doppler studies in lupus pregnancy. *Am J Reprod Immunol* 1992;28:172–175.

24 Harris EN, Exner J, Hughes GRV, Asherson RA. *Phospholipid-binding Antibodies.* Orlando: CRC Press, 1991.

25 Staub HL, Harris EN, Khamashta MA, *et al.* Antibody to phosphatidyl ethanolamine in a patient with lupus anticoagulant and thrombosis. *Ann Rheum Dis* 1989;48:166–169.

26 Rauch J, Murphy E, Roth JB, *et al.* A high frequency idiotype marker of anti-DNA autoantibodies in MRL-lpr/lpr mice. *J Immunol* 1982;129:236–241.

27 Bevers EM, Galli M. Co-factors involved in the antiphospholipid syndrome. *Lupus* 1992;1:51–54.

Specific immunotherapy for systemic vasculitis

C. M. LOCKWOOD

INTRODUCTION

There is growing evidence that the primary forms of systemic vasculitis such as Wegener's granulomatosis and microscopic polyarteritis are autoimmune diseases in which both humoral and cellular mechanisms may play a role in pathogenesis. Thus, the finding of circulating autoantibodies to neutrophil cytoplasm antigens (ANCA) in many patients with untreated vasculitis was the first substantial pointer to an autoimmune aetiology [1]. Subsequently research has shown that these autoantibodies have the ability to activate neutrophils [2] and promote cytotoxic effects on cultured endothelial cells *in vitro* [3]. More recently further clues have been provided about how vasculitis might be initiated by the demonstration in several laboratories that neutrophil adhesion is increased through upregulation of the β-integrin, CD18 [4]. Thus, these findings provide a rationale for directing therapy toward control of autoantibody production and *inter alia* for using autoantibody levels to monitor treatment.

There is somewhat less evidence for the role of cellular mechanisms in the production of vasculitis. Antigen-specific T-cell responses have not been easy to identify in experimental or human vasculitis and thus demonstration of their direct involvement in pathogenesis has remained elusive [5]. However, products of activated T cells have been measured and correlated with disease activity thereby giving indirect evidence for a T-cell association with disease [6, C.M. Lockwood *et al.*, unpublished data], although whether this is a cause or consequence of the inflammatory process remains unclear.

Whether considering humoral or cellular mechanisms in the generation of autoimmune vasculitis, perhaps the best clinical evidence for the importance of either has been provided by the response to immunotherapy. Thus, empirically it has been found that the most effective treatment for vasculitis consists of a combination of cyclophosphamide and steroids, at dosages which, in other autoimmune diseases, together with plasma exchange, synergize to suppress autoantibody formation [7]. Furthermore, for severe vasculitis affecting the kidney, a randomized prospective study has shown that the direct plasmapheresis treatment of the humoral compartment, in association with cytotoxic drugs and steroids, carries greater benefit than drug therapy alone [8]. As far as cellular responses are concerned, there is some evidence that specific therapy directed toward T cells can be effective. There are a few case reports citing the value of cyclosporin A in treatment [9] and there is also our own experience of one patient whose systemic vasculitis (which had a substantial lymphocytic component) showed a striking response to monoclonal T-lymphocyte antibody therapy [10].

We have explored two new forms of immunotherapy directed towards regulating the autoimmune responses at B-cell and T-cell levels respectively. The first, high dose pooled human immunoglobulin given intravenously (IVIg), has effects predominantly on B-cell production of autoantibody, while the second, humanized monoclonal antilymphocyte antibody, has effects mainly on T-cell function.

MECHANISM OF ACTION OF IVIg IN AUTOIMMUNE DISEASE

A wide range of autoimmune diseases have been treated by IVIg, and a number of possible mechanisms have been described which might explain the therapeutic effects observed [11]. In clinical studies reversal of monocyte and endothelial cell activation has been documented after IVIg administration with a consequent fall in monocyte-derived interleukin 1 (IL-1) secretion and endothelial leucocyte adhesion molecule 1 (ELAM-1) expression respectively [12]. *In vitro* experiments have shown IVIg to reduce monocyte IL-6 release and to inhibit uptake of C3b and C4b through the mononuclear phagocytic system, as well as having a non-specific effect on Ig production by lymphocytes [13]. That there may be a direct effect on T cells was suggested by the ability of IVIg to inhibit the development of diabetes in the non-obese diabetic mouse [14] and by the normalization of T-cell subsets after IVIg therapy in Kawasaki disease [15].

However, it was the influence of IVIg on the idiotypic–antiidiotypic network regulation of the immune response [16] and our finding that idiotypic–antiidiotypic interreactions were demonstrable in patients with ANCA-positive systemic vasculitis which led us to explore the use of IVIg for these conditions [17]. We had found ANCA antiidiotypic activity in sera of patients with systemic vasculitis who were in remission which could inhibit the ANCA binding in pretreatment sera as well as the ANCA activity of sera from other untreated patients. Similar inhibitory activity was demonstrable in IVIg. Furthermore, this could be enhanced 10-fold by affinity chromatography purification of the $F(ab)_2$ of IVIg on a column made from the immobilized $F(ab)_2$ of an ANCA-positive serum

[17]. These studies suggest that remission sera and IVIg contained regulatory factors (antiidiotypic antibodies) which might be useful for treatment and furthermore that these might be prepared using simple procedures such as affinity chromatography.

TREATMENT OF SYSTEMIC VASCULITIS BY IVIg

We have carried out an open study of IVIg in systemic vasculitis [18]. There were 14 patients of whom 13 had the diagnosis of either Wegener's granulomatosis (WG) or microscopic polyarteritis (MP) (Table 1). The remaining patient had an ANCA-positive rheumatoid vasculitis. Nine had disease which was refractory to steroids and/or cytotoxic agents; five were untreated. All patients received IVIg (Sandoglobulin) at a dose of 2 g per kg, as 0.4 g per kg each day for 5 days. There was a reduction in disease activity in 13 out of the 14 which led to clinical remission in eight. Laboratory investigations confirmed the response seen clinically, with falls in the mean erythrocyte sedimentation rate (ESR) and C-reactive protein (CRP) values from 52 mm and 44 mg per litre to 43 mm and 16 mg at 8 weeks respectively. Abnormal pulmonary infiltrates, present on chest X-ray in seven, resolved in four and quantitative assessment of inflammation as judged by paired indium-111-labelled polymorph scans showed that seven of nine patients with abnormal imaging before IVIg had benefited from treatment. At follow-up after 10 months two patients had relapsed but benefit was maintained in

Table 1 Treatment of 14 patients with intravenous immunoglobulin (IVIg)

Patient	Diagnosis*	Organ involvement†	Pre-IVIg‡ activity	Drug treatment§ (mg/day)	Post IVIg activity	Follow-up (months)	Time of relapse	Follow-up activity	Follow-up treatment
1	WG	URT, K, L, E, J	2	C100, P10	0	12	9	0	C100, P10
2	RV	J, S	2	P10	1	9	—	1	P10
3	WG	URT, L	2	—	1	12	2	0	C100, P10
4	MP	K, L, S, N	2	—	0	18	—	0	—
5	MP	URT, L, K	2	C100, P10	0	12	6	0	C100, P10
6	WG	URT	2	A150	0	12	—	0	A150
7	WG	URT, L, E, H	2	P40	0	12	—	0	—
8	MP	E, J	2	—	1	12	—	1	—
9	MP	L, N	2	A150, P20	0	7	—	0	A100, P8
10	WG	URT, L	2	C100, P30	0	7	—	0	C100, P12
11	WG	URT, L	2	C200, P20	1	8	—	0	C100, P10
12	WG	URT, L	2	C100, P10	1	6	—	1	C100, P10
13	MP	L	2	—	0	6	—	0	—
14	WG	L	2	—	1	5	—	1	—

Clinical findings, disease activity and immunosuppressive therapy in 14 patients with systemic vasculitis treated with intravenous immunoglobulin (IVIg).
* WG, Wegener's granulomatosis; MP, microscopic polyarteritis; RV, rheumatoid vasculitis.
† URT, Upper respiratory tract; K, kidney; L, lung; J, joints; E, eye; S, skin; N, nerve; H, heart.
‡ 2, Active disease; 1, partial remission; 0, complete remission.
§ C, Cyclophosphamide; P, prednisone; A, azathioprine.

Table 2 Effect of IVIg on laboratory indices in 14 patients

Index	Pre-IVIg	8 weeks post-IVIg	Follow-up
ANCA % binding	10/14 positive	9/14 positive	7/14 positive
(normal <16%)	55%	27%	32%
CRP mg/l (normal <6)	44	16	11
ESR mm/h	52	43	31
Indium-111 leucocyte scans	Nasal uptake 8	Nasal uptake 7	Not done
(paired in 11)	Lung uptake 7	Lung uptake 3	
	Subglottic uptake 1	Subglottic uptake 0	

the remaining patients with continued falls in ESR and CRP (Table 2).

Serial ANCA measurements showed a paradoxical rise in levels at approximately 10 days after treatment commenced and four patients noted a transient exacerbation of their systemic symptoms at this time. Subsequently ANCA levels fell to approximately 50% of their pretreatment values. Three patients became ANCA-negative. $F(ab)_2$ fragments of IVIg were shown to inhibit ANCA binding of 10 patients pretreatment and preliminary studies have shown that this *in vitro* effect correlated with the amount by which ANCA levels fell by the 8 week assessment stage *in vivo* [18].

There have been reports to suggest that IVIg treatment might have adverse effects on renal function in patients with glomerulonephritis or with systemic lupus erythematosus [19,20]. On the other hand beneficial effects have been reported in membranous glomerulonephritis [21] and no disturbance of renal function was seen in our patients. However, because of the efficacy of standard therapy, our study deliberately excluded patients with rapidly progressive glomerulonephritis, the most acute and aggressive renal injury. The beneficial effect of IVIg in systemic vasculitis has subsequently been reported in two other studies, the first describing remission in two patients with WG [22], the second documenting improvement in five of nine also with WG (C. Richter, personal communication). We have given IVIg alone as first line treatment for two patients with WG and circulating ANCA. There was disappearance of ANCA in both and resolution of radiological abnormality in the one patient with a pulmonary lesion.

RATIONALE FOR MONOCLONAL ANTIBODY THERAPY IN SYSTEMIC VASCULITIS

A small group of patients with vasculitis was identified in which the individuals were characterized by abnormal T-cell infiltrates at vasculitic biopsy sites, absence of ANCA and progressive disease, despite therapy with high dose steroids accompanied in turn by either cyclophosphamide, azathioprine or cyclosporin A [23]. Their referral coincided with the

Table 3 Treatment of four patients with monoclonal antibodies (mAb)

Patient	Diagnosis*	Clinical vasculitis†	Biopsy sites showing abnormal T-cell infiltrates	Dose of mAb in mg (days) CDw52	CD4	Remission (months)	Need for further mAb treatment
1	MP	S, J, Scl, Pl, Per	Rash, nerve, artery	2 (8)	20 (12)	42	No
2	MP	S, J, Pl, Per, GB	Synovium	12 (5)	20 (5)	7, 3, 12	Yes
3	Sjögren's syndrome	S, J, Pl, Per, GB, Pan, K, optic neuritis	Lung, kidney	40 (5)	—	13	No
4	Behçet's disease	S, J, V	Vein, lung	10 (5)	20 (10)	3	No

Clinical findings, biopsy details and monoclonal antibody therapy in four patients with intractable vasculitis. All patients were refractory to prednisolone, cyclophosphamide, azathioprine and cyclosporin A. In addition patients 1, 2 and 4 had failed treatment with plasma exchange and high dose pooled IVIg; patient 4 had also received total lymph node irradiation before referral.
* MP, Microscopic polyarteritis.
† S, Vasculitic rash; J, arthritis; Scl, scleritis; Pl, pleuritis; Per, pericarditis; GB, acalculous cholecystitis; Pan, pancreatitis; K, nephritis; V, phlebitis.

availability for therapeutic use of humanized monoclonal antibodies (mAbs) with specificity for lymphocytes, particularly T lymphocytes. Considerable experience has been gained of the use of mAbs as therapeutic agents in experimental autoimmune diseases [24]. However, experience of their use in humans for such conditions is still limited. We have now treated four patients with intractable vasculitis achieving remissions of 7 months or longer in three. The clinical details of the patients and relevant laboratory investigations are given in Table 3.

Monoclonal antibodies

Three mAbs were used for these studies. The first, CAMPATH-1H, a 'humanized' antilymphocyte antibody, is genetically engineered to have a rat hypervariable region grafted into a human immunoglobulin framework region. The CAMPATH-1H antigen, CDw52, is predominantly expressed on human lymphocytes, macrophages and monocytes. Antibodies raised against this antigen efficiently lyse lymphocytes but not monocytes in the presence of human complement. Within the lymphocyte population the major effect on CAMPATH-1H appears to be on T-cell numbers and T-cell function, with depletion of both CD4 and CD8 subpopulations being reported after its administration in humans [25]. The other two monoclonal antibodies recognize the CD4 antigen present on human T-helper cells. Initially only a rat IgG 2b CD4 antibody was available but later a humanized IgG1 CD4 was engineered in the same way as CAMPATH-1H [23]. The mode of action of the antibodies is different: CAMPATH-1H is lytic whilst the CD4 antibody has a blocking effect. Either mode of action avoids the cytokine release phenomenon seen with other anti-T-cell antibodies, such as OKT3. The mAbs were given intravenously in doses up to 40 mg per day for up to 10 days.

Effect of mAb therapy

Two of the four patients achieved substantial and sustained remissions of 48 and 20 months to date, while a third patient needed further treatment after 8 months and thereafter has had courses of mAb therapy on two further occasions. In this patient the development of antiidiotypic antibodies to CAMPATH-1H necessitated their removal by plasma exchange. In the fourth patient remission was for only 3 months and subsequently mAb therapy was ineffective. In this patient persistent high levels of interferon, which were unaffected by mAb therapy, raised the possibility that a CDw52-negative population of lymphocytes, such as natural killer (Nk) cells, might play a role in his vasculitis. Treatment with thalidomide, which can inhibit interferon-mediated tumour necrosis factor (TNF) release by monocytes *in vitro* and *in vivo* [26], proved successful in controlling his disease long term. There was in each patient an impressive lowering of the number of circulating CD4 cells, and counts greater than 0.2×10^9 per litre did not return for 3 months (one patient), 11 (two patients) and 12 months (one patient). However, no patient experienced systemic opportunistic infections and the one patient who developed oral candidiasis responded to appropriate antibiotic treatment. This was encouraging considering the extensive immunosuppression all four patients had received.

Although humanization is designed to reduce the likelihood of antiglobulin responses occurring, an antiidiotypic response did occur in the second patient after a second course of CAMPATH-1H therapy. However, intensive plasma exchange lowered the levels of antiidiotypic antibody sufficiently to enable mAbs to secure a third remission successfully. The CD4 antibody was not available at the time this patient first needed treatment. Whether the development of the antiidiotypic response can be avoided in the future by the early combination of CD4 with CAMPATH-1H remains to be evaluated. There is evidence from experimental studies that this might be the case since combination treatment can achieve better tolerance than that achieved with individual mAbs used alone [27].

The combination of CAMPATH-1H with CD4 antibody was effective in the first patient and in this patient CAMPATH-1H alone had only a transient effect. It had been our intention to treat our subsequent patients in this manner but the limited availability precluded the implementation of this strategy in our second and third patients. Experimental studies have demonstrated that a combination of two mAbs with similar specificity to those we used can synergize to achieve control of an ongoing autoimmune arthritis, whereas either alone can prevent its induction but not its progression [28]. We believe such a strategy may offer additional benefits in some patients, although in others, as exemplified by the third patient, CAMPATH-1H alone was effective long term when a sufficient dose was used. Whether this reprogramming of the immune system effected by mAb treatment can have sustained effects, independent of the treatment, or whether as in our second patient it makes the patient more sensitive to lower doses of conventional immunosuppressive drugs remains to be seen. Nevertheless, further studies to explore the use of these monoclonal antibodies in other autoimmune diseases seem warranted.

CONCLUSIONS

These studies have illustrated the possibility that human or humanized immunoglobulins may be utilized as safer and more specific forms of immunotherapy than conventional treatment for autoimmune systemic vasculitis with steroids and cytotoxic agents. Their usefulness to the clinician will depend on how long-lasting is the reprogramming of the immune system they achieve.

REFERENCES

1 Woude FJ van der, Rasmussen N, Lobatto S, *et al.* Autoantibodies to neutrophils and monocytes: A new tool for diagnosis and marker of disease activity in Wegener's granulomatosis. *Lancet* 1985;i:425–429.
2 Falk RJ, Terrell RS, Jennette JC. Antineutrophil cytoplasm antibodies induce neutrophils to degranulate and produce toxic oxygen radicals *in vitro*. *Proc Natl Acad Sci USA* 1990;87:4115–4119.
3 Ewert BH, Jennette JC, Falk RJ. Antimyeloperoxidase antibodies stimulate neutrophils to damage human endothelial cells. *Kidney Int* 1992;41:375–383.
4 Keogan MT, Rifkin I, Ronda N, *et al.* ANCA increase neutrophil adhesion to cultured human endothelium. Proc 4th ANCA Int Workshop, Lubeck, May 1992. *Adv Exp Med Biol* 1994 (in press).
5 Mathieson PW, Lockwood CM, Oliveira DBG. T and B cell responses to neutrophil cytoplasmic antigens in systemic vasculitis. *Clin Immunol Immunopathol* 1992;63:135–141.
6 das Neves FC, Kaskas B, Hartley B, Cameron JS. Interstitial cellular infiltrate and soluble interleukin 2 receptor in patients with renal vasculitis. *J Am Soc Nephrol* 1991;2:592(Abstract).
7 Savage COS, Pusey CD, Bowman C, *et al.* Anti-glomerular basement membrane mediated disease in the British Isles 1980–1984. *Br Med J* 1986;292:301–304.
8 Pusey CD, Rees AJ, Evans DJ, *et al.* Plasma exchange in focal necrotizing glomerulonephritis without anti-GBM antibodies. *Kidney Int* 1991;40:757–763.

9 Gremmel F, Druml W, Schmidt P, Graninger W. Cyclosporin in Wegener's granulomatosis. *Ann Intern Med* 1988;108:491.
10 Mathieson PW, Cobbold SP, Hale G, *et al.* Monoclonal antibody therapy in systemic vasculitis. *N Engl J Med* 1990;323:250–254.
11 Dwyer JM. Manipulating the immune system with immune globulin. *N Engl J Med* 1992;236:107–116.
12 Leung DYM, Cotran RS, Kurt-Jones E, *et al.* Endothelial cell activation and high interleukin-1 secretion in the pathogenesis of acute Kawasaki disease. *Lancet* 1989;i: 1298–1302.
13 Andersson JP, Andersson UG. Human intravenous immunoglobulin modulates monokine production *in vitro*. *Immunology* 1990;71:372–376.
14 Forsgren S, Andersson A, Hillorn V, *et al.* Immunoglobulin-mediated prevention of autoimmune diabetes in the non-obese diabetic (NOD) mouse. *Scand J Immunol* 1991;34:445–451.
15 Leung DYM, Burns JC, Newburger JW, Geha RS. Reversal of lymphocyte activation *in vivo* in the Kawasaki syndrome by intravenous gammaglobulin. *J Clin Invest* 1987; 79:468–472.
16 Sulton Y, Rossi F, Kazatchkine MD. Recovery from anti-VIII:c (anti-haemophilic factor) autoimmune disease is dependent on generation of anti-idiotypes against anti-VIII: c autoantibodies. *Proc Natl Acad Sci USA* 1987;84:828–831.
17 Jayne DRW, Esnault VLM, Lockwood CM. ANCA anti-idiotypic antibodies and the treatment of systemic vasculitis with intravenous immunoglobulin. *J Autoimmunity* 1993;6:207–219.
18 Jayne DRW, Black CM, Davies M, *et al.* Treatment of systemic vasculitis with pooled intravenous immunoglobulin. *Lancet* 1991;337:1137–1139.
19 Schifferli J, Leski M, Favre H, *et al.* High-dose intravenous IgG treatment and renal function. *Lancet* 1991;i:457–458.
20 Jordan SC. Intravenous gammaglobulin therapy in systemic lupus erythematosus and immune complex disease. *Clin Immunol Immunopathol* 1989;53:S164–S169.
21 Palla R, Cirami C, Panichi V, *et al.* Intravenous immunoglobulin therapy of membranous nephropathy: efficacy and safety. *Clin Nephrol* 1991;35:98–104.
22 Moudgil A, Tuso P, Kamil E, *et al.* Treatment of Wegener's granulomatosis with pooled intravenous immunoglobulin. *J Am Soc Nephrol* 1991;2:600(Abstract).
23 Lockwood CM, Thiru S, Isaacs JD, *et al.* Humanised monoclonal antibody therapy for intractable systemic vasculitis. *Lancet* 1993;341:1620–1622.
24 Waldmann H. Manipulation of T cell responses with monoclonal antibodies. *Ann Rev Immunol* 1989;7:407–444.
25 Isaacs JD, Watts RA, Hazleman B, *et al.* Humanised monoclonal antibody therapy for rheumatoid arthritis. *Lancet* 1992;340:748–752.
26 Sampaio EJ, Morera AL, Saron EN, *et al.* Prolonged treatment with recombinant interferon induces erythema nodosum leprosum in lepromatous leprosy patients. *J Exp Med* 1992;175:1728–1738.
27 Chen Z, Cobbald S, Metcalf S, Waldmann H. Tolerance in the mouse to major histocompatibility complex-mismatched heart allografts and to rat heart xenografts using monoclonal antibodies to CD4 and CD8. *Eur J Immunol* 1992;22:805–810.
28 Hom JT, Butler LD, Riedl PE, Bendele AM. The progression of the inflammation in established collagen induced arthritis can be altered by treatment with immunological or pharmacological agents which inhibit T cell activities. *Eur J Immunol* 1988;18:881–888.

Index